Musings of a Medical Dinosaur

Who we are, how we got here, and where we are going

J. Barry Engelhardt, MD

Copyright page

©2017 James B. Engelhardt
All rights reserved. Published in Canada.
Printed in the United States of America.

www.jbarryengelhardtbooks.com

Cover illustration by Carol Brodkin-Sang
Cover design by Nancy Halpin, Lara Bednarz, and Julie and Scott Brandon

No part of this book may be used or reproduced in any manner whatsoever without the prior written permission of the publisher, except by a reviewer who may quote brief passages in a review.

Musings of a Medical Dinosaur / written by James B. Engelhardt
Issued in print and electronic formats:
ISBN 978-0-9917574-3-5 (pbk.)
ISBN 978-0-9917574-4-2 (electronic)

Dedication

For my father, Norm, who is my inspiration for these musings.

He taught me to question everything and to search for better answers.

I wish I could have known him better.

Contents

PREFACE vii

PART I: WHO WE ARE
    Chapter 1: Incontinence 1
    Chapter 2: Mind Game 10
    Chapter 3: The Phone Call 20
    Chapter 4: Fear 25

PART II: HOW WE GOT HERE
    Chapter 5: In the Beginning 33
    Chapter 6: Knowing Me, Knowing You 43
    Chapter 7: Hockey 51
    Chapter 8: The Myth of Objectivity 60
    Chapter 9: The Way We Are 73
    Chapter 10: Facing Our Fears 95
    Chapter 11: Neuroplasticity and the Mind 104

PART III: WHERE WE ARE GOING

Change: The Universe's Only Constant
    Chapter 12: Change and Growth 127
    Chapter 13: Jane 133
    Chapter 14: Love 141
    Chapter 15: Motive and Mind 153
    Chapter 16: Maturity 162
    Chapter 17: Paradox 181
    Chapter 18: The Medical Tribe 200

Endless Possibilities
    Chapter 19: Thought Experiment 1 215
    Chapter 20: Values 218
    Chatper 21: Thought Experiment 2 227

Chapter 22: Death 232
Chapter 23: Complexity: Ethics 242
Chapter 24: Complexity: Decisions, Decisions!. 251
Chapter 25: Complexity: The Black Box. 270
Chapter 26: Teaching and Learning 291

Never Say Never
Chapter 27: Intimacy 317
Chapter 28: Blame and Shame 338
Chapter 29: Asymptotes 353
Chapter 30: Paradox Revisited 374
Chapter 31: Bucket List 383

Acknowledgements 399
About the Author 400
Other books by the author: 401
Appendix 1: Fifty Things I've Learned So Far in Medicine 402
Appendix 2: Thoughts for Patients 407
Appendix 3: POEMs 410
References 420

Preface

ON MY SIXTH birthday I became very annoying. You know how most six-year-olds continue to ask "Why?" no matter how many successive answers you give them? Well, I did that to an extreme. I always wanted to dig deeper.

I am now nearing my sixtieth birthday, and things haven't improved. In fact, they may have gotten worse. I don't want to be annoying just for the sake of being annoying (well, maybe once in a while). It just turns out that getting to the bottom of things can make people irritable.

I used to feel badly about this until I read that all great truths contain paradox, and I think this is what makes people feel unsettled.

For example, as most people know, a great truth of life is that it involves pain. Pain is nature's way of warning an organism that its survival is in question, and living things are programmed for survival. So, all living things work to avoid pain. On the other hand, we humans come to realize that in situations involving pain (physical or emotional), we often grow the most. Losing weight to improve our health is painful; breaking up with someone when we are in an unsatisfying relationship hurts. So the paradox is that although we are programmed to avoid pain, we accept that this thing we are supposed to avoid can help us. Weird, eh?

So, you see, in writing this book, I want to make you feel uncomfortable. Because when we feel uncomfortable, we know that we are dealing with stuff that both matters to us and challenges us. We are delving into the great truths, into the heart of paradox. And that discomfort and challenge tells us that we are attempting to grow.

On the surface, this book is about the practice of medicine from the perspective of a family doctor who has been doing his shtick for about thirty-five years. In this day of such rapid changes, thirty-five years makes me a dinosaur. Personality-wise and physique-wise, I see myself more as a brontosaurus than a tyrannosaurus or velociraptor, hence the book cover. I am large and plodding and am working on becoming a vegetarian.

I have been, more through good luck than management, fairly healthy, so I can speak more from one side of the stethoscope than the other. This is most fortunate for me because I am quite a wimp. However, at times I have been a patient, and I will share that experience as well.

On a deeper level, this is a simple man's struggle to make sense of nearly sixty years of life and thirty-five years of sharing patients' journeys. Something along the lines of Søren Kierkegaard's words that "Life can only be understood backwards; but it must be lived forwards."

But be warned, as a family doctor I am an expert in nothing, and I like it that way. In fact, I never want to be an expert. I am a generalist, and that is both my greatest strength and greatest weakness. Paradox, you say?

That is why I called this book "musings," not "treatise." I will be thinking out loud, not offering a definitive tome. When I offer answers, they invariably will lead to more questions. Annoying, yes; blame the six-year-old still inside of me. But those questions will be at a higher level than the answers, so I trust it will be worthwhile.

So what am I going to muse about?

One of the many things I wanted to understand when I was six years old was how I "worked." What was going on inside of me? That's probably what drew me to medicine. I enjoyed medical school for that very reason—I was finally learning about the human organism, and it was fascinating.

In 1985, I completed a three-year residency in family medicine that included extra obstetrical training, six months of anaesthesia, and three months of work in an intensive care unit (ICU). My first years of medical practice were filled with interactions with patients in which I could apply my training, and much of it was technical in nature, such as giving anaesthetics and caring for patients in a small ICU.

I assisted at hundreds of births, witnessed the deaths of a number of patients, and shared everything in between. It was busy and stressful, and I loved it!

But slowly over time I realized that my career felt incomplete. Like a scientist studying lab subjects, I had come to understand the human *organism* pretty well. I felt comfortable with all aspects of the human body, even ones that made most people feel uncomfortable or squeamish. But I wasn't sure that I understood human *beings* nearly so well. I was confused; we appeared to be living paradoxes.

Each of us, myself included, seemed regularly to plumb both the heights of altruism and the depths of narcissism, inspire with stunning insights amid surprising naïveté, and occasionally make leaps of maturity in a setting of nearly unrelenting stubbornness.

So, after years of thinking that I was done studying "us," I started over again and explored the human species from a different perspective, this time trying to figure out what made us tick.

I have shared with thousands of patients the births and deaths, joys and tragedies, and hope and despair that define our lives. In doing so,

I have both observed and wondered, and my musings revolve around three questions:

1. If we understood ourselves better, could our lives be better?
2. If we understood ourselves better, could our world be better?
3. If we understood better how we got to where we are now, might it provide insight as to where we go from here?

In seeking answers, I have read from a wide variety of sources. When sharing this wisdom with you in this book, I often forget where I heard or read it. If I remember, I tell you; I don't want to take credit for someone else's work or ideas. My sincerest apologies to those I don't identify; I can assure you that memory, not malice, is the culprit (I am, after all, an old brontosaurus).

Also note that I have changed the names and some characteristics of the people featured in the stories I tell, in order to maintain confidentiality, without compromising the essence of their teachings.

One of the important themes in this book is the concept of "having enough." In keeping with this theme, since I have enough money, all profits from this book are being donated. Because addictions are conditions in which an individual can't seem to get enough, I am offering the profits to addiction centres to assist individuals in obtaining treatment.

I appreciate you reading this book. Thank you. I hope some day we can share our thoughts and grow together.

Barry

PART I: WHO WE ARE

Chapter 1

Incontinence

Incontinence: (noun) the inability to maintain control; (medically) the inability to contain bodily waste; involuntary urination or defecation

INCONTINENCE MAY SEEM a pretty odd title for the opening chapter of a book, and you are right. But there is a method to my madness, so hang in there.

In the first months of life, we are all incontinent, and in the absence of disease or illness, we gradually mature to continence and maintain a measure of control over our urine and bowels for the rest of our lives. Unfortunately, a wide array of illnesses and conditions can sometimes play havoc with this desired state of affairs, even if only transiently.

Now, it's time for us to be honest with each other, okay? Tell me, since childhood, have you ever been incontinent? I am a doctor, sworn to confidentiality, so I promise I won't tell a living soul. Well?

Specifically, have you ever been incontinent of stool? You know, had a poop at a time or place when you are not supposed to have a poop, all without expecting it? Maybe you picked up some bug while holidaying in Mexico and then rolled over in bed or strained to pick up your luggage and, oops, stuff happened?

Or maybe you have just had a really scary experience where you pooped yourself?

If you are too embarrassed to admit to it, I understand. Well, I had an episode at work where I came as close to incontinence as you can get without actually being incontinent.

I know I am not alone in this regard. I am sure many of you have had these near misses, even though you may not care to remember or share your story with me.

Most of us practising any acute-care medicine have had at least one of these experiences. In pseudotechnical jargon, we refer to what bails us out from experiencing the humiliation of a full-blown, five-alarm loss of bowel control as "sphincter tetany." That is, the muscles that constitute the "last line of defence" in our anus go into hyperdrive and save us from impending disaster.

So if you won't tell me about your brush with the unmentionable, I will.

As I mentioned in my preface, in my early career I was very interested in the biomechanical aspects of the human body and disease, which is why I was attracted to doing general practitioner (GP) anaesthesia. As a family doctor (a.k.a. GP), I had taken nine months of extra training—six of anaesthesia and three of the intensive care unit (ICU)—in order to be pronounced competent to provide anaesthetics for people undergoing surgeries. So I worked part time as a family doctor seeing patients in my office and part time as a GP anaesthetist.

I was trained to give basic anaesthetics to *low-risk* patients undergoing *low-risk* surgery. Full-time anaesthetists are board-certified as specialists who train for five years or more and are capable of providing anaesthesia to more complex patients having more complicated surgeries. I do the low-risk work, and the big shots do the high-risk cases, or at least that's the theory.

The problem is, high-risk situations sometimes pop up suddenly and unexpectedly, and it may simply be impossible to have a full-fledged anaesthetist available. So, occasionally, we GP anaesthetists have to do our best in situations beyond our control and at the limit of, or beyond, our comfort or expertise. There is a certain adrenaline rush involved in that, and perhaps that is what draws us to it. Adrenaline, of course, cuts two ways.

Many years ago I was on call when a cute six-year-old boy was brought by his parents to the emergency department of our rural hospital. He was suffering from a sore throat and had trouble breathing. There is a long list of causes (referred to as the "differential diagnosis") of a child at this age having trouble breathing, and some can be quite serious. The emerg (emergency) doctor had called in our local otolaryngologist (ear, nose and throat specialist), a good friend of mine, and he in turn called me in to help out.

It was obvious that this child needed to have some help with his airway because he was struggling to breathe and was not improving. Based on the story his parents had provided and the examination of the young lad, the differential diagnosis included two serious possibilities: epiglottitis and bacterial tracheitis. Both are serious infections that cause swelling and secretions to block the airway, either at the level of the epiglottis, just above the larynx (or voice box), or at the level of the trachea, the large cartilaginous tube below the larynx leading directly to the lungs.

It is important in these situations, when the child is quite sick and scared, to proceed very cautiously because upsetting the child can suddenly make his breathing much worse, to the point of complete obstruction, and that is bad news. Needless to say, time did not permit us the luxury of transferring the child in an ambulance hurdling down a bumpy highway to an urban hospital where specialist anaesthetists were available. In this particular circumstance, as one of a handful of GP anaesthetists at our hospital, I was part of a small cadre of people who were the best our hospital could offer to this child and his family.

As a resident, I had seen one case of epiglottitis and had been handheld through the process of securing the child's airway in the safest haven of the hospital for performing such a feat—the operating room. That particular case, five years earlier, had gone well. In my second year of practice, I saw my second epiglottitis and managed it as an independent physician, not as a resident with a staff person overseeing my work, prepared to bail me out if I screwed up. That case, too, went well.

So I was feeling scared but confident that I could handle the challenge, particularly because my good friend, the otolaryngologist, would be there to perform an emergency tracheotomy if I could not intubate (place a plastic tube through the mouth into the trachea) the child to secure his airway.

Everything went very well, initially. We took the child to the operating room and very gingerly began to anaesthetize him in order to insert the airway-preserving endotracheal tube. When the child was sufficiently "deep," in other words, well anaesthetized, I looked down his throat with a laryngoscope, and the diagnosis was clear: bacterial tracheitis. After aspirating the copious secretions that had been making his breathing so laborious, I inserted the endotracheal tube relatively easily and stabilized it so that it would not become dislodged. With the diagnosis confirmed and airway secure, we could now safely transfer him to a specialized children's hospital, which would continue the treatment and assure complete recovery. The worst was over, or so I thought.

The plan was for me to fly down with the patient by helicopter to that facility, but of course, it takes time to make all of the arrangements and have the chopper come to our hospital. We had an adult ICU, but no paediatric ICU. We simply did not have the volume of patients nor staff at a small rural hospital to maintain one. No problem. The helicopter team would be there within an hour, and we could certainly manage to take care of the little lad until they arrived as he was now safe and stable.

Unfortunately, at six years of age, a child's airway is not that large, nor is the endotracheal tube we put into the trachea. The young boy continued to produce copious secretions, and eventually it became more difficult for him to breathe again. He became restless and was "bucking the tube," clearly struggling. I used an Ambu bag (a compressible bag attached to a tube or mask to blow air into the lungs) to help him breathe, but it was necessary to frequently suction the secretions to keep the tube patent. Eventually, though, the thick secretions began to take their toll, and it became very difficult to maintain his breathing comfortably.

I knew that I would need to replace the tube. He was still asleep from the anaesthetic, but not enough to change the tube because that is *very* irritating for the patient. Our airways have some of the most sensitive nerves in our body; it's nature's way of keeping our airways open, by getting very upset if anything gets in the way. If we don't keep them open, we can die very quickly. Even the smallest bit of unwanted material will make us cough and hack uncontrollably for that reason, as any of us who have had a postnasal drip will testify.

It is said that the art of anaesthesia is 95 percent boredom and 5 percent panic. That may be a bit of an exaggeration, but it hammers home the point that bad things can happen in a hurry when you are dealing with airways, so preparation is critical. You learn to have a carefully crafted routine that provides the tools to deal with whatever is thrown at you. You always do it the same way, and you check and double check. You leave yourself margin, and you make sure that you have extra amounts of everything, just in case. Your routine gives you confidence and comfort. Naturally, losing that routine can throw you off.

I had already brought lots of equipment with me when we moved from the operating room to the ICU, in case something went wrong during the transport. So I was well prepared to change the tube in the ICU; everything I had had in the operating room was with me still, including a large selection of different-sized endotracheal tubes (you never know exactly what size tube you will need until you get in there).

I set up as I usually did and proceeded to give the child intravenous medications, both to paralyze him and keep him unconscious enough to intubate him and keep him comfortable until the helicopter team arrived. I would then breathe for him with his new secured airway using the Ambu bag.

As he drifted into a deeper sleep, breathing for him with the Ambu bag became a little easier, but I knew I still had to replace the tube. So I calmly placed the laryngoscope in his mouth with my left hand, and with my right hand removed the mucous-filled tube, suctioned the remaining secretions in his throat, and then reached for one of the new endotracheal tubes I had placed on my right side two minutes earlier.

But when I reached for one of the tubes, there was nothing there. The child was incapable of breathing for himself, given the drugs I had administered, and all of my tubes had vanished!

Even as I type the details of this story twenty-five years later, I can feel twinges of the terror I felt. It was horrible. My safe, dependable routine was disrupted, and I wanted to run and hide or just disappear into thin air. I wanted to be anywhere but there. I experienced an intense nausea and a nearly overwhelming sense of foreboding. That's as close as I ever came to incontinence (and believe me, it was close), and I never want to get that close again.

Fortunately for me, my friend the otolaryngologist, himself shaken, pulled me back from the brink, reminding me that I could probably use the Ambu bag and just a mask, without the tube, at least long enough until someone could find some paediatric endotracheal tubes (there were none normally in the adult ICU, and the operating room was two floors down). After all, I had cleared the secretions, and the swollen airway would not collapse down immediately, having been stented by the first tube during the previous hour.

Fortunately, the boy's airway retained its patency. I used the Ambu bag and mask until some new tubes magically reappeared. Then I successfully reintubated the still-paralyzed and unconscious little boy.

As I taped that new endotracheal tube solidly in place, my thoughts and fears, including my sphincter tone, gradually returned to a more tolerable, near-normal level. The team arrived, and we transferred over to the chopper and had an uneventful flight to the paediatric hospital and its ICU. By the time I made it back to home base, it was around two in the morning.

So, what had happened to the original extra tubes I had brought up to the ICU, the ones with which I was going to do the second intubation? Was I not as well prepared as I thought I was?

Well, in fact, I had done my usual preparation, but it turns out that before I realized that I would have to change the original tube, the staff had suggested that we have the parents come up and see their son. We had already told them that the initial operating room proceedings had gone well, so we thought it important for them to see their son now that things were stable.

However, after many of these challenging cases, things often get a little messy with tape and sheets and other stuff strewn all over. The staff had simply thought that a little tidying up would be in order before the parents came into the room, and that included getting rid of my extra endotracheal tubes just before I was forced to do the second intubation. Oops!

No one ever admitted to taking them from where I had placed them. And I have no idea how long it was before they were returned to me; it seemed like years but was likely only a minute or two. The child was unaware of it and suffered no ill effects. My nerves seemed to have been the only casualty.

It would be easy to blame the staff for what happened, but this was a rare situation for them—an intubated child in an adult ICU.

But more than that, the hard lesson was that, ultimately, it was my responsibility. I had made the decision to change the tube, I had given the medications, and I had taken the tube out. The buck had to stop with me, the doctor, as terrifying as that may be.

I never told the parents what had transpired during that second intubation. In part, I felt that they had had enough worry for one night. Their child was going to be fine (and he was), and the miscue, although it could have been lethal, caused no harm to anyone but me. But of course, in part, I didn't tell them because I really didn't know how to articulate to them that I had almost killed their child!

After I had arrived back at our hospital around one in the morning, I returned all of the equipment I had taken with me for the flight. I was physically tired and mentally drained. I prayed that there would be no more pager calls for me for the rest of the night. As I walked out to my car in the emerg parking lot, something very strange happened.

Initially, I felt a sense of contentment. I had ultimately done a good job, rebounding, with the help of my friend, from a near catastrophe. A "that which does not destroy you makes you stronger" kind of moment.

But then I felt a profound weakness. There was a deep fatigue, of course, but it was more than that. Reviewing the case, as I usually did after a challenging one, I wondered what I would have done if the tubes had not been found in time. What if his airway had become blocked? The otolaryngologist would have had to do an emergency tracheotomy, a challenge at any time, but particularly on such a small airway in an adult ICU with staff who likely had never seen one (nor had I!).

That's when it really struck me: the child could have died, and I would have had to explain to his shocked and grieving parents that it was my fault.

I knew that if it had happened, I would have manned up; that wasn't the problem. The problem was, I was now heading home to see my two children and pregnant wife. How, had I killed this couple's only child, could I simply have gone home, kissed my children snuggled asleep in their beds, nuzzled up beside my wife, and carried on with my usual life?

That's when the profound weakness hit me. I staggered toward my car, collapsing onto the concrete curb before getting there. Sitting there, heart pounding and nauseated, I realized that had that child died because of me—if it had been my fault—I wouldn't have been able to live with myself. Had the little boy not been allowed to see his family again, I would have made sure that I would not allow myself to see my family again either.

Chapter 2

Mind Game

DESPITE THE DRAMA of the story I related to you in the first chapter, there really was nothing unduly complicated about what I did. Anyone with reasonable dexterity and enough training can learn to intubate; I did!

After all, a laryngoscope is a pretty simple device. It has a handle with an articulated flange, in which is embedded a light source to allow for visibility in the back part of the throat, the laryngopharynx. There aren't a lot of buttons or switches; it has only one function.

There are times when other factors involved in preparing a patient for intubation, in terms of the status of their heart and lungs, as well as head and neck issues, can make it significantly more challenging and, hence, nerve-racking. But the process of intubation itself is usually not tremendously difficult. When you look down with a laryngoscope, there are only two holes to put the tube in: the larynx leading to the trachea, where you want the tube to go, and the esophagus, the tube our food goes down, where you don't want the tube to go.

Occasionally, someone's anatomy can make intubation very difficult. There was one patient I simply could not intubate. I could not see his larynx leading to his trachea, and all attempts to intubate him blindly failed. For the elective surgery he was undergoing, I had the option of simply using a bag and mask for the anaesthetic delivery, which I did without incident.

But when you must get a tube down to obtain or secure an airway and can't, it is a terrifying experience. As with the little boy in the last chapter, the only option remaining to prevent asphyxiation is a tracheotomy: making an artificial opening through the front part of the neck into the trachea directly and inserting an artificial airway into it. This procedure is technically challenging at the best of times. But when done as an unexpected emergency, where the time constraint is mere minutes before brain damage begins, less than perfection can be catastrophic for the patient.

This brings me to an important insight: a lot of medicine is in our mind. It is all about how we perceive reality. By that I mean, what makes medicine very different from a lot of things we do in our lives is what hangs in the balance: someone else's life. It's not so much that it is complicated but that the stakes are high.

We like to think that what we do is incredibly complex, requiring a phenomenal IQ and extraordinary technical skills. It seldom requires either. I am quite sure that any seamstress or experienced knitter could technically do very well in the operating room. I suspect that excellent mechanics would also make excellent orthopedic surgeons. A wise and thoughtful hairdresser, who often listens to people's sad stories supportively, with the right training, could become a reasonable psychiatrist. The crucial differences, of course, are that you are sewing the flesh of another living human being, not cloth; or operating on a machine that is always living and you can't turn off while you manufacture new parts;

or the person you are counselling may commit suicide, and you will be held accountable.

True, there is a lot to learn about the human organism, and for that you need a reasonable intellect and memory. Like any field of study, a passion for the work is important too. But I seriously don't think you need to be a genius or a sleight-of-hand artist, or anything close to it, to train as a medical practitioner.

Certainly, the admissions process to medical school requires stellar academic performance, proof through references that you are a reasonably functioning and civil person, some evidence that you have at least a modicum of social and nonacademic skills and are not just an accomplished bookworm, and life experience that indicates interest in aiding humanity.

But it may come as quite a shock to most of you that when we are screened for entry into medical school, or residency, we are not screened at all for any physical aptitudes. Our hearing is not evaluated to determine that we can differentiate the midsystolic murmur of aortic stenosis from the pansystolic murmur of a ventricular septal defect. Our vision is not assessed to confirm that we can distinguish a benign from a malignant mole. Our touch sensation is not tested to assure that we can detect a worrisome nodule on a prostate. Like everyone else, it is simply assumed that if we do something often enough, we'll get better at it.

Nor is our ability to handle stress screened. I am not even sure if or how one could be screened for stress-management capability since the stress of dealing with someone else's life is hard to approximate, and few life experiences a twenty-two-year-old would have had can provide much insight in this regard.

However, once you are in medical school, the mystique begins. You are now part of the tribe, that valiant group of very special people who devote their lives unwaveringly to the enhancement of human life. You can deal with misery and misfortune, blood and guts, and do it all on little sleep and still keep smiling. Well, at least that's the persona we are encouraged to adopt as members of the medical tribe.

I once led a hands-on seminar for some first-year medical students dealing with injections, suturing, and other minor technical procedures. They were excited but also very nervous. I began by showing them a photo on a large screen of a narrow, winding road going up the side of a mountain. There were no guardrails on this road, which meant that a moment of inattention might result in one toppling over the edge to a near-certain death hundreds of metres below. Oohs and aahs filled the room.

I then asked them why they should feel any different driving on a road at ninety kilometres per hour, where all that separated them from the people going in the opposite direction at the same speed was a single yellow line. Surely, a very similar moment of inattention, crossing the yellow line and colliding at essentially 180 km/hour with an eighteen-wheeler, would leave you as dead as the fall off the cliff?

The light went on for them. It's all how your mind interprets it. The same is true of the practice of medicine. Injecting a human with a syringe and injecting an orange are different, not so much in the technical or intellectual aspects but in the psychological aspect. The same holds true for the seamstress and the surgeon, the mechanic and the orthopod (orthopaedic surgeon), and the hairdresser and the psychiatrist.

I frequently think back to a most amazing man I met during medical school. His name was Harry Whittaker, and when I knew him, he was in his sixties and had been working as a laboratory technician for almost fifty years. In his teens, he had begun his career by taking care of the microscopes in the histology laboratory (histology is microscopic anatomy, as opposed to gross anatomy, which is the anatomy we can see with the unaided eye). I doubt that he even had a grade ten education; people in those days seldom did.

Over the years, as part of his job, he attended all of the histology lectures that all of the medical students attended. Despite his lack of formal education, he was quite a clever fellow, so, not surprisingly, he learned a lot about histology.

He was perhaps the most humble man I have ever met. He was

always smiling as he shuffled around the classroom in his white lab coat, offering assistance and gentle encouragement to us like a mother hen tending to her chicks.

During medical school, at the end of each formal histology lecture, our learned professor would leave the room. Then the real teaching began—by Harry. In a simple and folksy style, he explained to us what was going on in the slides, how to recognize what we were looking at (stacks of Big Macs were red blood cells, for example), and how to make sense of it all. If it weren't for Harry, many of us would have had a much harder time passing the histology exam.

The first thing to learn from this is that anybody, in my opinion, given enough interest, time, and support, can learn to do most things to some degree. Do something often enough with a little coaching and you will get better at it, perhaps even quite proficient. Maybe not to the point of being well paid for it, but enough to enjoy it and be helpful to others.

The second thing learned from Harry is what he used to say to us around exam time. He would profess his perpetual amusement that nearly every medical student ran around frantically at exam time, moaning like Chicken Little that they would never pass and become a doctor one day. Perhaps to reassure us, but I suspect more likely in an attempt to keep us humble, he would remind us that despite our angst, the day would arrive when we would receive our diplomas and be called "doctor." And on that day, everything would change. Magically, not only would we be doctors, but now we would also know how to fix fridges, invest wisely, have great political insights, and more. People would seek our counsel on no end of topics, because, after all, we were doctors.

I got his tongue-in-cheek message, and have retained it ever since. I am not sure that all of my colleagues did. So it turns out that Dr. "Bones" McCoy on *Star Trek* had it right, after all: "Damn it, Jim, I'm a doctor not a _____" (I'll let you fill in the blank).

Memorizing a pile of big textbooks about how the human body functions (and hopefully understanding them) is a wonderful achievement. But all it means is that you have memorized and understood a pile of big textbooks about how the human body works. That's it. It doesn't give you better fine motor skills. It doesn't necessarily make you a morally better person, or a more mature and wiser person either. And it doesn't necessarily mean that you understand how human beings work, including yourself.

As my first chapter illustrates, it doesn't mean that you know how to handle real-life stress, especially life-and-death-type stress, even though you may know how to intubate. Despite the fact that everything turned out all right in the end, does my thinking process at the end of the last chapter, about what I would have done if things had not turned out all right with the little boy, mean that I shouldn't have become a physician? That I didn't have the right stuff?

From a purely intellectual perspective, I think medicine was a good choice for me. I have always enjoyed learning, and the sciences were a passion for me. I wanted a job that was interesting and contributed something useful to the world, made it a better place. To be honest, I am not sure what else I am suited for. Perhaps teaching. But from a nonintellectual perspective, I am not sure I am cut out to be a physician. It's not that I doubt myself so much as I doubt whether I know what qualities one should have for being a physician. And it's not clear to me whether anyone else knows either.

Since there seems to be no universally agreed upon, dependable screening process for determining what makes a good doctor, we often resort to using surrogate markers. In other words, we examine and measure identifiable markers in the hope that they will give us some insight into the things we really want to know about. They are, at best, just approximations.

For example, if someone can do well under the stress of exams, maybe that means they'll be wonderful at telling a patient that they have terminal cancer?

Maybe if someone is a really good musician or athlete and has done so competitively, that means they have exceptional manual dexterity and the mental toughness to handle a difficult intubation?

Perhaps if they have a really pleasant personality, they will not succumb to the lure of greed in a profession that earns more money than most people make?

There was a time when people had little formal education, which meant that becoming a doctor was exceptional, primarily in its rarity. Today, lots of people have multiple years of postgraduate education, as physicians do. We are no longer exceptional. Many people have stressful jobs and work long hours, including blue-collar workers. Many times in winter, I have looked out from my comfortable office to see a crane operator climb ten or more floors to operate a large crane carrying many tons of materials. In her line of work, a moment of inattention could cost lives, and I have secretly hoped that she was getting paid at least as well as I am. How do they determine if crane operators have the right stuff?

I must admit that I have never been comfortable being called "doctor." I am not entirely sure why. I think it's because I feel that it puts a wall between the person for whom I am caring and me; that somehow I'm special and deserve a special appellation.

During residency, I struggled with this physician persona. Wearing a tie and a white lab coat and introducing myself as doctor just didn't feel right. I was blessed to have Ernie Haynes as my staff supervisor at the time. He was a wise sage who recognized my struggle and quite literally changed my life with three simple words. He took me aside one day and said, "Barry, be yourself."

It amazes me how compassionate interactions change us; how much we need one another. How three such simple words, offered lovingly to me, changed for the better not just how I looked at the world but, more importantly, how I looked at myself. I never got a chance to thank Ernie for saving my career. I suspect he knew, nonetheless, because he saw me grow so much afterward. I think it was then that I got my first few insights into how we humans tick.

I understand that the profession likes to be called "doctor" as a sign of respect for the hard work, knowledge, and sacrifice that comes with the career. Fair enough. But I suspect the real motivation is that it helps us put a protective wall between our patients and us. Let me explain.

Patients quite rightly want us to be kind and compassionate and sensitive to feelings, but often only to their feelings or feelings that help them. In other words, patients want us to be very sensitive and kind when dealing with them, but when our endotracheal tubes go missing and we are just about to fill our diaper, they want us to be as cold as ice. "Doctor, tell the previous patient you saw that they have terminal cancer in the most compassionate way you can, but then come into my exam room like nothing happened, and focus all of your attention on my problems, no matter how trivial by comparison."

In other words, have a huge reservoir of compassion, but be able to turn it off and on instantly and effortlessly. Don't let it get to you on a personal level because that might adversely affect your treatment of me. And while you are at it, don't let your personal struggles or your own medical conditions compromise your care of me either.

I know that I am sounding, perhaps, somewhat harsh here. Many patients do care about their doctor's feelings, and I am always very moved by that. And the truth is, when you are scared, in pain, or suffering, it's hard to care about what the doctor is feeling at the moment, and I get that. It's perfectly reasonable to expect your doctor's undivided attention when you see her or him; it's just from this side of the stethoscope, it can be very difficult.

So the paradox is, we want a sensitive and an ice-cold doctor, all in the same nicely wrapped package.

In all of my years of practice, I have never been given any time or assistance in dealing with any of the numerous stresses I have faced. I have had to resuscitate, unsuccessfully, a young man involved in a severe motor vehicle accident, share the horrible news with his family that he had died, and then go right next door to deal with someone upset because they have had to wait four hours to be seen for a sore throat.

I have been at the deaths of hundreds of patients, been sued a few times (doing high-risk work like anaesthesia and emerg makes it unavoidable), and worked for twenty-four hours straight (or more), and there has never been any acknowledgement of the emotional toll it takes nor any assistance for that. No critical incident counselling. We patients want sensitive physicians, empathetic and compassionate physicians, but on our terms.

This is why we medical people build these walls—like being called "doctor." Benign enough, but some of the behaviours we adopt to cope with this emotional residue are not so benign. We get sidetracked by alcohol, drugs, or affairs, or by the money, the prestige, or the mystique. It's not because doctors are *bad* people. It's because doctors *are* people. We are not special; we are not exempt, no matter how many textbooks we memorize.

The profession tries to pretend that we are exempt, of course, by having very strict admission criteria, but none of those criteria really have much to do with the really important issue: that medicine is not so much an intellectual game or a talent game but a mind game.

I suspect that if I were to apply to medical school today, I would not be granted admission. The standards are so much higher in the sense that the profession wants to give the impression that those admitted are *Übermensch*—superwomen and supermen. They want to brag that they accept only individuals who have not just great academic gifts but are also exceptionally talented and successful in multitudinous ways. They have excelled in athletics or music or the arts, for example. And they have demonstrated a profound ability for caring for others by becoming involved in some humanitarian effort, often in a remote and underprivileged part of the world.

All of this sounds wonderful, except it means by definition that medicine is becoming a profession of the elite. Perhaps it always has been, to some degree, but with such expensive tuition, and the need to demonstrate proficiency in so many other aspects of life, one has to be very well off financially to develop the resume needed to prove that you have the right stuff, that you are an Übermensch.

I came from a middle-class family. We did not have the money to nurture any other talents, if I had had any. I had to find a job every summer to pay for university, any job I could get my hands on. I could not afford to travel to exotic lands and do volunteer work, as much as I might have wanted to.

But this admission process brings me back to one of my original questions. What surrogate markers are we using to identify the people we think will make the best physicians? Will such wildly talented people be able to handle the stress of life and death better? More importantly, can they relate better to their patients, most of whom are mere mortals? Do they have the compassion to care for people who are much less accomplished? Are they any less prone to the psychological foibles we are all subject to? Are they better balanced people, able to avoid the pitfalls that prestige and wealth expose us to?

As my career unfolded, I reflected upon my training and how incomplete it seemed in terms of understanding how human beings really worked—how I worked. Sure, I had gained the technical and intellectual skills to do my job, but was my mind ready for it? Had it matured enough to deal with all the stuff that lay beyond the technical and intellectual?

So I read more about philosophy and psychology; I wanted to understand better how my patients and I function at a deeper level. And I read about evolutionary neuropsychology because I needed to know more about our evolution to the pinnacle of nature's cognitive pyramid as the species with the fullest consciousness and sentience.

Chapter 3

The Phone Call

DURING THE TIME that I was reading more about philosophy and psychology, I interacted with many patients in many different circumstances, and each time I learned a little more about our minds. Let me share with you a story about a good friend and patient of mine, Joe. His mind surprised me one day in a way I never expected, from which I learned a great deal.

I had known Joe as a patient for about eight years. He was in his midsixties. He had a great sense of humour and was very down-to-earth. He kept abreast of how my kids were doing. I considered him a good friend.

Joe's life had not been an easy one. In the 1950s, when psychiatry was not as sophisticated as it is today, he had been admitted to psychiatric institutions several times for anxiety and depression. Back then, there were not as many effective drugs, so he had received electroconvulsive therapy (ECT). This is a brief procedure performed under general anaesthesia, during which electrical currents are passed through the skull and, hence, to the brain to trigger a brief seizure. In doing so, brain chemistry is changed, resulting in improvement in some mental illnesses such as severe depression. Joe had received at least one full course of ECT, with good results according to him.

But his journey, naturally, had left some scars. He functioned at a reasonably good level but knew that he would never be free of his anxiety completely. There was a strong history of mental illness in his family, and some traumatic life events as a youth contributed to his fragile emotional state. There would be times of relative psychic stability, but he and I both knew that he would likely never be cured.

I always looked forward to seeing Joe, but don't get me wrong, he could frustrate me as well. Like many anxious people, he worried about his health in particular, sometimes to excess. It might not be an exaggeration to say that he was a little hypochondriacal. But the beautiful thing about Joe, which made me so fond of him, was that he recognized this in himself. This meant we could have a very honest dialogue about his health. He knew that he had a tendency to blow minor symptoms out of proportion (termed "catastrophic thinking"), so he learned over time to trust my judgment with respect to when to simply watch and wait and when to investigate further. Well, most of the time.

Every once in a while, he would get himself so worked up that no amount of rational thought on my part could settle his angst. I would be forced to relent and order some test to prove to him that nothing serious was going on.

There is always a risk involved in doing tests, in looking further. In general, in medicine, you ought to order a test very carefully, understanding the purpose of the test before you do it. In other words, you have to have some idea what you are searching for; otherwise, you'll end up ordering the wrong test that can't possibly answer your question. For example, an ultrasound is not the best test to look at a bone, and a plain X-ray is not the best to look at nonbony structures.

Then you have to ask yourself if there is any point in doing this test if you are not going to do anything about a legitimate result, either because you can't or you won't? It's true, there are times when you won't do anything *directly* about the test result, but it is still worthwhile doing. For example, if you find out that you have terminal cancer, you might not want to have a hip replacement since the recovery from such surgery might steal what little precious time you have left. But in general, it is common wisdom that you don't do a test just for curiosity's sake because tests can be expensive, uncomfortable, and risky.

People often forget about the risks of tests, and some tests carry more risk than others. Any time a test is invasive—that is, it involves entering into your body (e.g., scopes, X-rays, needles)—there are risks.

There is always the risk that a test result comes back and you are not sure of its significance. There is something abnormal, but does it mean anything? Does it really relate to the patient's symptoms, or is it a red herring, an "incidentaloma" as we like to call it?

There is also the risk of the false-positive result. In other words, because no test is ever 100 percent accurate, sometimes a test says that you have something wrong, and it turns out on final analysis that you don't. That means that you have taken the risk of the initial test for no benefit; but worse still, in order to prove that the test was a false positive, you have to undergo further tests, all of which may be painful, anxiety-provoking, and risky as well.

Now getting back to Joe, he had been having some vague abdominal discomfort, and on the first visit, I reassured him that there appeared to be nothing seriously wrong and that the best thing to do was to monitor the situation for a little while. I explained to him that there were no red flags, worrisome signs, or symptoms, but if such arose, then to come back to see me.

None arose, but Joe worried nonetheless. He was noticeably more anxious on the second visit, and although nothing clinically had changed, I realized that he would only be reassured if I ran some appropriate blood tests.

The tests, of course, came back normal, but on the follow-up visit, his third visit about the discomfort, Joe was not reassured. I have always made it a rule not to take a patient's intuition lightly, so even though I was convinced that there was nothing wrong, I relented and ordered an abdominal ultrasound. Just like everybody else, I can make mistakes, and it's easy to be dismissive of someone's symptoms just because they have worried excessively in the past for no justifiable reason. The truth is that even the most hypochondriacal patient eventually dies.

The result, unfortunately, came back abnormal. The difficulty was that the radiologist, understandably, could not be sure what the exact problem was or if there was one at all. What the radiologist had seen was a mass somewhere around the head of the pancreas. The pancreas, which is the organ deep in the abdomen responsible for producing both digestive enzymes and insulin, is so far back in the abdomen that it can be hard to see in detail, particularly if the patient is at all chubby, which Joe was. (Radiologists euphemistically state that the accuracy of the report is limited by the patient's body habitus—"yellow muscle" the surgeons call it.)

The worry was that this could be pancreatic cancer—a disease that often has no symptoms until it is quite far advanced. The position of the pancreas deep in the abdomen is part of the problem. But my reading of the ultrasound was that the mass did not seem to be part of the pancreas but in front of it, although it was hard to be sure. I was concerned, but Joe was near panic. I arranged for an urgent CT scan, which would elucidate the truth for us. The scan was scheduled in two days, on a Friday, and I would hopefully have the result by Monday. I did my best to allay Joe's fears and urged him not to get ahead of himself, as difficult as I knew that would be for him.

He told me he would hang tight over the weekend, and I promised that I would call as soon as I knew the result.

I received a call about Joe Monday morning before I started to see patients. But it wasn't the call I was expecting from the radiologist.

It was a call from the coroner.

The previous evening, Sunday night, Joe had been sitting with his spouse watching their favourite TV program. During a commercial break, shortly before the end of the show, Joe got up and went to the bathroom. He returned in time to see the end of the show. As was usually their routine, his spouse went to bed ahead of him, kissing him good night beforehand.

The next morning, his partner awoke to find that Joe was not in bed. Entering the living room, his partner found him sitting as he had the night before, lifeless. Joe had taken an overdose of his psychiatric meds and various over-the-counter medications during that bathroom break and had died during the night.

The phone call from the coroner was devastating for me. The news of a patient committing suicide is one of the most gut-wrenching experiences I think a physician can have, second only to the death of a child in their practice.

I had lost a good friend, and I hadn't seen it coming. I thought I had allayed Joe's anxiety sufficiently for him to get through the weekend, and that together we would deal with whatever the CT scan revealed on Monday.

But the saddest part of the story came thirty minutes later. The radiologist called and was completely convinced that the mass was a benign lipoma—a collection of fat in front of the pancreas. The autopsy later that week confirmed the diagnosis.

Chapter 4

Fear

I OFTEN TELL people that I am blessed to be a family doctor because I have the most interesting job on the planet. Since entering medical school in 1978, I have spent my life studying the most complex, most varied, and most intriguing thing in the known universe: us!

Every day I have the privilege of interacting with my fellow humans about so many things that are central to our lives: pregnancy, birth, illness, disability, happiness, sadness, death, and love.

And the one experience that brings people to see me more than any other, of course, is fear.

That's what brought Joe to see me about his abdominal pain. I suspect that Joe committed suicide for the same reason that all people who commit suicide do: fear.

As a youth, I had always been taught that nature imbued all living things with two overwhelming instincts, both of which are necessary if a species is going to survive and flourish.

The first instinct is for survival of self. Every creature does whatever it takes to stay alive. Death is to be avoided at almost all costs, with few exceptions such as protection of offspring. All species have developed internal mechanisms to maximize life expectancy, each according to their environment, but all sharing many similarities, like the fight-or-flight reflex. Evolution depends on survival of the fittest, necessitating a continuous process of adaptation to an ever-changing milieu in order to simply live.

The second instinct is for reproduction so that the species as a whole survives. This second instinct, paradoxically, can clash with the first. During copulation, a creature is often at its most vulnerable, so these affairs are often brief for that reason. Although there are lots of exceptions, thank goodness!

I don't know if animals ever commit suicide. Like blushing, it may be something peculiar just to humans. If that is the case, how do we explain suicide—the overriding of the one universal, self-preserving instinct that seems to make such basic sense?

The answer is fear. Human beings, when we developed our substantial frontal lobes, developed the ability to think about the future in a way that animals cannot. Our greatest fear is not the fear of death. (In fact, in many studies, people have ranked public speaking as a greater fear than dying!) No, our greatest fear is the fear of future pain that we cannot control. We fear overpowering, endless suffering.

What kind of pain are we talking about? Physical pain is one type of pain, no doubt. But more often, it is a psychic pain that strikes in us the greatest fear: the fear of humiliation or shame or inadequacy and, particularly, the fear of loneliness.

It's because we are communal beasts; we are hard-wired to interact with one another, to care about, and for, one another. It is astounding how many of our senses and how much of our developed brain have to do with some form of communication.

I remember reading a book by a reporter held as a political captive for several years. He described brutal torture, but the most painful experience he had, paradoxically, was solitary confinement. Why? Because when we are rejected and ignored, we feel unworthy of that one thing we all need: love. I can imagine the hopelessness that reporter experienced. He must have felt so worthless, ignored, and insignificant because he wasn't even worth torturing.

Look at how many people end their lives during financial crises or after losing their jobs. They feel lost and hopeless because they think that their drop in social status or monetary stability will render them unwanted, that they don't matter or belong any more. Witness how many people become depressed or die shortly after retirement, perhaps in part because their sense of belonging, of being needed, can decrease so dramatically. Social factors, especially isolation, are strong predictors of suicide.

I suspect that Joe experienced an insurmountable peak of fear that Sunday evening. He felt so afraid of the future—the pain of cancer, the lack of control, the sense of losing who he was, and ultimately the loneliness of a prolonged dying process—that he simply chose to avoid it with the easiest, quickest, and most painless process he could find.

This primal emotion—fear—has more control over us than we often recognize. Thich Nhat Hahn, a Vietnamese Buddhist monk, explores this in his wonderful book *Fear*. We want to see anxiety as a mental illness that afflicts only an unfortunate few, but we are all controlled by it, often more than we like to think.

This, quite frankly, is why I have a job. Let me explain.

Occasionally, a stranger will ask me what I do for a living, and I will give them the most honest answer I can. I tell them that my job is to predict the future.

They often look startled; I don't look at all like a fortune teller. No matter what problem a patient comes to see me about, ultimately what they care about most is the future.

Suppose right now you are in horrible pain. Think of the worst pain you have ever had or the worst that you could imagine. However, suppose you also know that it will completely disappear very shortly, and it is not a manifestation of any serious disease. In other words, very soon it will be gone, and you will be back to your previous health, never to be bothered by that discomfort again. Would you really come to see me? Not if you were completely sure that it would be so brief that you could not get to me in time for me to do anything helpful. You wouldn't waste your time if you knew the pain would be gone before any of my interventions could become effective.

Even if you did, you know I cannot take away the pain of the past or present, just your future pain. The pain you say you are experiencing right now is already in the past by the time you recognize it and share it with me. It is always future pain that is your concern.

When is my pain going to end? Is it going to come back again? Does it mean I have some serious underlying problem? Is the quality of my future life compromised? Is the quantity of my future life compromised? Will I suffer with this alone? All are questions about the future—your future.

Just as guilt is always about the past, fear is always about the future. And with the rise of our consciousness, we humans have developed a very profound appreciation of the concept of time, as well as a substantial propensity to be concerned about the future. We plan, and we enjoy planning. We prepare for the future. We have expectations of the future; we care about it to a much greater degree than most of the other species on the planet. I don't think frogs and chipmunks make retirement plans. And when signs or symptoms arise that worry us that our vision of the future is in doubt and not within our control, fear is generated. And this is what prompts people to visit doctors. Animals don't visit doctors or financial planners, at least of their own accord.

So I have come to appreciate that my job is to try to predict a patient's future. Of course, I can't; no physician can with any great certainty. We can only give probabilistic guesses based on studies, experience, and intuition. We'll talk about that later in more detail.

But for the moment, the important point is that fear of future suffering is a universal experience that drives each and every one of us, some more than others. There is no escaping its clutch completely.

How did this come to pass? How is it that the human species seems more affected by this than any other species, to the point that it can occasionally cause us to override one of nature's most powerful instincts for survival?

Medical school and residency never gave me these answers, and I wasn't sure where to look. As is often the case, when you are lost, the best place to go in order to find yourself is back to the beginning.

Yes, I went right back to the big bang.

PART II: HOW WE GOT HERE

Chapter 5

In the Beginning

PERHAPS IT IS paradoxical that a man of faith, Jesuit priest Georges Lemaître, developed the big bang theory (the cosmic event, not the TV show). In any event, his theory has permeated modern culture in a way similar to how Charles Darwin's theory of evolution influenced his era and is still influencing us today.

Surprisingly, in order for me to grasp how we humans work, I had to go right back to the beginning of time and explore the development of the universe (cosmology). I am no cosmologist, so please bear with my, perhaps, simplistic understanding. What little I know I have gleaned from the fascinating series *Cosmos*, hosted by Neil deGrasse Tyson, as well as from books I have read, including Brian Greene's *The Fabric of the Cosmos* and *The Hidden Reality* and books by Stephen Hawking.

The Big Bang

The crux of the big bang theory is that in the beginning, there was a small and very dense blob of primordial plasma that for some reason expanded suddenly and very quickly. Science cannot explain how nor why it got there. In fact, such speculation is beyond the realm of science. It's just there, and that's all there is to it. I guess we have to take it on faith, given that it is Georges' theory!

Nevertheless, during the initial expansion, the primordial plasma was thrown apart at speeds faster than the speed of light under the influence of a repulsive gravity. As the universe cooled in the first little while after the big bang, subatomic particles like protons came into existence as expansion slowed. Then attractive gravitational forces began to dominate, causing the simplest atoms, the element hydrogen, to be drawn together into nascent structures that eventually became stars.

Over many millions of years, inside the incredibly hot cores of these primitive stars, other elements like helium and lithium formed from the fusion of hydrogen atoms. All of the elements we are familiar with today have been formed in this way, which means that all of the chemicals that constitute you and me have been made inside of the stars we see when we look skyward at night. We are literally manufactured from the very stardust of the universe.

How is all of this relevant to Joe's fear?

If we pay close attention, this story of the big bang, and what followed over the billions of years since, can teach us a lot about how we have come to be and how we function in the world. And that includes the role that fear has come to play in our everyday lives. So let's dig a little deeper.

Ken Wilber, a brilliant modern philosopher, elucidates in his books *A Theory of Everything* and *A Brief History of Everything* the various levels of complexity of the universe: the physiosphere, the biosphere, the noosphere, and the theosphere. He explores the evolutionary process whereby the universe makes rather unexpected and monumental transitions from lower levels to higher levels of complexity. Each level includes and transcends the levels below it. This point is key.

These transitions, however, are rather inexplicable. For example, at the big bang, something mysterious happened. This amorphous blob of very tightly packed stuff blew apart and eventually formed protons and neutrons and all of the other elementary particles and energies that are the fundamental building blocks of the universe. Up until that point, the universe was very simple. All that existed were a few dozen types of fundamental particles racing around independently. The physiosphere sprang into existence as these particles interacted with one another and formed more complex structures. There were no longer just a few dozen types of things out there, but a massive number of things out there.

Guided by the laws of the physiosphere, the limited number of elementary particles gathered together to form simple hydrogen atoms and then more complicated atoms that then coalesced into stars that then made even more new atoms. These atoms were flung out into space and interacted to make complex molecules that eventually became planets. The universe evolved from a handful of elementary particles racing about independently to a place with myriad structures, some very small like atoms and molecules, and some very large like stars and galaxies that interacted with one another in very complex ways. And we haven't got a clue how or why this event occurred.

The development of the physiosphere highlights the process of evolution: the universe goes from being less complicated (a few types of particles) to more complicated (lots of different particles and the new structures they produce). It also became more complex, meaning more interactivity between particles and structures. In other words, the contents of the universe become more interdependent, more *relational*.

Over the hundreds of millions of years that followed on earth, molecules and the structures that molecules formed became even more complex. Then, once again, something mysterious happened.

Some of these chemicals, under just the right circumstances, did something unique. They grew and morphed into structures that could interact with their environment, move, and then eventually become self-replicating. A primitive type of awareness evolved. Inanimate chemicals crossed a mystical boundary and became *life*. The biosphere manifested itself.

We know that this happened on earth, although we don't know exactly when or how. We suspect that it may have happened elsewhere in the universe, and we keep looking for evidence. This thing called "life" functions under all of the rules that govern matter and energy, but it has also developed some new principles of its own that could not be derived simply from the laws of the physiosphere. The biosphere includes the physiosphere but transcends it with its own unique rules of engagement. No understanding of quantum mechanics can fully explain the concept of reproduction or the coursing of blood through arteries. If you are doubtful, ask yourself, "Is the principle of survival of the fittest, which seems to guide evolution in the biosphere, a principle we apply in the physiosphere?"

The Brain

On earth, over many millions of years, life continued to grow more complicated and complex. Single cells developed defence mechanisms for survival, including receptors for detecting danger and machinery for either fighting or fleeing. An embryonic type of fear entered the repertoire of life.

Over time, some of these apparatuses evolved into more sophisticated sensory organs, like ears and eyes, that offered a survival advantage. In the animal kingdom, one of these organs developed a central role, one connecting and coordinating all of the others: the brain. These structures, particularly the brain, allowed for even more possibilities for interactions to occur between living things and their environment and, even more importantly, among living things themselves.

Very primitive brains are seen in fish and reptiles. In these creatures, the brain is essentially a relay station for autonomic and reflex activities. It consists of the brainstem (pons, medulla, and cerebellum) and lower parts of the midbrain with strong connections to the spinal cord. These structures control the function of internal organs as well as movement and basic senses. Here powerful reflexes for survival reside. We refer to them as "instincts."

It is important to realize that the brain and body are intensely enmeshed. Hormones—chemicals secreted from body organs like the thyroid, parathyroid, and adrenal glands—bathe the brain through the rich blood supply it receives; in turn, nerves—extensions of the brain—permeate the body. There are multiple feedback loops, so the brain controls the body, but the body also controls the brain. The organism as a whole is constantly reacting to its environment with literally lightning-fast speed through these nerves that mediate their effects in both the brain and the body.

If you have ever tried to catch a frog, you know how fast these reflexes are. Sneak up as slowly and quietly as you like, but only the quickest and slyest among us can move as swiftly as the frog can when it senses its life is in danger. These primitive reflexes may not be highly selective or refined, but they are extremely intense and highly effective.

Over time, this reptilian brain became more complex as the reptiles evolved slowly into mammals. In the lower mammals, the brain expanded beyond the brainstem and midbrain to develop what is referred to as the "limbic system"—amygdala, hippocampus, thalamus, hypothalamus, and the basal ganglia, among others—and the neocortex (more on this later). The limbic system's functions include the mediation of emotion, behaviour, motivation, and memory. The neocortex, the "new brain" above it, is where more cultivated processing of information occurs. In lower mammals, the neocortex remains rather small, but in higher mammals it becomes massive, taking up by far the largest share of the cranial cavity.

The primitive reptilian reflexes of course remained, but added to them is a vast repertoire of even more sophisticated behaviours, courtesy of the limbic system and early neocortex. Anyone who has pondered the idea of petting a lost bear cub knows better than to do so, even if momma bear appears to be absent. The limbic system and neocortex are responsible for this more sophisticated reflex of protecting one's young, something reptiles do not do. The embryonic brains of reptiles are simply not programmed for it. So in lower mammals, fear advances to another level. No longer purely self-protective, fear evolves into a nascent form of altruism, if only a proximate one (such as their own offspring or family).

As these lower mammals evolved into higher mammals, one genus distinguished itself above all of the others: the hominid. Not only did their cerebral hemispheres grow substantially, their frontal lobes did so in particular. This growth culminated in a species referred to as "*Homo sapiens.*"

Then, once again, something mysterious happened.

Consciousness

This brain, with its large hemispheres and frontal lobes, did something no lesser brain could do: it achieved full consciousness, including the abilities of introspection and self-reflection, and from there the noosphere became fully manifested. Yet again, the level of complexity of the universe had expanded. All living things had had within them some level of awareness. But as life evolved, so did this awareness, culminating in the full self-awareness of humans, who could not only contemplate abstract thoughts, but they could interact with their fellow humans far more profoundly and so discuss these new thoughts as well. The mind was born.

Similar to the big bang and the appearance of life, we don't understand exactly how human consciousness developed, nor when.

As a boy, I remember watching Stanley Kubrick's movie *2001: A Space Odyssey*, based on Arthur C. Clarke's book of the same name. It was the myth of my childhood and hypothesized an alien intervention, using a large black monolith, to accomplish this metamorphosis.

Of course, *2001: A Space Odyssey* is just a modern-day movie from a science-fiction book. But in fact, most cultures throughout history have developed their own narratives to explain this transformation to full consciousness.

In the Judeo-Christian tradition, Genesis explains not just how God created the universe in six days, but how he also imbued humanity with this gift of consciousness.

Eve eating the forbidden fruit of the tree of knowledge is the mythical story describing how humans evolved into sentient beings. Once Eve and Adam ate the fruit, they gained the full consciousness that their fellow inhabitants of the garden lacked. They were then self-conscious of their nakedness and covered up. As sentient humans, they then knew the difference between right and wrong and had to live with the responsibility that that entailed. They had a conscience. They had fully conscious minds, not just brains.

Rabbi Harold S. Kushner explains this well in his wonderful book *Nine Essential Things I've Learned About Life*. In the book of Genesis, God declares that there are repercussions for humanity after Eve and Adam shared the apple. Women would suffer pain during childbirth, pain they would feel for the rest of their lives because consciousness would keep them connected, as parents, to their offspring in a fashion unlike all other animals in paradise. Men would be forced to labour for their existence. They would be aware of their responsibility for their family's future. They would have to consciously work for their family's survival, not simply graze for their own sustenance.

Of course, Genesis is just a story. But one thing is clear: there will be no going back. Humanity will forever be saddled with the joy and sorrow of consciousness. Paradox?

Part of this sorrow is an escalation of pain. We are still subject to the physical, painful stimuli and the reflex behaviours to deal with them that the reptiles have. Try not taking your hand off of a hot stove. And like dogs and cats, we protect our young and those closest to us. Ask any parent what their greatest fear is. No matter what the age of the parent (or their progeny), it will almost invariably be about the lives and health of their children, not themselves.

But as humans, the ante has been upped even further. We have a conscience that can care beyond the immediate family, even beyond our tribe or species. Altruism has arisen within us.

And we have a mind that can contemplate not just the immediate pain threatening us, but can consider future pain as well. And to make matters worse, we can have psychic pain—existential pain—not just physical pain.

Is it worth it? The famous philosopher John S. Mill stated, "Better a human dissatisfied than a pig satisfied." I think he is right. But in the middle of great pain and suffering, like the kind that Joe must have been experiencing, it can be hard to believe that.

Make no mistake. The various chemicals of our nervous system—acetylcholine, norepinephrine, dopamine, GABA, serotonin, and others—that mediate communication among nerves in our brains and with the rest of our bodies, are powerful. It is said that we have billions of neurons—nerve cells—in our brains and spinal cord that can each have up to several thousand connections—synapses—with other neurons. The communication between them is constant and near instantaneous.

The deep reflexes of our brainstem are life-saving and are not easily countermanded. How long can you hold your hand on a hot stove? The limbic system operates equally quickly and powerfully. Try not being upset when a stranger threatens your two-year-old.

And despite the power of our cerebral hemispheres, they still use the same chemicals with equal rapidity. Further, they remain deeply wired to the same more primitive pathways of frogs and grizzly bears. When we are told by a partner that they no longer love us and want to end our relationship, our heart pounds, our breathing becomes laboured, and we feel nauseated and dizzy in a way similar to physical pain. We want to run away from our lives, from the pain and impending loneliness. We may even be at risk of incontinence. That's because our cerebral hemispheres still manifest through our limbic system and brainstem as well, and these neural connections result in the same physical sensations in our bodies as physical pain would trigger.

Ideally we would like to utilize these deep, ingrained neural networks only when they are of immediate advantage to us, like when our hand is on the hot stove. But the process of evolution has prevented that. In fact, it has made it even more convoluted. How so?

Reptiles tend to be solitary critters for the most part. They don't operate in herds as mammals do. So their instincts revolve primarily around self-preservation, as we have seen. Their reproductive habits reflect this as well: there is little, if any, direct contact with their mates. When there is, it is generally quick and to the point.

But lower mammals, with their burgeoning neocortex, socialize. They raise their young; they often travel together. Their reproductive habits mirror this: their copulation involves foreplay and direct physical contact.

That sociality changes things for mammals. True, a deer does not want to be eaten by the hungry wolves any more than a frog wants to be eaten by the bird. And being the weakest deer in the herd does increase the likelihood that it, not one of its compatriots, will be eaten. But for a social creature, it is more than just about being eaten. Being the weakest deer in the herd means you risk the possibility of being alone, of not being able to be with your mate or raise your young, and for social creatures that matters a lot.

This is even truer for *Homo sapiens* because so much of our brain is directed toward communication and socialization. It, too, is reflected in our reproductive habits. We are one of the few species who mate facing one another. We communicate during mating—with our eyes, our face, our touch, and, of course, our speech. We value and enjoy intimacy.

So it should come as no surprise that it is not just death or physical suffering that triggers intense, painful, and deep-seated angst. Being abandoned, like solitary confinement, does too, in a very primal way. It wallops us from the top of our brain down to its very core.

Furthermore, this leap to consciousness provided us with two other assets: the ability to think critically, located usually in the left hemisphere, and the ability to be creative, usually on the right. With the development of these assets, we came to understand the concept of time and could now ponder the future and try to control our environment and, hence, our destiny to a remarkable degree. We came to value control, and we do not like to lose it. That is why, beyond the messiness of it, incontinence is so disarming. We crave control in our lives, and losing it can terrify us. It leaves us vulnerable to the vagaries of the harsh world around us. That's why panic attacks are no fun. Interestingly, control is the central focus of the present assisted-suicide debate.

So I have no doubt that despite my reassurances, and likely those of his spouse, Joe experienced irresistible, raw fear that could not be comforted by any neuronal influences from his cortex, at least for a brief period. That fear was born from at least three sources: the fear of future pain, the fear of abandonment, and the fear of loss of control. Fears so entrenched and powerful that they overrode his most basic instinct for self-preservation.

After Joe's death, the annoying six-year-old inside me kept asking, "How did Joe acquire such fear? Did I not see it because I was afraid of something too? If so, what?"

As I said earlier in chapter 4, I had always understood that fear can motivate patients to see doctors. However, my inquiry into this business of fear intensified after my experience with Joe. Fear was clearly significant in conditions that threatened our survival; but I wondered if it was more pervasive than that, perhaps a fundamental, unavoidable constituent of the human condition.

Over time, I began to see fear as an integral part of my profession, in the very nature of medicine, in the work I did daily, in every patient I saw. I saw it as the primary source of our insecurities and, hence, the cause of many of our behaviours, wise and otherwise.

And I had to find out more.

Chapter 6

Knowing Me, Knowing You
(with apologies to Abba)

I REMEMBER A day about twenty-five years ago when I found out a lot more about how humans work. It was a Saturday in the winter, a time when there are more than an average number of infectious diseases permeating communities, and ours was no different. I was scheduled to work a shift at our local walk-in clinic.

The shifts can be very busy, and unpredictably so, because they often tend to operate, as the name suggests, on a walk-in basis. The doors open for a certain period, but as long as you are in the door by the time it closes, you will be seen. I suspect that having scores of people, many of whom are there because of a concern about having a potentially contagious infection, crammed together tightly in a small room for hours is not the most sophisticated way of practising medicine. Be that as it may, many clinics still operate using this method.

Nevertheless, in the rural community in which I practised, we all had to take our turn to provide health care in the off-hours to our fellow community members.

Many of us don't find these clinics to be the most rewarding medicine to practise for a variety of reasons. People who are already not feeling well and not in the best of humours wait for hours sometimes to be seen. Given the jam-packed lives everyone leads, patients just want to get the quick fix and be gone. So there is a lot of pressure to "grind them through" and give them what they want, which means that we use shortcuts to get the job done. Pleasantries are abbreviated, and we cut to the chase pretty quickly. I think that's why a lot of us don't particularly enjoy the shifts—it's too much like an assembly line, and we don't feel that we have the time to really explain things well to the people we see. (I think that there are better ways to provide such a service, but more on that later.)

Around the time of this particular shift, there had been, as there is from time to time, a lot of chatter about the overuse of antibiotics, particularly during flu season. I decided on this particular shift that, despite the usual busyness of such clinics, I would make a concerted effort to take more time explaining to patients in reasonable detail the rationale for *not* prescribing antibiotics in cases where I felt that they likely had a viral illness for which antibiotics could not possibly help. I was hoping that by doing so, I would provide a better service and that patients would appreciate this effort. In return, although I would be there for 50 percent longer (and I was), I would enjoy a more satisfying day.

Let me give some background information first. We do not have medications for *most* viral illnesses. There are exceptions, for example, like herpes. But for most viral infections, which comprise by far the majority of respiratory infections ("upper respiratory," meaning the nose and throat, as well as "lower respiratory," meaning the lungs), and in the Western world, also the majority of gastrointestinal infections, we have no specific medications to eradicate and thus shorten the duration of illness. (Paradoxically, viruses are much harder to kill because they are *simpler* than bacteria!) We can only offer what is referred to as "supportive care." In other words, we provide general advice about how to minimize symptoms (and contagiousness) and aid your own body in eliminating the virus as quickly and effectively as possible. This includes such measures as resting, eating well, and drinking more fluids.

Now the word "flu," like many words used to describe medical conditions, has two meanings. There is the general public's meaning, which is often a vague catchall, and then there is the specific medical profession's meaning of the word. However, we physicians often succumb to the generic use of these terms to simplify things, although sometimes it simply serves to confuse.

For example, people will talk about a "stomach flu" or a "head flu" or a "cold flu." I understand what they mean, that some part of them is under the weather, but "flu" really is a short form for influenza—a very specific type of virus with very specific, and sometimes lethal, symptomatology. The true flu—influenza—often leaves people feeling very miserable, far worse than the average "flu" people complain about. And it illustrates a point that patients sometimes don't understand: just because you feel *really* lousy doesn't mean that you must have a bacterial infection. All that said, a flu can be very serious and epidemic—millions of people died of the Spanish influenza at the start of the last century.

It is true that there are some medications available to treat influenza, but for most of us, they will only shorten symptoms by a day or two (if that). They can be of use in some populations more than others and are probably most useful for *prevention* in those exposed to, but not yet sick from, the influenza virus.

Given this state of affairs, it is important to try to determine if someone who is complaining of what could be an infectious disease has one that is viral, for which we can most often suggest only supportive measures, or bacterial, for which an antibiotic may be very helpful. (There are other infectious diseases that are neither viral nor bacterial, for example, fungal, but for the sake of this discussion, I will limit the boundaries.)

So the assessment seems to be a straightforward binary one: do the symptoms (complaints) and signs (objective evidence) the patient displays collectively point toward a viral or bacterial cause?

The first challenge is that although, ultimately, one must decide one way or the other, medicine is, by its very nature, a probabilistic endeavour. As I explained before, doctors are trying to predict the future from a range of potential outcomes. It is much more like a light switch with a dimmer control than a light switch with a simple off-on mechanism; it's a matter of degree.

For example, a classic streptococcal pharyngitis (streptococcus being the commonest *bacterial* cause of a sore throat, commonly referred to as a "strep throat") has quite a number of symptoms (e.g., fever, headache, sore throat, absence of cough, difficulty swallowing) and signs (e.g., enlarged lymph nodes; swollen, red tonsils with whitish pus on them). But many of these symptoms and signs are not specific to strep throat. And not everyone exhibits all of them or exhibits them the same way. Treating children poses special challenges because it can be difficult for them to tell us how they are feeling.

Equally, the symptoms and signs may not all be fully present at all times in the illness, especially in the first few hours. There are also a number of symptoms and signs that would rule against a strep throat, for example diarrhea is not common with strep throat. So like most illnesses, and most things in life, symptoms manifest along a spectrum. Most people will have the common constellation of symptoms, but there will be atypical presentations too; "canary presentations" as we call them.

To make matters worse, laboratory testing is never 100 percent accurate either. Throat swabs, for example, depend a lot on the quality of the swab done, which can sometimes be difficult (for example, in young children). Beyond that, every lab test has its limitations because they are limited by humans and their technology.

So at the end of the day, based on all of the available data (symptoms, signs, and investigations), we make a probabilistic determination (one might want to go so far as to say "guess") about whether the patient's sore throat is viral or bacterial. You can rarely (if ever) say 100 percent it is bacterial or not. We can only give probabilities along a spectrum. That's true for all of medicine, not just sore throats.

I'll discuss ethics a bit later in the book, but for now let me offer that our job as physicians is to educate patients with the most accurate information and analysis (based on our knowledge and experience) available at that time, in a manner that they can process, such that they can make a (hopefully) wise decision regarding treatment (or further investigations perhaps).

Patients (except in rare circumstances of mental incapacity) are free to choose how they want to proceed. Equally, physicians are under no obligation to provide to patients something that would cause more harm than good (e.g., an immediate tonsillectomy) or no good at all (e.g., an antifungal medication for a strep-throat bacterial infection).

Now, let's return to that shift many years ago at the rural walk-in clinic, when I took extra time to explain to each patient who likely had a viral illness why an antibiotic would be of no help. In these types of clinics, the majority of patients who present with infectious disease symptoms have viruses. So, for an adult who appeared to me to have a viral sore throat, I would say something like the following: "You have had no fever, your tonsils appear normal, and you have multiple symptoms that do not fit with strep throat—such as diarrhea and a hoarse voice—and for that reason I think the likelihood of you benefiting from antibiotics is less than five percent since there is a ninety-five percent chance that this is viral."

However, if I thought the infection was very likely strep, I would say, "Your child has a high fever, headache, and pussy tonsils—all of which point to a ninety percent or more chance that this is strep for which antibiotics would be very helpful." (Children tend to benefit far more from antibiotics for strep throat than adults do.)

Now remember, this was twenty-five years ago, and times have changed somewhat. What do you think the response was to my endeavours?

Not good. Oh, a few people (around 20 percent) appreciated the education and chose, because of the low odds, not to go ahead with a prescription but to keep an eye on things and return if symptoms or signs changed in keeping with a bacterial infection (waiting, perhaps, for the result of a throat swab). The majority (70 percent) at the end of my exposition simply looked somewhat dumbfounded at me, wondering when they were going to get the prescription. My lecture appeared erudite and irrelevant to them; they had simply come there for a quick fix. A few people (10 percent) were quite upset and cut me off, demanding the prescription because they had waited already long enough.

I wasn't angry. It was an experiment, and like any true scientist, I simply wanted to know what effect taking the extra time would have, one way or the other. I accepted any outcome because all outcomes teach us something. In fact, I found it all rather amusing. Okay, I'll admit, it was a little depressing too.

Now it would be easy to generalize that the 80 percent who simply wanted antibiotics were abusing the system, were not very sophisticated, and were worrywarts, but that would be not only unkind but unduly simplistic and unhelpful. The truth is, I don't blame them. The medical profession has not always done a good job at educating patients. In fact, at times we have misled them into believing that we can do more than we can. If I were a patient, I might not understand either.

I believe things have improved since that day twenty-five years ago, but perhaps not as much as you might think. Why is that? We should know better—we hear a lot about the overuse of antibiotics and the rise of resistant strains—we are all *reason*able, aren't we, and yet the overuse persists.

But where does *reason* fit into the picture? The Greeks, led by Socrates, worshipped reason, and their influence is still powerful today. But is reason the whole picture?

Clearly, fear is playing a major role here. We know how miserable, disabling, or even lethal bacterial infections can be, particularly from stories of the preantibiotic era not so many decades ago. We want to be safe.

And our lives are busy. We don't have time to be sick; our lives are already maxed out. As doctors, we hear, "One more night of this cough interrupting my sleep will break me; give me an antibiotic just in case." Many people are living paycheque to paycheque and can't afford to miss work or compromise what little job security they have. The theoretical risk of antibiotic resistance sometime in the *future* pales in comparison to their real fear in the *present* moment that their child could get very sick or die, or they could mess up at work because they feel so lousy and subsequently lose their job. Deep visceral pain and fear can have a tendency to win out over rational thought, especially when we are feeling vulnerable and compromised.

A couple of years ago, someone put a poster on the door of one of the exam rooms I was using. The poster was an attempt to educate young people about the risks of excess alcohol intake. It contained a long list of scary statistics about the increased likelihood of multiple diseases correlated with alcohol abuse. Most of these diseases would take thirty or more years to manifest.

I suppose that all of the people involved in the design, production, and placement of this poster had their hearts in the right place. It is quite likely that they sincerely cared about these young people and desperately wanted them to change their behaviours in order to improve both the quality and quantity of their lives. Clearly, they felt that a very effective approach was to appeal to the *reason* of these bright university students by simply presenting the facts objectively. Their rational intellect would do the rest, and voila, they would stop drinking to excess.

But I wondered to myself, is it realistic to think that reason is the final common pathway these students use in making decisions that affect their health, especially when it comes to alcohol? I suspect that the majority of the young people the poster was targeting used alcohol as a way of coping with their loneliness, their anxieties (especially social anxieties), their depression, and their insecurities, as well as multiple other stressors. They wanted to fit in. They wanted to feel "okay." They wanted to dull their pain. What is the likelihood that the powerful emotions they have *in the here and now*, that drive them to drink, are going to be overruled by rational concerns about the theoretical risks of diseases they *might* experience many decades hence? Very unlikely, I suspect!

The perspective of the people involved in the poster campaign belies a common mistake we make about ourselves: that we are purely rational creatures.

Perhaps the most fundamental error we make in any discipline of human behaviour—be it medicine, law, education, politics, or business—is failing to understand how humans really work. We develop theories about how to engage a discipline (e.g., politics) in the real world that seem to ignore a fundamental, very practical truth: humans are not computers. We do not behave like Mr. Spock from *Star Trek*. In real life, we don't act like the textbooks say we ought to. As Yogi Berra said, "In theory there is no difference between theory and practice; in practice there is."

So, given humanity's penchant for not always relying on reason for decision making, do we simply throw up our hands in frustration and give up? Or do we use the oldest coping mechanism in the book—denial—and just deceive ourselves that such is not the case and soldier on in feigned ignorance? We often do choose one or the other, but we don't have to. Twenty percent of the people I saw that day in the walk-in clinic chose otherwise.

As is usually true in life, few challenges have binary outcomes; there are almost always more than two possibilities, and often many more along a wide spectrum. And as it turns out, our complex brains are up to the task of finding them, *if we let them.*

I found out over the subsequent years of practising medicine that nurturing our brains to do that is the tough part. Sometimes the answers are found in places we least expect them. To my surprise, I began to understand more about decision making when I looked at something I learned to do as an adult that had nothing to do with medicine: the game of hockey!

Chapter 7

Hockey

I PLAY ICE hockey. For those of you who are not familiar with hockey, I will provide you with a quick primer.

Hockey is a sport involving two teams playing against each other. Each team has one net at opposite ends of the playing surface. There is a solitary object (a puck or a ball) that the teams try to control and propel into the opponent's net using hockey sticks (a process called "scoring a goal"). There are three types of players on each team: three whose primary role is to put said object into the opponent's net (forwards), two whose primary job is stop the opposition's forwards from putting said object into their own net (defence), and one individual whose sole job is to guard his team's net (goalie).

Hockey can be played just about anywhere, including your kitchen if your parents will let you. When it is played on ice, with players wearing ice skates, it is referred to as "ice hockey," and the object used for scoring is called a "puck." It is a round disc consisting of six ounces of hard, vulcanized rubber.

I am one of those very odd individuals who enjoys being a goalie. I would play every day if I could. Yes, I know it's hard to believe, but I *like* trying to get my body in the way of very hard pucks shot at high speeds by very good players toward the net I am defending. The harder the shot, the better.

That is not a *rational* way of thinking or behaving, which is what makes the people who play the position of goalie so odd (every hockey player knows that goalies are, ahem, "different"). However, neither is it *irrational*. It is *nonrational*, meaning that one cannot use *reason* to make a decision for or against being a goalie.

That is generally true for most of our *aesthetic* likes and dislikes. Our senses and feelings tell us what we happen to find pleasurable, what feels right, but we often can't explain or justify them or find a reason for them. We do not need to universalize them either. I don't know why I like vanilla ice cream, rock-and-roll music, and impressionist art, and just because I do does not mean that you have to as well. Beauty is in the eye of the beholder, not in the "reason" of the beholder. As we will find out later, logic and reason seem to reside in our left hemisphere, creativity and imagination in our right.

I'll talk more about the difference between aesthetics and ethics later, but for the moment I will simply point out the distinction. *Aesthetics* is about what *I* find enjoyable and pleasurable. It's all about me and my feelings. I like the taste of vanilla ice cream because *I* like it, not because *you* like it, and we don't have to agree; enjoy chocolate if you'd rather.

Ethics is quite different. It's about how I ought to *behave* and how I ought to *treat others* (and, of course, how others ought to behave and treat me). We do want these beliefs about behaviour to be universalized because we believe they are rational not whimsical; that they are reasonable. The rules I use to treat you, I would also like followed by you in your treatment of me. Even if we disagree about our favourite flavour of ice dream, we ought to agree on rules of human conduct. It is an integral part of the concept of fairness, something we appreciate even when we are six years old. Enjoy your chocolate ice cream, but please don't smush it in my face unless I ask you to (which is unlikely because I would prefer you smush vanilla ice cream).

Something is *irrational* when it contradicts reason, like telling me that you are my friend then angrily smushing ice cream in my face when I ask you not to. Now, let's go back to goaltending for a moment.

I simply like playing goalie a lot and have been enamoured by the idea of doing so since I was a youngster, though I didn't start until my midforties. Why I have been drawn to the position of goalie is a complete mystery to me. Of course, for the life of me, I cannot figure out what is so exciting about shooting a puck into a net (there is nothing uglier than a puck in the net!). Wanting to score goals is also *nonrational*. Nonrational thoughts, like aesthetics—wanting to stop the puck versus wanting to score—can't be reasoned for or against and don't have to be agreed to by everyone. Thank goodness, because if we were all goalies, hockey wouldn't be much fun, and conversely, shooters hate when there is no goalie.

Don't get me wrong; I don't like pain and don't want to get hurt (I told you I was a wimp in the foreword, remember?). So I wear good equipment, and I don't do stupid things like expose my back to the puck, where I have little protection. That's *rational* thinking and behaviour.

What would be *irrational* is to say that I don't want to get hurt but then proceed to play goalie with very good players and *not* wear equipment. It is self-contradictory. It defies reason.

To summarize:

- nonrational—mysteriously enjoy being a target
- rational—wear good equipment because I don't want to get hurt
- irrational—claim to hate pain but behave to maximize it by not wearing equipment.

Now, what has all this got to do with antibiotics and a walk-in clinic? Or posters about drinking too much alcohol?

Well, as it turns out, lots. Because we all have parts of us that are rational, parts that are nonrational, and parts that are irrational, no matter how much we want to deny it. No exceptions. And the source of our irrational thinking and behaviours tends to be fear.

As we have seen already, thinking at the level of our brainstem, like reptiles do, is not very sophisticated. It's binary—fight-or-flight—and by definition, there is no time for contemplation and, hence, reasoning. Any time you have an immediate, visceral, and emotion-laden response to a stimulus, assume the brainstem and lower brain are involved at least to some degree and *be careful*. If you are really in a life-or-death situation, then the response generated at this level may be the right one. But unless it is life-or-death, check it out with your cerebral hemispheres first. That's what my otolaryngologist friend helped me to do, and because of it I avoided incontinence!

I have frequently been amused when people who rarely get sick show up at a walk-in clinic explaining that they are not one of *those* people who run to the doctor for every little cold, demanding antibiotics inappropriately. They don't succumb to the same fear as *those* people do. They are purely rational: they *really* are sick, and they *really need* the prescription. Of course they seldom do. But in fairness, when you rarely get sick, you can't realize how bad you can feel with any one of the myriad, relatively benign, garden-variety viruses out there. And feeling really sick, knowing that there are serious bacterial (and viral) infections out there, is scary.

If you have never had, or witnessed, really serious bacterial diseases like bacterial tracheitis or epiglottitis, it's easy to be fooled. It's tempting, too, to think that the doctor you are seeing is not taking you seriously, or not compassionate, because he is not jumping to give you a prescription. Of course, patients may forget that the doctor has seen serious bacterial infections and knows that you don't have one of them.

The important point is that the world is not divided into *those* people and us. We are all part of *those* people insomuch as we all behave rationally, nonrationally, and irrationally at times.

Going back to my walk-in clinic experience, it is easy to dismiss the 80 percent who wanted antibiotics in situations where they were likely to be of little benefit as acting completely irrationally and *solely* out of fear. But remember that medicine is about predicting the future; it is a probabilistic endeavour. So opting for antibiotics when the likelihood is only, say, 5 percent is not *irrational* necessarily. After all, there are 5 percent who don't appear to have a bacterial infection and who, in fact, will have a bacterial infection. But it is more complicated than that. Deciding to treat can also depend on context.

Several years ago I did an exercise with family medicine residents, and it was quite an eye-opener for some of them. The scenario was as described above with a person with a sore throat whose probability of having strep was 5 percent. I asked them, "If you were a patient, what would you do?" Without hesitation, they all agreed that they would forego the antibiotics and opt for supportive treatment only. Fair enough.

But then I added context to the equation, which meant that we needed to avoid the trap of binary thinking (simply fight-or-flight):

- What if you were a single mother running a daycare?
- What if your spouse was going through chemotherapy?
- What if you were just about to leave on a trip to exotic locales, one that you had been planning for some time to celebrate a major life event?
- What if you had brittle diabetes?
- What if you had upcoming major surgery that you simply could not postpone?

You get the picture? They did. In all of these situations, the repercussions for missing the 5 percent are more significant. Context matters.

Yes, the probability of strep lies along a spectrum, but there is more than one spectrum to consider.

Life is seldom a linear experience. Life is complex; we interact with one another. Understanding context means understanding that in a complex, interdependent universe, there are other spectra to consider. You may infect many children in your daycare or your immune-compromised spouse, ruin your once-in-a-lifetime holiday with your spouse, destabilize your diabetes, or complicate your recovery from surgery. Sure, lots of time 5 percent is so low and the implications for not treating are trivial enough that you don't treat, but not always.

Acknowledging the low probability but opting for the antibiotics anyway might be quite rational in some of these circumstances, despite the odds. One has to weigh not just the likelihood of something happening but also the significance of it happening. Life presents lots of nonbinary, nonlinear problems for patients and doctors alike. A rare but lethal event should be approached more seriously, perhaps, than a benign but common event.

Taking the antibiotic when there is a 95 percent chance of your symptoms being bacterial in origin is rational, and there are times when taking the prescription when the chances are only 5 percent can be rational as well.

Flipping a coin would be a nonrational approach. You are not using reason to come to a decision (although you could argue that flipping a coin to make a decision is irrational in itself!).

Taking antibiotics knowing that you have less than a 5 percent chance of a bacterial infection and that the diarrhea you have, which further confirms the presence of a virus, will likely be made worse with the antibiotics, is irrational when there are no mitigating circumstances. It's primarily binary, fight-or-flight fear.

It is important to remember that humans are not reptiles even though we maintain fight-or-flight hardware, and we are not machines, even though we can be logical. We are capable of working through problems with our entire, complex consciousness. We don't always have to succumb to fear generated in our brainstem and limbic systems and live in a world with only two choices. Equally, physicians cannot be ruthlessly cool and calculating like the ultimate binary tool—a computer—and act in a purely linear and mechanical fashion, ignoring context.

Both patients and doctors must weigh the evidence in a compassionate, human fashion and strive to make the right decision in the context of the probabilistic science called medicine. We ought to use our grey matter to manage the grey zones (which is where most of medicine, and life, resides).

Ideally, then, we should carefully evaluate the evidence, holistically contemplating the benefits and risks.

But that's hard to do, and we should not disparage ourselves on this point, because in truth we are very motivated by pain and fear of pain, more so than pleasure. It's in our DNA. Perhaps it's because we often find that pleasure is not as good as we thought it would be, and that it is often mixed with some pain.

However, it's more likely that pain motivates us more because it has the potential of lethality about it. We can survive and continue to experience pleasure in the future if we forego pleasure now, but maybe not if we ignore pain. This is why we prefer to avoid difficult discussions and painful topics—elephants in the room. And we don't always welcome or appreciate individuals who don't avoid these things and want us, or force us, to address them. We get angry at doctors who don't give us treatment we want, even though it is highly unlikely to help. Historically, we have even tortured or killed people who tell us things we don't want to hear.

It's in our nature. In fact, it's in nature itself.

I am always amused when someone with whom I am sharing a cottage or campsite, while looking out at the sun setting on a calm lake, comments how peaceful it is "out in nature."

Next time you are at a cottage or camping, just observe how peaceful nature is. I have. That cute chipmunk is a bundle of nerves, a tightly wound ball of fur. Play vanishes the moment any one of a plethora of triggers—a loud noise, a shadow overhead—presents itself. Without thinking, shelter is found in a burrow or up a tree instantly. Far safer to evaluate threats from there than out in the open.

Fear, like so many things, lies along a spectrum. At one end of the spectrum is a reasonable fear, an apprehension that is justifiable given the circumstances. A small rodent in an open field sees a shadow upon the grass that seems to be getting bigger and decides, shrewdly, to head for cover. Little is lost by assessing the shadow from the safety of a burrow, even if it is not a predatory bird. My hand feels painfully sore; better take it off of the hot stove element right now before I suffer third-degree burns.

At the other end is fear that is not reasonable. Fear that is not supported by any reasonable evidence. Irrational fear. Like mindlessly taking an antibiotic for what is almost surely a viral illness. Or like wanting to run away because your endotracheal tubes are missing—it's not going to help.

Believe it or not, the greatest challenge I faced in the walk-in clinic that day was not an academic one (what are the diagnostic differences between strep throat and viral pharyngitis), but a behavioural one: fear. It's the greatest challenge I face every day in medicine. And not just patients' fears, but mine as well. No matter what your symptom, there is some potentially serious or even lethal disease that could be causing it. A sore throat could be epiglottitis or bacterial tracheitis, and they can kill if misdiagnosed or mismanaged. So I, too, have fear: what if I guess wrong and someone gets really sick, or dies?

So we need to be gentle with one another. That doesn't mean that we give up, nor retreat into denial. We remain tough on the issues but soft on each other as we use our grey matter, our full humanity, to explore the grey zones, forgiving one another when pain or fear gets in the way of doing that.

Given that neither patient nor physician can escape fear completely, can we at least mitigate its potential for harm? Is it possible to limit ourselves only to rational fear?

As a doctor, in order to answer these questions, I had to study them like the scientist I was trained to be, by examining them like bacteria in a petri dish or a rat in a laboratory.

Or so I thought.

Chapter 8

The Myth of Objectivity

MY STUDY OF human behaviour, fear in particular, technically began before I became a doctor. I was in fourth-year medical school, which at the time was referred to as "clerkship," and we were referred to as "clinical clerks." On the totem pole of medical hierarchy, we were just above lab rats, and only because we could feed ourselves. So, you guessed it, I was the subject of my own experiment.

It involved my first bone marrow aspiration and biopsy on a real, live person, and in retrospect, it is rather humorous, but it wasn't at the time. A patient I was following had an undiagnosed anemia (a lower-than-normal number of circulating red blood cells, the cells in our blood that carry oxygen to all of the other cells of our bodies). We needed a bone marrow sample in order to elucidate the cause of the anemia (in adulthood, our red blood cells are made in the marrow of our large bones; earlier in our life, they are also made in our spleens). My staff physician directed me to perform the marrow aspiration and biopsy and suggested I obtain the sample of marrow from the patient's pelvic bones, the commonest location from which to do so. Sometimes we use the sternum, but as you shall see, it was lucky for me that she told me to use the ilium (a bone of the pelvis).

I had never done the procedure nor had I seen it done, but I had read about how to do it. My staff doctor assured me that she would walk me through it. That made me feel a lot better. Until she told me that four of my colleagues were going to watch. Okay, no big deal, we had all watched each other do procedures for the first time before. But then she told me that the patient had generously agreed to allow a gaggle of young nursing students to watch as well! I mean, sure, I was single, and it would be nice to impress some female students, but come on, this was my first time doing the procedure—way too much risk of complete humiliation!

However, being only slightly above the lab rat meant I had no say in the matter. I put on the sterile gloves and began to prep the patient. Thank goodness I was using the ilium, because it meant that the patient was lying on their stomach and could not see the shear terror on my face.

As I started to inject the local anaesthetic agent, I began to sweat. I don't mean a couple of sexy beads on my temple; I mean dripping sweat. On what was supposed to be a sterile operating field (after I had prepped it). I dared not make eye contact with any of the nursing students. I tried to move with authority as I injected the local anaesthetic, despite the tsunami of perspiration. I then drove the long thick needle through the bone into the marrow. The patient only screamed once, briefly thank goodness (my staff doctor explained to all present that this was not uncommon, whew!), and fortunately for both me and the patient, I had obtained an excellent sample of marrow.

The patient actually thanked me, as did the nursing students as they left. I tried to adopt an "aw-shucks, it was nothing" demeanour as I ogled them during their departure. They seemed more focused on the gallon of sweat I had secreted, however, and giggled as they left.

How often have you thought about your doctor's fear? Well, I am sure that you must have realized that during our training, we get scared, but what about once we are full-fledged doctors, not just high-level lab rats?

Well, it's more common than you might think. Barring psychopathic tendencies, most people are going to be scared when something bad is happening to someone else, especially if they are responsible for fixing that something bad and, particularly, if they are responsible for creating that something bad ("iatrogenic disease," as it is referred to in medicine, more on that later).

It is not common, however, for physicians to acknowledge, let alone discuss, those kinds of emotions. It's why we don't talk about death much, often using euphemistic language like "pass on," just like everyone else in society does.

In fact, as far as I am aware, there are no courses or even lectures on death itself in medical school or residency. Oh yes, we talk about the *fact* that people die and explore the detailed *physiology* of it, but we do not explore it as an *experience* with the attendant emotional content. We don't talk about what it feels like as you are dying (e.g., from experiences of patients who relate this to us before they die). We talk a little about the emotions loved ones have, but mostly the obvious ones (e.g., sadness, anger, confusion, relief). We don't often speak much of the other emotions that can complicate the dying process.

For example, sometimes loved ones are not so much relieved because the patient's suffering has ended, but rather because their own suffering has ended (on many levels potentially).

In particular, we do not talk about *our* emotions. It took quite a while before I told my wife about the emotions I experienced after the case of the near-failed intubation. And until I wrote that story (more than twenty-five years after the incident!), I had never told anyone else: not my friend the otolaryngologist who had been with me, not my family doctor, not any of my friends or colleagues. Seems rather bizarre, doesn't it?

The universe is a complex place: we don't know all of the answers, we cannot predict the future, and we are all human. So, no matter how good a physician may be, and no matter what discipline of medicine he practises, he is dealing with situations on a daily basis that have potential to be matters of serious disability or death. What sounds like a trivial complaint—a sore throat—can be epiglottitis.

So as long as one practises medicine, one is at risk of having bad things happen, and sometimes when bad things happen, patients or their families sue doctors. For a long time, we were not allowed to discuss lawsuits with anyone other than our legal counsel, for reasons of confidentiality. This meant that we suffered with the pain, shame, fear, and humiliation alone. Lawyers do their best to support you, but they are not therapists. We are simply expected to "suck it up." Rather unhealthy, and frankly unrealistic, isn't it? Doesn't sound like wise advice from a profession that is supposed to understand how people, including doctors, work, does it?

Of course, this "moral residue," as ethicists refer to it, will take its toll, and we try to find ways of dealing with it. All too often, we utilize the oldest mechanism we humans have always used to deal with unpleasant realities, something I alluded to in the last chapter: we use denial, in one form or another.

Denial can be a useful psychological tool in the short term, but long term it is not a wise tactic. Pain needs to be acknowledged and processed for it not to pathologically affect our psyche.

In his wonderful book *Denial*, Ajit Varki explores denial as a necessary coping mechanism in our development as humans. Briefly, his thesis is that at the time of the earliest hominid species, the world was, as it is today, full of risks. At that time (and still true today), all living things were in potential peril from a multiplicity of lethal events, including from other living things (in fact, most often from other living things!). A creature attaining full consciousness would go insane quite quickly if it appreciated this riskiness completely. It would be psychologically overwhelmed by the shear magnitude of the potential for harm, and death, over which it often had little control.

Without denial and its attendant gift of allowing us to ignore all but the most proximate threats to survival, the creature would psychologically be unable to function, integrate with its fellow creatures, and copulate to advance the cause of consciousness in the species. In other words, it would be a complete basket case! I think that there is a large level of truth in his reasoning, and it likely gives some understanding for why we use denial so extensively in our lives today, despite the fact that we are considerably more sophisticated and have significantly more control of risk than our progenitors did.

It also brings us back to the concept of fear. It was fear that nourished denial at the dawn of humanity, and it still does so today. Yes, we may be clad in chic attire, have many letters after our names, drink fancy wine, speak with calm authority, and appear to have life "by the tail," but we are all afraid to our very core, and we all use denial on a daily basis to cope with it.

In that same clerkship year, I experienced my first patient death. I had admitted an elderly woman from a nursing home with decreased level of consciousness, likely from sepsis (systemic infection). Her prognosis was quite poor. I was attending rounds (where the staff physician would go "round" with his group of underlings on his team, including clerks, interns, and residents, to examine the patients under their collective care), when the nursing staff paged me. I was directed to come immediately because my elderly sick lady was having a seizure.

I raced to her room and found her seizing and administered diazepam intravenously. At that time, it was the drug-of-choice for stopping a seizure, but it was not good for preventing them. Unfortunately, although the drug worked, she began seizing again, so I had to administer a different drug, phenytoin, to both stop her present seizure and prevent her from having more.

However, phenytoin has risks (as all drugs do), and one of them is that it can adversely affect the cardiovascular system and cause it to collapse, especially in the sick and the elderly, and she was both. In order to minimize such risks, one must inject the drug very slowly, which I proceeded to do at a rate twice as slowly as recommended, just in case.

She stopped seizing and seemed stable, so I returned to the rounds. About ten minutes later I was paged again: the patient had died.

I was devastated! I had been so careful administering the medication, but had I been careful enough? My senior resident could see my anguish and so accompanied me to the bedside to make the official pronouncement of death (the patient had previously requested *not* to have any resuscitation in the event of sudden death).

I had never seen a newly deceased person before, and I was not sure what to do. With encouragement from my resident, I respectfully approached her, put one end of my stethoscope in my ears and the other on her chest, listening carefully for any heart sounds. I closed my eyes (as I still do to this day when I use my stethoscope) to improve my concentration.

At first I heard nothing, and I was concerned that my emotional state was affecting my hearing. Then I focused more intently, and to my shock, I heard a rhythmical thumping in her chest. I happily opened my eyes and looked up at my resident with glee, explaining that she was not dead, that I heard heart sounds! As I did so, I saw a wry smile appear on his face, but I didn't know what to make of it. He didn't seem to be sharing my excitement and relief, exactly.

Then I clued in. I looked down and saw him tapping his fingers on the far side of the patient's chest where he was sitting. I had not heard heart sounds because there were none; I had heard his tapping! As soon as I realized his little prank, he chuckled. He had tricked the gullible little lab rat!

I will admit that it relieved the terrible tension I was feeling, the guilt I had laid on myself. She had been a very sick, old woman whose time had come, and fortunately she had died with a nurse present and relatively comfortably. My administration of the antiseizure drug likely had little to do with her death, and treating her seizures warranted the small risk. The resident took me aside later and explained that people die, that I wasn't to blame, that we can't cure them all, and that we just have to move on. It did help a little.

But it also revealed for me the way we deal, or rather don't deal, with death, or more generally, the way we don't deal with emotion in our line of work. So why don't we address feelings better? I think it is because we do not know how.

I don't think we as a species have quite figured out how to reconcile being an independent human being, replete with our individual emotions, values, and ethical frameworks (which, among other elements, combine to form our individual agency), with the roles we play in our society.

When we don the white coat and take on the role of doctor or researcher (or lots of other roles in society), we hide ourselves behind the persona, and it seems as though society wants us to do that, at least Western society does. We pretend to adopt an objective stance, one that reflects our present social ethos (and, hence, its morals, perspectives, and values) so perfectly that we simple blend into it like a neutral watercolour. We become strictly a representative of the collective, deferring to the wisdom of the collective, sacrificing our own unique humanity in the process.

As I mentioned earlier, I had a difficult time with that in residency; I didn't feel comfortable "playing the role." And during my career, I have struggled more candidly with the barrage of pain, suffering, and death inherent in our work than some of my colleagues, which perhaps explains my pursuit of palliative care, philosophy, and ethics.

As evidence of this, my own evolution as a physician has taken some interesting twists and turns. In my early years, I was enthralled with the biomechanical aspects of medical science, so I became very procedure-oriented. I saw physical interventions as what medicine was all about, in part because we do have an impressive array of procedures (administration of drugs, as well as more strictly mechanical methods, like surgery) to assist the lives of our patients. Many procedures, like intubating a sick boy with a sore throat and breathing problems, are impressive and life-saving.

I remember the first cardiac arrest I dealt with as staff physician in my first few months of practise. The buck stopped with me, and it was very different than being a resident. The patient survived and recovered completely, and I thought to myself, Barry, it's all paid off—all the work, study, and sacrifice—because you can save lives!

Over the ensuing months, the next six cardiac arrests I dealt with were all unsuccessful. I did exactly the same thing as I had done in the first one. I thought, What's the matter? What's going on?

Slowly I came to realize that I wasn't quite the miracle worker I thought I was and that there were all kinds of variables that I, like every doctor, had no control over. The universe is a complicated and complex place, and we have only a wisp of understanding about how it all works.

That was a humbling, not humiliating, insight. Humbling means that you are brought back down to earth to see your rightful place in it. Humiliating means that you are made to feel less significant than you should. We often confuse these two concepts, which is unfortunate. We benefit and grow from humbling, not from humiliation.

I slowly came to realize that health-care professionals can *occasionally* assist nature, but we can *always* interfere with it, and the wise practitioner learns when to get out of the way and simply observe nature's miracles with a sense of awe. When we suture a laceration, we assist nature in healing. No magic potions leak from the suture material to make tissues mend. Sutures simply bring separated tissue back into apposition to assist nature's healing. Ditto for casts on broken limbs, salves for rashes, and antibiotics for infections. Many patients are surprised that we can fight off bacterial infections without antibiotics. For example, adults with strep throat usually gain only a day or two of reduced symptoms with antibiotics. Equally, if your immune system is sufficiently compromised, antibiotics may not successful.

Given this reality, it important not to fall prey to the misbelief that doing something is always better than doing nothing. Our fear prompts us to "just do something," but sometimes the best, yet hardest, thing to do in medicine is nothing (and often true in other areas in life as well). It's hard for doctors, and especially hard for patients and their families, to simply be present for one another in our collective fear.

One of the best examples I had of this was in my second year of practice when I was working in a somewhat isolated, small Ontario town. A little girl, daughter of a couple with whom I eventually became friends, presented with a very high fever. After completing my examination and finding no source for the fever, I was sure it was roseola—a generally benign viral illness of childhood that can give very high fevers without many other symptoms. There is no specific investigation to confirm the diagnosis; it is a clinical diagnosis, and the only treatment is supportive.

I explained the reasons for my diagnosis to the nervous young couple, and at an intellectual level, they understood and agreed. But it was difficult for them, and me, to see their daughter have such a high fever for so many days, even though she seemed otherwise well. Fortunately, as I expected, on the fifth day the fever disappeared, the classic roseola rash appeared, and the diagnosis was confirmed. But boy, was it hard waiting and doing next to nothing!

Objective scientist

As a youth, I was very influenced by the hit TV show *M.A.S.H.*, and I am sure that many of us entered medicine at least in part under its trance. One episode in particular stands out for me. Colonel Blake took Hawkeye Pierce aside after the tragic death of a young soldier and said, "Son, there are two rules in medicine: Rule number one is that patients die. And rule number two is that doctors can't change rule number one."

I thought back to that after my sixth failed cardiac arrest. The colonel in *M.A.S.H.* tried his best to help Hawkeye deal with death, but the insight he offered, although true, didn't reduce the sting and sadness that much, any more than my resident's droll attempt did in dealing with my angst after experiencing my first patient death.

Some have come to believe that we don't need to deal with it, that once we adopt the persona of the physician, we neatly compartmentalize any emotional or moral residue within it, and we are henceforth able to completely disconnect it from the human being we return to when we are off-duty.

It paints us as being, perhaps, superhuman, like the Übermensch medical schools are searching for. Because we have memorized some textbooks or mastered some physical skill like suturing, we are now able to do the "grand disconnect" from our own humanity. Or, perhaps, magically by accumulating enough data and seeing enough suffering and death, that we come to understand suffering and death, process them and come to peace with them. We become resilient to them, almost like we are outside of it all from this high perch looking down on the struggles of our fellow humans.

It evolves, or perhaps devolves, into a subtle, or not so subtle, parentalism. We put ourselves (and are put) above the fray, so to speak, like parents overseeing children consumed by something only children would be consumed by. Please don't get me wrong: parentalism is not something that doctors unilaterally foist on an unsuspecting public. The public craves it, in fact, to a certain degree, demands it. It's a coconspiracy driven by fear. Doctor and patient alike want to believe that there is always something we can do to make things better. And that, as I have said earlier, is simply not true. No antibiotic will help a viral pharyngitis, no matter how sore the throat. And roseola just takes time to pass.

So we try to adopt the role of objective scientist. But science discovered almost a century ago, when it discovered quantum mechanics, that scientists are never outside the experiment. In the famous electron experiments, quantum mechanics describes the position of an electron using a probability wave function, a spectrum, not as a constant and discrete point in space-time. The electron is not in any particular location until we look for it, and then the probability wave function of the electron collapses to one specific point depending on how the physicist does the experiment.

The scientist is part of the experiment, and there is no escaping it. Pure objectivity is a physical impossibility. And not just in physics but in all of life. In a sense, we are all entangled, although in a different sense than the quantum entanglement of electrons that Einstein referred to as "spooky."

Ethicists use the adage "there is no view from nowhere." We cannot be objective, neutral, dispassionate, or whatever other term we may want to use.

This chink in the armour becomes more obvious when physicians or their loved ones become ill. We are just as scared as everyone else. Sometimes, when we have knowledge and experience the lay public does not have, we can recognize when worrisome symptoms and signs are absent and "maintain an even strain" (from the movie *The Right Stuff*).

For example, I am always surprised that patients seldom ask their attending physician, "Doctor, when you get a sore throat exactly like mine, what do you do?" Most of the time, we don't take antibiotics. In thirty-five years of clinical medicine, having seen literally thousands of patients with infectious disease and having picked up a fair number of "bugs" from them, I have taken antibiotics exactly twice: once for illness, once for prevention after being exposed to meningitis.

But knowledge is a double-edged sword. We also recognize the significance of some signs and symptoms (or lack thereof) that the less educated would not notice, let alone appreciate, and those will trigger fear. We may have seen or heard of a rare case that went sour that shares similarities to the present case, and we may worry more than we ought to. Such anecdotal cases, experienced or learned, can mislead us into "catastrophic thinking" (more on that later).

Of course, we never want to admit that we worry. We euphemize it more as legitimate concern, which sounds less fearful. Or else we try to justify our concern as rationally defensible, not at all like that irrational worry only the less-sophisticated public falls prey to (*those* people).

Hogwash! When the poop hits the fan, we worry and panic and fret just like everybody else. All of our textbook expertise and experience turn to smoke when our own health and survival (or a loved one's) is at stake. When the white coat is off, we are just as frail and vulnerable as any patient (and their family). Physicians often want to, or do, jump the queue under the pretense of rationality when they get sick. After all, as physicians they know better, right? They don't succumb to fear of pain, suffering, and death like the rest of us mere mortals, do they? Let me give you an example.

Many years ago, "Larry," a family doctor, saw his family doctor regarding some symptoms that sounded mildly worrisome. Although Larry had been under some unusual stress, he was generally healthy, so he was not used to feeling out of sorts. To compound matters, a slightly older colleague and friend of his had recently died of cancer, a cancer that would give symptoms similar to what Larry was experiencing. Anxious, he visited his family doctor convinced that he had the same serious illness and would require some invasive investigations in order to confirm, or hopefully deny, the ominous diagnosis.

Wisely, his family doctor did a thorough history, and together they realized that nothing serious was likely going on. Larry had been under more stress than he had realized, had not been taking care of himself, and was clearly very affected by the death of his friend. The wise family doctor not only didn't order any fancy tests, but he didn't even examine the patient. They made a plan that if things did not improve with better self-care and appropriate grieving, then in a couple of weeks they would reconsider. Larry's symptoms settled in short order.

You are probably thinking that I was the wise family doctor, and I am just being modest, right? Wrong! I was the patient! (I thought the pseudonym "Larry" might give it away.) I took my colleague's death very hard as he had been on the finest people I had ever known. He also had a young family as I did. But his death was a bit of a canary, and my fears got the better of me.

So, sorry to burst your bubble, but physicians worry and fret like everyone else, me included. And I have seen numerous other examples.

That persona we adopt when it is someone else who is sick and dying fades pretty quickly when that someone is us (or someone we love). There is a fragile veil between our humanity and our persona. The intense visceral fear of pain, disability, and death, universal to all living things, is what shatters it. And we don't like to talk about it. We maintain an even strain.

So it turns out that from both sides of the stethoscope, fear and denial are two of the most important realities of our existence.

I have been able to understand this from the patient perspective. After all, many times I, or my family, have had symptoms, and had I not been a physician I might have been quite worried. I might have wanted an antibiotic too. Ignorance is not always bliss.

But why is it that given all of the books we have read, all of the patients we have seen, and all of the life experiences we have witnessed (birth, suffering, death), we still fall prey to the same emotions, the same traps of fear and denial?

Because, my friends, it turns out Alexander Pope was right: *errare humanum est*.

To err *is* human.

Chapter 9

The Way We Are
(with apologies to Barbra Streisand and Robert Redford)

IF YOU EVER want to understand human error, take a psychology course. I did in my first year of university, and I have been fascinated by human behaviour ever since. The Milgram experiments were probably the clincher for me.

You have likely heard of a disturbing experiment performed by Stanley Milgram in the early 1960s in which he examined behaviours of individuals who were engaged as volunteers in a psychology experiment. Briefly, he set up an experiment involving unsuspecting volunteers to test the limits of trust that these volunteers would manifest in the context of "scientific research" under the auspices of authority figures, who were psychology research scientists.

The volunteers were told that the purpose of the experiment was to test the effectiveness of negative reinforcement on the learning process. They were led to believe that all volunteers were relegated to one of two groups: one group, the learners, and a second group, the monitors, who would apply negative reinforcement—electric shocks—to the learners when they made a mistake.

This, of course, was *not* the case. The individuals who *appeared* to be doing the learning were not volunteers at all but were actors fully aware of the ruse. The only real volunteers were the ones responsible for delivering the electric shocks to these actors, under the supervision of the scientists, the authority figures, overseeing the experiment. The purpose of the experiment was, therefore, not to explore learning and negative reinforcement but rather to explore the behaviours of the volunteers in such contrived situations, although they were not made aware of this until after the experiment was over.

The actors (pretending to be learner subjects) were in one room and were able to be heard (but not seen) by the real volunteers and scientists (the researchers running the experiment), who were in another room. The actors seemed to be hooked up to a device capable of delivering electric shocks to them under the complete control of the real volunteers. In truth, there were no such devices; the actors simply acted as though electric shocks were being delivered.

Before the experiment began, the volunteers themselves were given a sample of a *low-level* electric shock to demonstrate its unpleasantness. The volunteers were then told by the researchers wearing official white coats to deliver increasingly powerful shocks, much more powerful than the ones they had received, whenever the subjects (actors) answered questions incorrectly. They were reassured repeatedly that the subjects, by volunteering, had agreed to this.

Despite the obvious and significant pain the subjects *seemed* to be experiencing, the volunteers continued to apply escalating levels of electric shocks under the direction, and support, of the scientists. For the most part, the volunteers either didn't question the process, or if they did, a significant number of them were very easily reassured by the authoritative voices of the scientists to continue despite their misgivings about the brutality of the process.

In some cases, this was true even when the control panel the volunteers were using to deliver the apparent shocks indicated that the shock they were about to deliver could be lethal! On many occasions, the subjects would no longer respond to inquiries by the volunteers as to their status (leaving the volunteers wondering what condition they might be in), and yet the volunteers would continue to apply near-lethal shocks at the prompting of the scientists.

Suffice to say that at age nineteen I was shocked when I read of these experiments (pardon the pun!). Sadly, having studied my share of human history I should not have been.

So what do our brains do to make us the way we are? Let's review brain structure again, and then explore the way it functions.

Using Our Brains

We have already explored the lowest levels of our brains, the brainstem and lower midbrain, which we inherited from our reptilian ancestors, and the upper midbrain, limbic system, and lower cortical structures, which we share with our lower mammalian cousins. These areas of our brain oversee all of the autonomic functions (e.g., breathing, heart rate, blinking) and also control many of our ingrained behaviours, like pulling our hand off of a hot stove. They are also responsible for fear and other deep-seated emotions we have explored.

We may not always be delighted with what these structures do for us (like when we are nearly incontinent), but without these critical parts of our lower brains, we could not function as an integrated, independent entity. Period.

So try as we might, use as much denial as we want, we can never be completely free of their literal millisecond-by-millisecond influence and control.

Above these more primitive structures lay the cerebral hemispheres—the highly complex structures where consciousness seems to reside, at least in part (more on this later). How do they work?

One way is to look at their gross structure. For most of us, our left brain—by that we mean primarily the left hemisphere of the cerebral cortex—is methodical, logical. It is more literal and likes to categorize things. It deals in language, both written and spoken, and is responsible for our explicit memory, where we consciously try to store new information. On the other hand, our right brain—the right hemisphere of the cerebral cortex—is more imaginative, creative, and nonverbal. It begins to function earlier in life and is more directly hard-wired to the limbic system, where emotion dwells. Our implicit memory (our subconscious memory) also resides in our right brain, where we maintain our autobiographical self.

Another way to look at our brain is to examine how we use it, how it can work for us. We can think in a very quick, reflex, and automated manner at a number of levels, including the brainstem. Other times, we process information more slowly and contemplate it before coming to a decision.

For example, we have implicit beliefs, beliefs we simply assume, prima facie, are true. Beliefs we simply don't question and act on directly. Green light means we can cross the stress. But we also have explicit beliefs, beliefs we derive for ourselves over time through learning, introspection, and experience. Beliefs developed because we *do* question. Although it is generally safe to cross on a green light, today the traffic is busy; it is dark, and the roads are slippery, so I will assess the situation more carefully before crossing. Many explicit beliefs can eventually become implicit beliefs over time, which can be both good and bad, as we shall see later.

In addition, there is inductive—bottom-up—reasoning, in which we make generalizations from specific observations, as opposed to deductive—top-down—reasoning, where we apply a general rule to a specific situation. Because it has rained a lot this April, I will continue to bring my umbrella with me to work (inductive). The sun always rises in the east, so we must be heading east as it is ten o'clock in the morning and the sun is in my eyes (deductive).

Are all of these ways of thinking innate—do we have them at birth?

Or are they learned? Perhaps this is a good time to look at human development and the stages we go through to become full-fledged adults.

Human Development

We start off our lives as newborns with what is referred to as "naive realism": we trust that the world is exactly as we perceive it to be. To best understand naive realism, consider your dreams. All kinds of ridiculous things happen to us in our dreams, and yet they seem so real and credible. They are so absurd that it is often hard to remember the details since they can be so incoherent. That's in part because our senses, which we use to validate our beliefs, are turned off for the most part when we sleep and because the conscious part of us that analyzes our thoughts is largely turned off as well. That's why we can feel ourselves flying even though we may have an inkling that it's too good to be true.

In the first few weeks of life, this naive realism is extreme, because as infants we cannot even differentiate ourselves from our environment. We do not realize that the breast we suckle from belongs to a separate entity, our mother. When we are hungry we scream and cry, and the food magically arrives. We run on raw instincts to feed, to sleep, and to dispose of bodily waste. So, if we experience something unpleasant (hunger, fatigue, messy diaper), with the higher brain not developed sufficiently to act as a censor, the lower brain feels quite free to express our displeasure liberally, no matter the circumstances. As insulting as this may sound, we are little more than cute reptiles.

Gradually, we begin to explore our body parts, differentiating our thumb from our foot. Up until this point, everything is just part of one thing in a sense; everything appears to still be *us*. We cannot understand that the breast milk we consume, the mother whose breast we suckle, and us (baby) are three different things. We are as narcissistic as we will ever be in our lives—we are the entire universe as far as we know! And the remainder of our lives is a journey of discovering that such is not the case, of experiencing progressive loss of this naive realism, this narcissism.

To clarify, narcissism is *not* selfishness. To differentiate, let me use an example. Imagine you are sitting at a table with five other people, and your favourite cake is brought in, and it is conveniently cut into six pieces, ideally one piece per person. The selfish person looks at the cake and says to himself, "That's my favourite cake, and I want more than one piece, which is going to be tough because there are only six pieces, and six of us present. I'll have to figure out some plan so that I can get at least one extra piece."

That's very different from the narcissist who looks at the cake and says to himself, "Wow, that's a lot of cake for me to eat! How am I going to do it?" The narcissist, like the young infant, doesn't realize that there are others in the room; he honestly thinks that the entire cake is for him. However, if a narcissist is willing to grow past his infantile narcissism, then one could say to him, "Excuse me, but did you notice that there are five other people at the table with you, which means that each of you should get one piece?" If the narcissist has matured or is willing to mature, he will eventually see that such is the case and gladly share the cake equally with the others present.

Selfishness is the less-than-admirable behaviour of a person who knows better and schemes to have more than his share; narcissism is the consistent behaviour of a less mature person who literally does not know any better. We understand and forgive the narcissism of the infant when she screeches at three in the morning for food. We are less tolerant of the competent adult who does the same.

So the natural evolution over time is to learn to differentiate "us" from "non-us." Slowly we come to realize that our parts are different from the things that are not us; our thumb is separate from our blanket. Then we start to recognize those closest to us, typically our mothers, and begin to see them as other than ourselves. After that, some primitive socializing—smiling, cooing—ensues to the delight of any onlookers.

The intense narcissism of infancy eventually gives way to a more accurate representation of the world, but it is a slow process. Playing peekaboo with babies is a good example of the persistence of naive realism. In their black-and-white world, you either exist or don't exist. That's why this game is so entertaining because babies are truly surprised when you magically reappear! (That's why most of us love magic so much, even as adults.) It is only in later infancy that they learn object permanence and, therefore, that there is a third option—you still exist even though they cannot see you. Equally, it takes time before they realize that even though they are not looking at you, you can still see them when they "hide" in the corner of the room or do something in private (like fill their diapers!).

By six months, we have a sense of bonding and do not like to be separated from our parents, who we have come to know and trust. Gradually, we evolve a very distinct sense of our physical selves, as we continue to identify images and other creatures around us as separate. Increasingly, we explore our environment, albeit with some trepidation. Around eighteen months, we don't always like to see new faces. We experience stranger anxiety as our unique sense of emotional self begins to blossom. The well-baby visit in the doctor's office at this age is always a challenge for this very reason. It's not difficult to sense the powerful fear arising within an eighteen-month-old as she clings desperately to one of her parents during the examination, screaming until they leave the doctor's office!

But eventually toddlers get over that and enter the "terrible twos." Although they are becoming emotionally attuned to those around them, they can't believe that what they want or are interested in isn't the same thing that everybody else, particularly mommy and daddy, are interested in. It's also the dreaded stage of learning the word "no." It heralds the process of separation from their parents, a process that will take, if done very well, the next twenty or so years. But in the early toddler years, humans behave, or misbehave, like adorable puppies.

However, in the later toddler years, their minds develop so that they are able to connect thoughts with images. They know what a picture of a dog represents, and that dogs bark. As they enter school, they begin to develop concrete thinking so that they are able to understand and generate concrete rules by which to classify the world. Dogs are dogs, cats are cats, and tables are tables. Dogs and cats can move and make noise; tables cannot.

As they finish grade school and enter high school, they enter the formal reflexive phase of growth, where they can think about thinking. They evolve past concrete to theoretical, abstract thought with an integrative logic. The concept of death and its ramifications enters their consciousness. It is the development of the observer self, the ability to see oneself somewhat objectively in the universe and to contemplate one's place in that universe. Here the seeds of altruism and self-sacrifice begin to mature. Anxiety, not surprisingly, frequently increases as well.

Sounds simple, doesn't it? What could possibly go wrong?

Making Sense of the World

In order to make sense of the world, we learn and develop internal theories to guide us, rules of thumb, or heuristics as they are known. They form part of our implicit memory. In truth, most of what we believe comes from someone else. Information that we avow as being factual is based almost always on trusting the authority of someone else. This statement is true for the entirety of one's life. The universe is so complicated, and life is so short that of necessity we must trust the opinions and thoughts of others, particularly those who have come before us. We cannot possibly check everything we believe, nor can we learn everything we know from first principles on our own, *de novo*. I have never seen China, but I believe it exists because a very large number of others say that it does.

This partly explains why implicit memory makes it easy to confuse "feeling that we know" with actually "knowing." Studies have even shown that we sometimes attribute to our own experience events we have heard others talk about in their lives, things we did not experience ourselves but feel like we did. Or we confuse what we experienced in our sleep with what occurs while we are awake.

As well, much of what you think you like, that you believe is strictly a reflection of your own individual tastes and is therefore generated solely inside of you, is in fact often told to you, one way or another. Don't believe me? Look at the clothes you are wearing, your hairstyle, the food you eat, the shows you watch, et cetera. Sure you aren't a little influenced by the society in which you live? Do you think if you lived in a different part of the world or at a different time in history that you would still be wearing the clothes you have on right now?

The reason why companies spend so much money advertising their products or services to us is because it works; they influence us tremendously. There is a daily bombardment of ads that tell you what you need, what is appealing, and what you should spend your money on. Corporations don't spend billions on advertising for no good reason. Do you think your teenage son would wear his pants below his buttocks if he had not been *told* to like that style? (I want to be around long enough to see the expression on their faces when they reach their forties. I suspect they will cringe as I did in my forties when I reviewed photos from my adolescence).

We trust our implicit beliefs because we trust, rightly or wrongly, the sources from whence they come: either our own life knowledge gleaned from our own explorations or, more commonly, from the life knowledge of others (even if we tend to confuse the two). Not surprisingly, that can lead to many errors, in part because those sources we trust, in turn, trusted their sources, and so forth, to a near-infinite regress. To make matters worse, our right brain can't generate rules or see patterns very well, whereas the left brain likes to come up with explanations no matter how ridiculous. We need both hemispheres to be working together to develop a coherent sense of the world. Otherwise, we are stuck with a childlike sense of naive realism—the right side—or we just make stuff up by inferring patterns and rules that can be grossly inaccurate—the left side.

We want to feel that what we believe is correct because we want control of our part of the universe, and we can't have that without an accurate picture of the universe around us first. Lack of understanding can lead to lack of control, and that leads to fear. The more ignorant we are of our surroundings, the more vulnerable we are, from reptiles all the way up.

Many years ago, I went to a meeting at my oldest daughter's grade school. It became obvious to me that a considerable number of parents believed that their children were like computers. As parents, they felt that their job was essentially to load as many of their programs as possible onto their children's "hard drives" before they left home. Give them clear decision-making rules for every situation imaginable, and they'll be just fine. They didn't seem to realize that their children were not machines but living things, and thus not only capable of developing some of their own programs but *needing* to do so as well. If children don't learn to do this while they are still at home under our care and influence, how will they be able to do so when they leave home and face unique situations we did not (and could not) anticipate for them?

These parents illustrated how much we don't like ambivalence; we don't like doubt. We want an antibiotic because we want to be sure. We don't want to be burdened with probabilities and statistics and take any chances. Best to dive for cover now and ask questions later. Cling to what has always worked before.

Sometimes we just fill in the blanks if we need to in order to make sense of things, to have a coherent basis upon which to act. We complete someone else's sentence before they can speak it. We look for, and find, patterns that may or may not be present: the sequentially illuminated lightbulbs in a neon sign appear to be "flowing" in a particular direction. We see images in Rorschach inkblots. Our perceptions, by definition, are *interpretations* of the world. Do I look fat in these blue jeans? Do I look thinner in black?

We receive sensory input from our various sense organs, but raw data must be processed within our brains to form an integrated, understandable, and ultimately useful *impression* of reality. Countless optical illusions attest to this truth, as do the tricks of magicians. We can be easily fooled. Some people are colour-blind. No two of us perceive the world with our senses exactly the same way. Beauty is indeed in the eye of the beholder. We each construct reality differently, and we reconstruct it moment by moment, based on new data and its interpretation. The signed playing card we thought the magician ripped and burned a minute ago is magically back again in one piece! We giggle in delight as we reexperience that naive realism of our childhood.

Many years ago, I had a delightful young married woman in my practice come into my office quite distraught. She said that her husband, also a patient of mine, was an alcoholic, and she needed my help or their marriage would be over. Knowing her husband, I was rather surprised at this sudden revelation, and I was also saddened because they were a lovely couple, and I hated to see their marriage on the rocks. To some degree, I felt embarrassment, too—how could this have been going on and I didn't see it?

I suggested that she ask him to book an appointment to see me and explain to him why. Several days later, he came in and he seemed rather calm, which surprised me. He stated that he sincerely did not think he had a problem with alcohol and proceeded to tell me that every day he had one regular beer, and only one beer, when he came home from work. I questioned him thoroughly, and his story did not waver. I reviewed his chart, including previous investigations, and nothing contradicted what he said. I was at a loss.

So I met with his wife again. She corroborated his story exactly—one beer every day when he got home. I asked her why she thought that made him an alcoholic. Her eyes welled up with tears.

When she was a little girl, her father was an alcoholic. He, like her husband, always drank beer from a can (the same brand, in fact). As soon as her husband cracked open his brew, that unmistakable sound of a beer can opening triggered a flood of terrifying memories and emotions for her. That, from her perspective, made her husband an alcoholic too. I gently explained to her that although his drinking was producing a problem for the two of them, he was not an alcoholic.

Her husband had never understood her seemingly irrational

response to his one-beer-a-day habit until the three of us met together. He immediately stopped having his daily brew, opting instead for a nonalcoholic beverage (and one not out of a can!). And she engaged in therapy to deal with the many painful and unresolved issues from her childhood. Our memories, especially implicit ones that are laden with significant emotion, can greatly affect our perceptions and their interpretations.

Although we are certain that our memories are like photographs, they are far from it. True, we can have a flashbulb memory occasionally, but this type of memory fades very quickly. For the most part, a memory is stored in multiple different locations in our brain as separate pieces that must be reintegrated when retrieved. This process is notoriously prone to error, as the practice of law can attest to. Eyewitness recollections, once the gold standard in legal cases, have proven to be far less reliable than once thought, hence the rise in use of DNA evidence. It is tragic to think of how many people (perhaps as many as 75 percent of those wrongfully convicted) have spent time in jails or prisons, or worse still, executed, based on self-assured but pitifully flawed recollections of (hopefully) well-meaning witnesses.

So in truth, we should really refer to memory as a bit of an illusion, much like optics can be illusory. And the more emotion is involved, the more inaccuracies can arise in perception, memory, and processing. If we are invested emotionally in a certain outcome, we can suffer from self-serving biases or outcome biases, in which we see what we want to see, remember what we want to remember, and conclude what we want to conclude.

And we don't like to admit to our shortcomings, to being wrong. It's not in our nature. Admitting we are wrong is uncomfortable; we feel threatened at a deep, reptilian level. Oops, maybe that shadow I assumed was a cloud overhead is, in fact, a hawk, and here I am still out in the open! My smoking can't possibly contribute to my breathlessness, can it? What does my weight have to do with my sore knees?

Oh, we might confess to an *insignificant* mistake, but we will confabulate all manner of elaborate sidestepping if we feel threatened. In so doing, we confuse justification with excuse making. Justification is a rational explanation for why we do what we do (or don't do what we don't do). "It's my fault. I let myself get so preoccupied with my thesis paper that I completely forgot to do the laundry." Excuse making avoids acknowledging our culpability by blaming someone or something else. Because we feel threatened, we are more interested in protecting ourselves than doing the right thing. "It's not my fault! If John weren't such a jerk, I might have remembered to do the laundry."

Admitting one is wrong becomes progressively more difficult the more there is at stake. Admitting to parents that you screwed up their child's intubation, resulting in the child's death, is more internally distressing than admitting to letting in a bad goal in a pickup hockey game. Professing to be an expert in a field (and being respected and compensated for that) and then having to admit to a fundamental and grievous error that casts doubt on that expertise feels so threatening that it can be near-impossible to do.

When we make excuses, we often engage in confirmation bias, skewing evidence to support what we already believe to be true. As John Kenneth Galbraith said, "Faced with either changing one's mind or proving that there is no need to do so, almost everyone gets busy on the proof." We reject counterevidence for no good reason other than the fact it is inconvenient to the theory we are trying to establish.

Many of us (myself included), when trying to slim down, sincerely forget to include the snacks we consume as contributing to our total caloric intake or minimize how much of them we gobbled. And we often overestimate how much exercise we really got that day to balance that gobbling. "I must have burned a lot of calories playing baseball tonight, so I think I'll have a second burger with those fries!"

Perhaps the most frustrating condition for me to deal with in practice is the opposite problem, anorexia nervosa. Patients afflicted by this can go to extraordinary lengths to become ultrathin. The mortality rate, especially among males, is quite high for that reason. More typically, the patient is an adolescent female, and she will exercise excessively, limit caloric intake, purge, use diuretics and laxatives, and wear large bulky clothing to hide her skinniness, all while being convinced that she is too fat.

If you point out another anorexic young lady who is hospitalized on the same ward as her for the same condition, she will agree that her compatriot is worrisomely thin. However, when you ask her to look at herself in the mirror (with the bulky sweater removed), she will say that she looks "fat", even though you tell her that her height *and weight* are identical to the other young lady. And she really believes she is fat!

When people doubt information that contradicts what they presently believe, they often defend their position by saying that they will believe it (the contradictory evidence) when they see it. The truth, however, is that we often only see it when we believe it, no matter how obvious it is. We often only see what we already believe. If we believe that we are fat, it doesn't matter what the scales say. In the words of Warren Buffett, "What the human being is best at doing is interpreting all new information so that their prior conclusions remain intact."

Part of the problem resides in our confusing correlation with causation. *Correlation* means that things are connected to one another, that there is some interdependence. There is a correlation between the sun disappearing and rain starting. *Causation* means that there is a correlation such that one thing is responsible for the other one. Clouds cause rain and cause the sun to disappear. The sun disappearing and the raining coming, although correlated, do not cause each other directly; they are both caused by clouds. We want to find causes for everything so that we can convince ourselves that we understand the world better, and that will keep us safe. For that reason, we are prone to seeing causation whenever we see correlation.

Because we tend to want to see the world in a binary fashion so that it is easy to understand, we can be tricked into thinking causation when we see correlation. Two things happen together; there may even be a temporal sequence, so clearly one must cause the other. We need to be keen observers and thinkers not to fall prey to invoking causation when it does not exist.

Medicine is particularly prone to this, sometimes in the form of wishful thinking. We take an antibiotic for a sore throat, and two days later we convince ourselves we are feeling much better so the antibiotic must have worked; it must have been a bacterial infection. From now on when I get those same symptoms, I *need* an antibiotic or else I won't get better. But it is quite likely that our sore throat was of a viral nature and just got better on its own. A possible mass near my pancreas seen on a CT scan may be the cause of my abdominal symptoms because it is something bad, or maybe it is an incidentaloma that is benign and not causative. Avoiding the confusion of correlation and causation can be life-saving.

We are very prone to deceiving ourselves in situations of social pressure, a phenomenon referred to as "groupthink." We are reluctant to go against the flow of the group. I can still hear my father say, "I guess if one of your friends jumped off a bridge, you would too?" whenever I let my hair grow any longer than his. (Of course, I dared not point out to him that he kept his hair short to fit in with his peers too!)

We suffer from the false-consensus effect. It is akin to the authority bias as manifest in the Milgram experiment, where we don't rock the boat for fear of being ostracized or made to look like a fool by an "expert."

There seems to be no end to our flawed thinking and perceiving. We often can't see the unexpected. It's why cars hit cyclists more often in countries where there are fewer cyclists—drivers are just not expecting them. Our intuition, our reflexive thinking, can lead us astray at times, but deliberation is only helpful if we have all of the necessary information, and skill, to deliberate well.

Oversimplifying a Complex World

Charles Darwin stated, "Ignorance more frequently begets confidence than does knowledge." It's easy to be confident without being competent, and it is easy to be fooled by people who are confident but who are not competent. We see this a lot in the world of politics. Those who want to lead often do so because they want to lead, not because they are any more gifted than the rest of us. The wisest person in the room is seldom the loudest or best spoken. We trust someone who looks or dresses a certain way. Charisma goes a long way in this world!

We are overwhelmed if there are too many choices—the paradox of choice. The reptile inside tells us to keep it simple and binary; that makes it easy. For that reason, we often don't look for alternative solutions or explanations. Hence, we are subject to the fallacy of the singular cause, trusting that a complex turn of events had only one cause and trying to find that cause or make it fit. Our retrospectroscopes always seem to have twenty-twenty vision, don't they? (Remind you of an investment advisor after your stocks have tanked? Be kind, please don't mention Bre-X!)

Default settings appeal to us for the same reason—they are easy and less threatening. Let's just keep things the way they are, even if that means that the digital clock on the electronic device we just bought blinks "12:00" forever.

We are often much more afraid of losing something than we are excited about gaining something, by what we should not do than what we should do. We tend to overestimate benefit and underestimate cost when engaging in activities because we want so badly not to lose.

Losing hurts. We want to avoid pain at all costs. We are more affected by the death of one person we know than a genocide involving a huge number of people who are strangers because we feel more threatened by the close *one* than the far *many*, especially if that number seems incomprehensible. It's impossible to be brutally objective and neutral, particularly with things we find hard to fathom (like large numbers).

In fact, like the paradox of choice, our difficulty with large numbers illustrates the challenge of dealing with the complex. As we develop, we learn concrete thinking (building a toy house with blocks) before we learn abstract thinking (writing a philosophy paper at university). We comprehend linear thinking (arithmetic) before we comprehend nonlinear thinking (calculus).

Understandably, we have a tendency to oversimplify, to keep things as binary as possible, because it's easier and less overwhelming. Per se there is nothing wrong with starting simple in order to appreciate complex things. But arrogantly mistaking a simple starting point as being the definitive end point is *simplistic* thinking that can do great harm because we assume that we know more than we do.

I see this a lot in medicine. The physical sciences—for example, physics and chemistry—examine and explain the functioning of the physiosphere and have devised laws and rules that have drastically changed our lives, much of it for the better. However, we frequently make the mistake of thinking that these physical laws can completely explain all aspects of the biosphere, and they cannot. For example, we try to explain atherosclerosis ("hardening of the arteries") by using the analogy of a clogged kitchen drain. It's a nice start, but we need to appreciate the severe limitations of the analogy. The PVC drain pipe is *not* a living thing, nor is the stuff we flush down it. But an artery *is* a living thing, and so are the cells floating in our bloodstream, and they interact as living things in a way that sink effluent and PVC piping do not.

Even when we can apply laws of the physiosphere to the biosphere, we must realize that many of these laws do *not* involve linear formulae. Linear is easy to see and comprehend because it is constant; nonlinear is far tougher.

Linear is easy because it is binary: something is either moving or it isn't. However, gravity, for example, is not a linear function; things go faster the farther they fall. If you look very carefully, like the Greeks did, you can prove it to yourself, but it is subtle and can be easily missed. Watch the next time it rains. The water pouring from the drain spout on your roof does something rather interesting. The water is a continuous stream just as it leaves the roof, but it has broken up by the time it hits the ground. That's because gravity is accelaratory, not linear. The rain at the beginning of the stream ends up moving faster than the water behind it all the way down, so the stream breaks up. You see it all the time, but did you realize that you were witnessing a nonlinear function?

It's also why falling from thirty feet is more than three times as bad as falling from ten feet. When pressure builds up inside of a closed space like our heads (for example, a hemorrhage inside of our brains), it does not do so in a linear way. Anyone who has ever blown up a balloon knows this. Each successive breath into a balloon is harder and harder until finally the balloon pops. Our default thinking that processes are linear is often wrong, despite the evidence that constantly surrounds us.

In our desire to understand the world, we constantly underestimate the complexity of the world and subsequently oversimplify, mostly, I think, because it fits with the simple heuristics we already know well and so requires no additional effort. We have a tendency to be frugal, and for good reason; life is tough enough without compounding it with make-work projects. Why labour harder than you have to? Always take the low-hanging fruit first; snatch the insect closest to you rather than farthest from you. Keep it simple.

This business of oversimplifying, of "dumbing things down," is a fundamental problem in science, and especially in the life sciences. We try to understand the complex whole by understanding the parts, by isolating individual components or factors. This may work in simple systems in the physiosphere. But in the complex systems of the biosphere, with its intense interconnections, this is more difficult.

It is difficult to be sure that by understanding the constituent parts that we can understand the whole. Changing one variable inevitably changes many other variables in ways we cannot always appreciate. We are only beginning to understand that when it comes to ecology. We change one thing in a closed ecosystem and invariably we encounter unpleasant and unpredicted (perhaps unpredictable) consequences. The impact of the very small temperature changes involved in global warming is having profound changes on all aspects of our weather.

Medical science is guilty of this as well, for example, when we equate arteries to PVC pipes. The sunscreen lotion we put on our children may control the one variable we want to control but may impact many other variables, some of which we may not be aware. How much research has been done on the long-term safety of slathering mountains of these chemicals on our children's delicate skin? And how much money is being made in doing so? Any chance that how we view sunscreen is affected by profit and advertising?

But beyond that is the reality that we are always *part* of the experiment. We are not, and cannot be, neutral. Our very humanity, with all of its shortcomings and limitations, influences how we do science, and we need to remember that. Every researcher who has ever lived, despite their protestations to the contrary, is prone to all of the distorted thinking and behaviours discussed in this chapter. It is impossible to escape fully, and that influences the results that they produce and how we interpret them.

And the idea that most of us can multitask is simply grandiose (less than 3 percent of us can truly do it, and I am not one of them). Our attention is very limited, and it, like memory, is more like an illusion than reality—we miss most things because we can only focus on a very narrow range. We remember the most recent things and the most stimulating things the best because they grab our attention best. The in-between and mundane stuff gets lost, no matter how important. Prove it to yourself the next time you are in a lecture hall.

Perhaps the most problematic of all of the errors we make is the attribution error. This is most commonly seen when we attribute all success we have to something brilliant about us or our actions, rather than to dumb luck. This happens a lot in medicine. We forget about the power of the placebo effect. We fail to appreciate the complexity of the human body. We think the cardiac arrest we ran was successful because we are just so good at what we do, and the failed resuscitations are simply "meant to be."

I look at it as a culmination of a number of biases, such as wishful thinking, hindsight, and the fallacy of the singular cause among others. We neatly reflect on our lives and draw what appears for us to be the single, inescapable conclusion that everything we did was brilliant because only that specific sequence of events and decisions could possibly have led to the wonderful outcomes we have enjoyed (and thus so richly deserve!). It conveniently denies the tremendous interdependency of the universe and attributes to us not merely superhuman powers but, more importantly, an indubitable worthiness of all that we have that is good.

The scary corollaries, of course, are that those who do not attain such vaulted successes quite simply did not deserve them, and that when things go south for us, clearly something is awry in the world because we certainly don't deserve such failure; it can't possibly be our fault.

It is not difficult to see that fear lies at the basis of many of these distortions. Deep in our brains, the reptilian and lower mammalian parts utilize simple binary functioning to reason through decision making. For those creatures, something is either safe or not safe, and they don't have the luxury of time or intellect to figure it out. If you don't hightail it as soon as that shadow appears overhead, you will be gobbled up. No time to analyze what the shadow is until after you are safe.

We instinctively find certain images pleasant and other ones unpleasant. The faces of panda bears make them look cute even though they can be quite vicious; looks can deceive us. We are inherently more afraid of something foreign than something known, no matter how benign it may be. That's why some computer-generated images used in animated films can seem spooky if they are close to, but not exactly the same as, the real thing. People all over the world find alien things interesting, but they also find them unnerving. We all have natural, inborn biases in favour of the familiar and against the unfamiliar. No exceptions.

This binary thinking is highly beneficial for all creatures. It can even be useful for humans at times, much in the same way that denial can be. But both are primitive and nonselective. Our brains can do so much more, if we let them. But we don't have to. We can continue to think in binary terms if we want, provided that we are prepared to live like frogs and chipmunks.

We can ignore pain or potential pain by using denial, but then we limit our ability to utilize our full powers of consciousness and grow. Helicopter parents soon enough find out that they deprive their children of life lessons and the growth of internal resiliency when every child always wins a gold star. Pain that does not produce serious harm helps us to grow by allowing us to get to know our present limits, test them, and push beyond them.

The truth is, with our large cerebral hemispheres and finely tuned sense organs, we are unavoidably capable of appreciating how complex the universe is in ways that our primitive earth-dwelling compatriots cannot. We can't completely escape knowing that there is more to our world than simply what we see or understand at the moment, no matter how hard we try to deny.

And the reality of that simply ups the ante in the fear department. We know that things are not so simple, that the world is never just black and white, but mostly grey. We would like to just have two possible solutions to choose from, but at a very deep level we know that such is not the case. So we only allow (or force) ourselves to think in binary terms and use denial to pretend that that is enough because it soothes us; it eases our fears. It tells us that everything is all right, that we are safe, because there are only two options, and we always choose the right one.

As with their narcissism, children fear out of ignorance and vivid imagination. Adults fear because we know at a deep level, no matter how strong our attempts at conscious denial, that we live in an inherently complex and threatening world, so we ratchet up our defence mechanisms to compensate. The more we deny, the angrier we get at the world, and particularly other people, when they reveal that our simplistic binary thinking is wrong.

This is why elephants in the room scare adults so much. Like a toddler in diapers who goes into the corner of a room to answer the call of nature "in private," adults can turn their backs on everyone to make them disappear and carry on as though nothing happened. After all, if we ignore things, they simply don't exist, right? But as adults we can't help but know the elephants are there, no matter how much we try to deny them. Often, anger is how we respond when we feel such deep, reptilian fear. Our limbic systems are tough to shut off.

Plato said, "For a man to conquer himself is the first and noblest of all victories." I would like to agree, but given how erroneously we function at times, how our fear and the other raw emotions seem to dominate our lives, how do we "conquer" ourselves?

Recall that at the moment of the big bang, the universe suddenly, and inexplicably, exploded from an incredibly dense blob into the fundamental particles of the universe, which evolved into present-day matter and energy—the physiosphere. When that happened, all of the rules and laws of the physiosphere came into play. Some time later, the molecules of the physiosphere evolved, again mysteriously, beyond their physiospheric limits to form life—the biosphere. New principles arose to guide it, such as survival of the fittest.

Further along in time, another mystifying transition occurred. The brain evolved to such complexity that it broke beyond its biospheric boundaries to form the *mind* and the noosphere appeared. At that moment we ceased to be defined in purely organic, biospheric terms. It is the same kind of evolutionary leap that occurred when life came into existence and was no longer defined simply by the inorganic dictums of the physiosphere.

The noosphere—the development of full consciousness—includes and transcends the biosphere. In it resides that enigmatic entity called the mind that Plato alluded to; that's where we conquer ourselves.

But first, I came to realize, we must face our fear.

Chapter 10

Facing Our Fears

HAVE YOU EVER heard of a fellow named Les Stroud? Perhaps you have seen his television show *Survivorman*. It's a fascinating show because this gutsy guy goes out in the wilds all over the world and makes do with a minimum of modern conveniences. Apart from a video camera to document his adventure, he seems to carry with him fewer tools than many of the explorers who discovered North America hundreds of years ago. It can be scary just *watching* his show.

It becomes obvious when you tune in that Les does not romanticize nature; he knows how unforgiving the wild can be. It's not that nature is mean, uncaring, or ruthless; in truth, it is amoral. Its duty is to its own flourishing, and part of that flourishing, as callous as it may sound, involves occasional purging. For example, most forest fires start naturally and are not man-made. It is a radical cleansing that nature does on a regular basis (there are lots of examples) to allow for new growth. Nature has been doing so in the biosphere for a very long time, and it seems to work pretty well. Over 99 percent of all of the species that have ever lived on the planet no longer exist; yet nature continues to truck along.

Apparently, there have been several major catastrophes on earth over the millennia like the one sixty-five million years ago that wiped out the dinosaurs (likely an asteroid hitting the Yucatán peninsula). If not for that event, from which, yet again, nature recovered, we humans might not be here. It's just unfortunate if you happen to innocently get caught in it. Alas, the poor brontosaurus! But don't get cocky: remember, hurricanes, lightning, and earthquakes are *natural* events too.

I fully realize that *Survivorman* may take liberties because it is meant for entertainment. Nevertheless, it illustrates the riskiness of being in nature. Unlike his counterparts hundreds of years ago, I suspect that Les has a backup plan in case things go south; Captain Sir John Franklin didn't when he explored the Arctic, and we know how that ended up.

It reminds me that when I am out in nature, it is not like it was for Captain Franklin. I, like most of us, drive there in my car and have a nice tent with a portable propane stove, battery-driven lights, a warm down-filled sleeping bag, lots of food, a water filter, and maybe even a cell phone. If I run into trouble, I have told people where I will be so that I can be rescued. I don't think they had highly trained personnel in helicopters back in Franklin's time.

I do hope that those of us who enjoy nature realize this. We are brave, but not that brave; few of us want to die, or be seriously hurt, doing something we love. If we are brutally honest with ourselves, we will admit that we have fear and act accordingly. Heroes are not reckless; they know the risks and proceed as carefully as the situation will allow, acknowledging that undesirable outcomes are a distinct possibility, and they are willing to accept them with equanimity. They may not be happy with a bad result, but they accept it graciously. That is facing your fear.

The other end of the spectrum from hero is pseudobravery. One pretends to be fearless by simply denying that bad things can happen (or denying that they can happen to us because we are special). Or because we kid ourselves into believing that should the undesirable happen, we will be okay with it, when in fact deep down we are not at all convinced that we will be. That is not facing our fears; that is denial.

Many years ago, I was working in a small northern community, and delivering babies was part of my medical practice. Outside of town was a small, devoutly religious community, who generally delivered their babies at home. A pregnant woman slightly older than me, with several children already, came to see me and asked if I would be interested in delivering her baby in her home. I had done my obstetrical training in a large community hospital and had delivered about 500 babies. On the one hand, that gave me a reasonable bit of confidence. On the other hand, that many deliveries had also offered the opportunity to get a tiny look at the very infrequent, but equally very terrifying, things that can go wrong with such a natural process.

I explained to this charming lady that I would love to deliver her baby, but the problem was that should something go wrong (e.g., placental abruption, cord prolapse, postpartum hemorrhage), many of the skills I had obtained during my training would be useless. In her home, I would not have the tools or assistance necessary to properly engage my skill set. I knew that the odds of me witnessing a beautiful and otherwise uneventful home birth were overwhelmingly good, but I was not prepared to take that chance. Why? Because although I would greatly enjoy the normal birth, I knew that I could not face the horror and guilt of seeing something bad happen and be helpless to do anything about it.

She smiled at me as tenderly as anyone has ever smiled at me. She was only a few years older than me but was clearly far wiser and more mature than I was or, frankly, still am. You see, because of her faith, she was completely at peace with whatever occurred, even her own death. I had seen this first-hand. The people in her community didn't panic when things went bad. For the most part, they lived on farms, and they knew death first-hand, not like us city folk. They didn't finger-point and sue everyone else when things went bad, especially if they knew it had been their decision. She understood my fear, and she forgave me for it, despite the fact that she did not share it. No one has ever been kinder to me in my life.

You may not agree with her religious beliefs or her decision to have her children birthed at home, but I hope that you respect her courage and her honesty. As Nassim Taleb would say, she had "skin in the game"; she had conquered herself. Contrast her with the CEO of a large bank, who takes big risks with your money, loses it, and then gets a government bailout so that they still end up with a $3 million salary. They have no skin in the game; they play games of risk with your money but are not prepared to lose theirs.

If I were still doing obstetrics today, I would be more willing, under low-risk circumstances, to do home deliveries, with one caveat: I would want to be sure that I was dealing with heroines and heroes like my patient above. I would need to know that the person was not using denial. That they truly recognized that no matter how low the risk, it is never zero. That should the unthinkable happen, they are okay with it. That their desire to sue would be based on incompetent practice *only*, not on unwanted, yet completely predictable, results. That they would not be expecting the conventional health-care system they shun to suddenly and magically bail them out when their decisions go awry. I would want them to acknowledge and face their fears, not deny them. But if you have never seen the death of a young mother or newborn, how can you know? I mean, *really know*?

It reminds me of the immunization debate. Let me first state that in no way do I want to judge anyone on the basis of their opinions on immunizations, especially when it comes to their children. Parents ultimately will have to bear the consequences of their decisions, good and bad; not the government, not the doctors, not me. And there is no more difficult or scary job than being a parent. Your children don't come with manuals. Just when you think you understand your five-year-old, she turns six. You're sure you have this parenting thing down pat after your first child, and your second child ends up being the polar opposite of your first, and you are starting from scratch all over again. There are no report cards to tell you how well you have done, no crystal balls to help you, and no awards or incentives.

So no matter what your opinions on immunizations or the reasons for those opinions, I understand, as a father of three, the stresses, doubts, and insecurities of the job of being a parent. Quadruple that if you are a single parent. The most you can hope for is that you do your best. And in a complex world full of uncertainty, that is all we can ask of you as well. But none of us can ever be absolutely certain of *anything*.

I think there are many legitimate reasons why people have concerns about immunizations. They mistrust large multinational pharmaceutical companies. They know that there is a lot of money to be made in immunizations, and that affects how people interpret data, no matter how scholarly or noble one's ambitions. They don't like politicians telling them how to raise their children. They know that no immunization is fully protective. The influenza vaccine is a good example because it requires making predictions about the future strains of the virus, and that is difficult.

Some people worry that we are giving too many vaccines and, like the overuse of antibiotics, not allowing our bodies to develop natural immunity or inadvertently promoting the development of resistant strains. I am always a little unnerved at how often the protocols and schedules for immunizations change. Each time we change, we are sure we have it right this time until, of course, the next time rolls around.

Others worry about the potential side effects of these interventions. Some are known and serious (rare anaphylactic reactions); others are speculative and, because of their rarity and delay in manifestation, are more difficult to prove. Of course, any side effect of any treatment is not a side effect in isolation; by definition, it involves a complex host as well. So unless absolutely everyone who undergoes the treatment has the same side effect, at least in part any side effects are manifestations of an intricate relationship between that specific treatment and that unique individual's makeup (more on this later).

On the spectrum of thinking, there is *rational thinking* (using reason to face our fears) at one end, and *irrational thinking* (using denial to avoid our fears) on the other. One could make a very rational case for not immunizing by saying the following:

"I am skeptical of the health-care system, particularly the pharmaceutical industry. I think when so much money is involved, it is hard to know the truth. I think a lot of these diseases are rare, and I believe that if my family takes very good care of itself, we can reduce the already low risk to something so low that I am comfortable taking it.

"However, I acknowledge that no matter how well we take care of ourselves, we are still at *some* risk, and some of these diseases happen *very* quickly, are hard to treat, and can be *very* serious, even lethal. I also acknowledge that to some degree, I am also relying on herd immunity to protect my family, meaning that the greater the number of people in the herd who are immunized, the less of that disease there is around so that even my family, who are not immunized, benefit from a lower risk of disease.

"Further, I will graciously accept that should anyone in my family contract one of these potentially preventable diseases, I will only expect the usual level of competence from the health-care system, not miracles. If I make the decision not to immunize, I will not then in retrospect sue everyone I can get my hands on for not warning me that this could happen and blaming them for the sequelae of my risk-taking."

That would be having skin in the game. That would be avoiding denial and facing your fears; that I can fully respect.

My worry, of course, is that people often operate closer to the other end of the spectrum where fear and denial dominate. Like the antibiotic conundrum, it's easy to think that these diseases only happen to *those* people, not my family. After all, we take care of ourselves, not like *those* people. They, well, kinda deserve it, but we don't, so it can't happen to us. Don't get me wrong; I am all in favour of taking care of oneself, and I am fully convinced that doing so will reduce your risk. But it will never *eliminate* it. Nature is far too complex for that kind of simplistic thinking.

Or it may be that people reason that if someone in the family gets one of these diseases, it will be easy to recognize so quickly that treatment can start virtually instantaneously and everything will be fine. However, some of these diseases are hard to spot really early on in their development and can proceed with lightning speed. And some simply have no cure once they begin to infect. Rabies, for example, is uniformly fatal if the vaccine is not administered soon after exposure.

I hope by now it is obvious that *we are all* built to fear. The reality is that when deciding about immunizations, most of us reside somewhere along the spectrum of rational-irrational, and that is completely understandable. Risk assessment is not easy to do. Probabilities are difficult to comprehend. It's hard to envisage disability or death if we have not seen it or experienced it ourselves, directly or indirectly.

In our modern lives, we are becoming progressively more removed from it. In the past when more of us lived on farms, we saw animals die, even during the process of giving life to offspring. Farms were (and still are) dangerous places to work; injury and potential disability were very real possibilities. When we lived in smaller towns that did not have as many nursing homes as we have today, our grandparents died in *our* homes, and we witnessed, intimately, their demise and death.

Less than a century ago, we experienced diseases like polio and measles, and not uncommonly people died of pneumonia. Today, we are relatively inexperienced in such matters, so they frighten us even more. This means that we avoid talking about them, but in the process become less capable of processing the possibilities of disability and death.

Over the years, I have become more skeptical of the benefits of modern medicine, but personally I have to admit that the one area of medicine I continue to believe in is immunizations. I think that the worldwide evidence of benefit for many of these is overwhelming. I personally have not seen, or even heard of, a case of epiglottitis since the newer vaccines have come out. Similar story for meningitis. I see fewer pneumonias too. My younger colleagues have likely never seen measles (I haven't seen one since early in practice). I hope to never see a case of tetanus. I have seen people afflicted by polio, though not an active case. If our great-grandparents were around, they would remind us of the great flu epidemic about one hundred years ago.

Part of the problem is, paradoxically, the very success of the vaccines themselves. They have been so effective in eliminating some diseases that we don't know anything about them, except for easily dismissed anecdotes from our elderly relatives. If you have never lived through a polio epidemic, you have no idea how bad that disease is. Meningitis is scary. Tetanus is not fun.

It is unrealistic to think that such upsides would come with *no price, no* downsides. I have no doubt that there may be risks to the vaccines, but as far as I can tell, they seem low, but again not likely zero. I don't blame people for being skeptical when no one will admit to any significant risks and pretend that immunizations are *completely* safe. I also understand, however, the reluctance to admit to risks—the binary thinkers out there will not balance the risks with the benefits, and their irrational fear could win out, and we could lose the one human intervention that has likely saved more lives than almost any other.

I don't know if we will ever have the final answer regarding a causative association between some vaccines and serious diseases. If we do find such an association, there should be assistance and compensation from the collective for the legitimate cases where there is harm. When we, as a collective, benefit directly (and particularly *indirectly* through herd immunity) from immunizations that cause harm to a few innocent individuals, we should take care of those individuals who are unintentionally harmed.

I find it rather amusing that sometimes people who are against vaccines bemoan the fact that there are still quite a number of nasty diseases out there—tuberculosis, AIDS, malaria, hepatitis C, herpes, and more—for which we have no vaccines. I guess it's easier to badmouth a vaccine for a disease you no longer see, one that now seems theoretical, than it is to badmouth a potential vaccine whose disease is actively wreaking havoc in your own backyard.

I think it is possible to face our fears and conquer ourselves; I have seen it in many patients. They have all inspired me. But it is not easy. I have not yet conquered myself.

So as a scientist trying to face my fears, I read more about the brain to understand better the macroscopic and microscopic structure and function of it, hoping it would give me some clues. In so doing, it became clear to me that there is a difference between the brain and the mind. A difference that not everyone agrees with, but for me one that evolution tells us is undeniably so.

Chapter 11

Neuroplasticity and the Mind

IN ORDER TO conquer ourselves, we must first understand ourselves. We are going to examine the brain and the mind. It is a little bit technical but only insofar as I think is necessary to allow us to grasp what it means to be a member of the species *Homo sapiens*. First, we will look at the brain in more detail on its own, then how it fits into the entire nervous system, and then finally examine how it fits into the big picture of a complete individual.

If you don't have a background or interest in science, don't feel overwhelmed; nothing I discuss is that complicated! But if you want, you can skip through to the subheading "Consciousness."

Before medical school, I took a course in comparative anatomy and got my first glimpse of evolution up close. The professor led us through the process of evolution by comparing the anatomy and physiology of fish, reptiles, and mammals, noticing the developmental similarities between them. With the eye of faith, one could see the continuity of structure and function as various organs and appendages evolved over millions of years from a lowly dogfish shark to a modern-day cat. Cat anatomy and physiology includes and transcends that of the species beneath it on the evolutionary ladder, such as the dogfish shark.

This was reinforced when I took anatomy courses in medical school that included studying the prenatal growth of humans from embryo to fetus to newborn to adult. One could see equivalences between lesser species and us. This pattern of including and transcending is the one Ken Wilber has observed occurring since the big bang, whereby a more complex species includes and builds upon elements of a less complex species.

This is no less true from the perspective of brain functioning. One can see, in the successive stages of emotional, psychological, and intellectual development of humans, an evolution similar to the physical evolution from fish to mammals. As we have explored earlier, a newborn's cerebral hemispheres are not fully developed, so they really have little more than the brainstem and the beginnings of the limbic systems to utilize. Hence, it is as narcissistic as any reptile, solely concerned with its own survival, using whatever mechanisms it has to ensure that its basic needs are met. And these means are primal and effective—ask any parent about their experience of a hungry baby crying at three in the morning. There is a reason why that crying is akin to fingernails on a chalkboard: it makes it impossible to ignore! Survival is paramount.

Gradually infants grow, not just physically but developmentally as well. What exactly is happening inside of their heads when this is occurring?

The Brain

In order to comprehend better what's going on, how evolution on a grand scale as well as evolution on a small scale within each of us proceeds, we need to have a shared understanding of the brain. I am not a neurologist, so I won't pretend that I know much about our brain, but let me share with you what I know.

We are going to look at the brain from three perspectives. The first two are more anatomical in nature: the *macroscopic* level and the *microscopic* level. The third is more a *functional* level.

The Brain from the Macroscopic Perspective

Let's start at the *macroscopic* level, the level we can appreciate without magnification. There are many ways to look at the structure of our brain, but for the sake of simplicity (but hopefully not to the point of simplistic) they are the brainstem at the bottom, the higher brain at the top, and then all of the other parts in between. We don't need to get into all of this, but let's take a brief look.

The brainstem consists of the medulla oblongata (the myelencephalon), the pons and cerebellum (the metencephalon) and the midbrain (the mesencephalon). The medulla oblongata connects to the spinal cord and lies at the base of our brain. It is where the most basic regulatory functions occur (e.g., breathing, controlling our blood pressure). We refer to these as "autonomic functions" since they are performed at a subconscious level, automatically. If the medulla dies, we die. The pons is above the medulla. *Pons* means "bridge," and the cerebellum sits on top of this bridge. The pons is involved in some autonomic functions, such as posture, and the cerebellum is involved primarily in coordination and balance.

Above the pons is the midbrain, which is involved in hearing, vision, arousal, and some control over movement.

Above the brainstem but below the higher brain lies the diencephalon, whose major components are

1. the thalamus, which acts as a relay station for many sensations including pain, vision, hearing, and other sensations, as well as being involved in memory, emotion, and wakefulness;

2. the hypothalamus, where the fight-or-flight response resides as well as our drives for food and sex; and

3. the pituitary gland, which oversees most of the hormone production (endocrine glands) in our body.

All of the structures I have described so far exist in all animals referred to as "vertebrates," the ones that have a brain within a skull and a segmented spinal column. This group includes fish, amphibians, reptiles, birds, and mammals like us.

Above the diencephalon is the upper brain or telencephalon. In nonmammals, this area is small and not well developed. It is larger in the lower mammals like mice and very much larger in higher mammals like dolphins and us.

The telencephalon, from bottom to top, includes some important structures such as

1. the olfactory bulb involved in smell;

2. the amygdala involved in attention, some aspects of learning, and emotion, especially fear;

3. the anterior cingulate cortex, involved in attention and motivation;

4. the hippocampus, involved in memory, both formation and retrieval, including spatial memory, and hence learning; and

5. the two cerebral hemispheres, left and right, including the corpus callosum, which connects the two sides.

The cerebral hemispheres have different areas, or lobes, each of which have specialized functions: at the back, the occipital lobes are involved in vision; on the sides, the temporal lobes are involved in language and hearing; on the top, the parietal lobes are involved in sensation; and at the front, apropos to their name, the frontal lobes are involved in movement as well as many higher-level functions such problem solving, judgment, and our social behaviour, to name a few.

Structures two to four above, along with the thalamus and hypothalamus, are sometimes vaguely referred to as the "limbic system," the part of the brain involved in emotion, behaviour, motivation, and some types of learning.

Lots of things can go wrong if disease or injury affects the brain, and the sequelae of such will depend on what part of the brain is affected and how badly.

The Brain from the Microscopic Perspective

Now let's look at the *microscopic* structure of the brain. It is important to understand this a little because it will help us better grasp how the brain grows throughout our entire lives.

There are a number of different kinds of cells that constitute our brain:

1. cells that make up the arteries, veins, and capillaries that carry blood to and from the brain;
2. glial cells that act as support structures, aid in tissue repair, and help to put myelin on nerves to make them work faster, among other activities; and
3. nerve cells or neurons, which we most commonly associate with the brain.

Each nerve cell consists of

1. a body;
2. an axon, a tube that extends from the body to reach other neurons; and
3. dendrites on the other side of the cell body from the axon, which interface with the ends of other axons of other neurons.

The places where dendrites come close to the ends of the axons of other neurons are called "synapses." The cerebral cortex, the surface layer of the cerebral hemispheres, contains nerve cell bodies and mostly unmyelinated axons, so it is grey in colour (hence termed "grey matter"). I have read that this layer, the cortex, is only six cells deep, which doesn't sound like much. However, the cortex is convoluted and has billions of neurons, each one estimated to have between one thousand and six thousand dendrites each. So despite the fact that it is only six cells deep, that's still a lot of connections!

Electrical signals, originating in the body of a neuron, travel down the axon at lightning-fast speeds. At the end of the axon, there are terminals packed with small sacs that are filled with neurochemicals, such as dopamine or acetylcholine, that release their contents when stimulated by the electrical signal. These chemicals are released into the space (synapse) between the end of the axon of one nerve and dendrites of a different neuron. The chemicals attach themselves to various receptors on the receiving dendrites, somewhat like a key in a lock, and this, in turn, stimulates the production of an electrical signal in the receiving neuron. Like the speed of the signal down the axon, this neurochemical exchange is also very fast because the synaptic space is so small that it does not take long for the neurochemicals to cross and complete their mission.

There are many different neurochemicals, each with different receptors throughout the brain, some used throughout the brain and some used only in specialized areas. This emitting and receiving of neurochemicals from one neuron to another is how neurons communicate. It is how all of the functions of our nervous system occur, whether in the brain, the spinal cord, or where nerves interface with muscles or other structures.

So when we have a thought, a sensation, or engage in an activity, it involves neurons firing in very specific ways, triggering a cascade of other neurons that eventually allow that specific goal—a thought, a sensation, or an activity—to be accomplished. Neurons tend to form networks with each other such that they can fire in a more efficient and reliable way to bring about these goals. It is said that neurons that "fire together, wire together." In other words, neurons become wired to each other in networks the more often they fire together by developing more axon-dendrite connections (more synapses) at which to transmit signals.

For example, if a hockey player shoots a puck at me, the retinae (which are really highly specialized neurons) in the back of my eyes send signals to my brain. This data in turn provides the necessary information to the motor neurons of my brain that guide my glove hand to (hopefully) make a brilliant save!

A food stimulates a taste bud on our tongue that in turn triggers neurons that send a message to our brain that informs us that we like this food and want more of it. The more often we taste that same food, the more synapses develop to transmit that signal and the more quickly we recognize its taste. The taste may eventually trigger a memory (wire with other neurons) of when we had it last and with whom we had it.

For the most part, the neurons and the neuronal networks of our lower brain, like the brainstem, are fully formed and functional when we are born (though not if we are born too prematurely). We don't need to learn how to breathe or dispose of bodily waste. (*Controlling* the disposal of bodily waste is another matter.) However, neurons and networks of the higher parts of the brain are not fully developed at birth. This should not be surprising given that it is estimated that we have so many nerve cells, each of which can have thousands of synapses with other neurons. It takes time to learn to become continent.

Part of this is done by adding myelin, a fat-based coating of material wrapped onto the axons of neurons (by glial cells). This process, called myelination, allows the electrical current in axons to flow more quickly. A lot of this myelination occurs in the first two years of life, which is why it is important for infants to eat well and have enough fats in their diet.

But there are even more impressive processes involved in developing neurons and their networks.

Shortly after the Stone Age ended, I entered medical school, and at that time we thought that all humans were born with all of the neurons they would ever have for the rest of their lives. If a neuron died, it was gone forever, and you were out of luck. It turns out that we were wrong (like we were about a lot of things way back then), and in addition to being able to repair neurons, new neurons can be also generated. But the most exciting part is that we have come to a fuller appreciation of how much individual nerves can *change* during our lifetimes. These discoveries are referred to as "neuroplasticity." The dendrites and their connections change throughout our lives.

When you learn to play guitar, brush up on your French, or rethink your perspective on mortality, you are changing your neurons: the cell bodies, the axons, and particularly the dendrites, as they interface with other neurons, can all change. You are altering their structure and their function when you learn to strum a new tune, recall the conjugation of *avoir*, or concede to the possibility of life after death.

We can change the way neurons fire and which neurons they interact with and therefore trigger. We can change the wiring. We can vary the wiring within a network or between networks by eliminating, modifying, or solidifying old ones or by establishing new connections between neurons and between networks.

The more often I practise hockey, learning and repeatedly rehearsing specific movements or skills, the more often those same neurons fire together. New connections between neurons are acquired or enhanced through development of more or stronger synapses between the dendrites of one neuron and the receptors of other neurons. With billions of neurons in the brain, and as many as six thousand connections each, the potential for forming new connections and networks is enormous.

It's a little startling that we didn't realize this sooner. After all, we have all learned skills during our lives that we didn't have at birth. What did we think was going on in there, anyway? It turns out we are constantly modifying our wiring by changing our firing throughout our entire lives.

So now let's look at how this wiring translates into our brain functioning.

The Brain from a Functional Perspective

From an evolutionary perspective, we can see the gradual development of the brain from reptiles to humans in terms of more neurons, greater complexity, and more intense wiring. And we can see the same thing in our own individual development. As I said earlier, watching infants grow is one of the most enjoyable and entertaining parts of my job. It's also what makes being a grandparent so wonderful as well!

As we explored earlier, very primitive organisms had only simple sensory apparatuses to warn them of impending danger. They gradually became more sophisticated until there evolved an integrating structure we refer to as the "brain." The brain itself continued to evolve. The primitive brain of the reptiles functioned predominantly in a binary fashion—fight-or-flight. Having a far simpler brain, primarily the limbic structures and the brainstem, fear of pain and death is the modus operandi of these organisms. Their emotional and cognitive repertoires are limited, which is why we don't, as a rule, have as many reptiles for pets as we have higher mammals. My pet turtle I had years ago either tolerated me for a short while or scurried away. It would not snuggle up with me like our dog did, and it never managed to fetch a tennis ball for me either.

As the brain evolved to greater complexity, it maintained these primitive lower brain structures and functions but added to it a far more complex network of neurons capable of doing more. That's when things got really interesting.

Now, instead of having a brain with sense organs that could only differentiate safe from unsafe, we expanded our catalogue of experience, and subsequently behaviours, by means of more complex sensory organs and a more powerful command centre. Dogs bond with us in a way that turtles never can. Cats are playful in a way my turtle never was.

In other words, as higher mammals with much more sophisticated sensory organs and a more profound processing centre, we now experience *pleasure,* engaging the world in a profoundly and qualitatively different fashion. Yes, we still have deep-rooted fear, but we have so much more.

We still eat to stay alive, of course, but we eat for pleasure as well.

Frogs differentiate flies from nonflies; we differentiate Camembert from brie, Chardonnay from Pinot Noir. I doubt that frogs reflect on the taste of flies in the same way: "My those large fat flies are rather tough and gamey! I think I prefer the smaller ones." We eat meals together as a social activity (or at least we used to!). We appreciate a glorious sunrise and understand that it marks the beginning of a new day. Our favourite music resonates with us, allowing us to vividly relive warm memories of past pleasures. We write and read books. We relish animated conversations. We enjoy laughing.

The breadth of stimuli that can produce pleasure for us seems nearly endless. On a regular basis, I am intrigued at the new activities people will invent to amuse themselves, including ones fraught with danger, such as BASE jumping!

We no longer behave simply to avoid pain or death; we consciously seek pleasure as well. Our desire to experience pleasure can produce its own set of problems, however. For example, it's at the source of all addictions (more on that later). It can seem, at times, that our lives are an unceasing search for more sources of sensory gratification, both quantitatively and qualitatively. I find this to be especially true when we are young and just beginning to discover our world and what our bodies are capable of experiencing within it.

Our desire to avoid harm and death is very deep-seated, rooted in the fight-or-flight response of the reptilian part of our brain. Although the quest for pleasure is not quite so primal, most of it still originates below the level of our cortex, particularly in our emotional centres associated with the limbic structures.

More importantly, at this level of our brain and its functioning, it is still all about us and our feelings; it is narcissistic. It is primarily in the highest level of our brain, at the cortical level, where we are capable of understanding complex and abstract ideas, such as caring about the sensations of people other than ourselves. Here, we have what are referred to as "mirror neurons," which can mirror the internal thoughts and actions of another human being. But we only develop these higher neurons to any great degree as we leave childhood and approach adolescence. And the process needs nurturing, mentoring. It is a crucial step on the road to "conquering ourselves."

To understand the rest of that road, we need to look beyond the brain.

The Nervous System

Up until now, we have been discussing primarily the brain, and although a very important structure, it is but one part of our *nervous system*, which is just one of many systems in our body. So I want us to now look at ourselves from a more holistic vantage point, as a complete organism. Let's start by looking at the entire nervous system the same way we looked at the brain, from the *anatomical* and then the *functional* perspectives.

Anatomically, the upper part of the system, the *central nervous system*, includes the brain, encased in the skull, and spinal cord, encased in the spinal column. The lower part, the *peripheral nervous system*, is composed of all of the nerves that go to and from the brain and spinal cord to the rest of our body.

Functionally, there are the *involuntary* and *voluntary* systems.

There is the *involuntary or autonomic system* that performs the "autopilot" functions (e.g., controlling our breathing, blinking). Most of this is overseen by our lower brain, but some at the level of the spinal cord (we refer to them as "reflexes"). We don't have to think about blinking or breathing, it just happens. We pull our hands off a hot stove without thinking. Our nervous system is very much involved, but not at a conscious level and not at a level easily controlled or overridden by our upper brain.

There is the *voluntary* system that is under conscious control. Most of our conscious thought, sensation, and behaviour originate in our upper brain, especially in the cerebral hemispheres. In other words, these are the experiences and activities we refer to as "thinking." Most actions, like taking a walk in unfamiliar woods, are done with a mixture of both the voluntary and involuntary systems.

Neuroplasticity

So what is wildly exciting about this concept of neuroplasticity? It offers us a perennial potential for near-unlimited growth. There is almost nothing about us that can't be changed. In fact, even some of the autonomic nervous system's hard-wired autopilot functions can learn to be controlled with conscious effort. There are people who have learned to control their heart rate and temperature regulation to a remarkable degree!

So all of us are hard-wired with some basic neural networks, many of which we have in common with each other and with other species, in fact. Some we have at birth, and some we acquire during our formative years. Some neural pathways we come to use without even thinking, like tapping our foot when our favourite tune comes on the radio. This is the basis for practising something over and over again. We do it so often that it becomes automatic because we repeatedly fire neurons together until they become wired together so efficiently that we can do them subconsciously, "in our sleep." It's how we learn to play a musical instrument or a sport or learn a language.

We also develop internal rules to guide us, heuristics, some to the point that we don't have to think much about them. We have mentioned some of them before, like not crossing a street on a red light.

But not all of the rules, the neural firing patterns, that we acquired are completely accurate or unfailingly helpful. A green light does not always mean it is safe to cross; we ought to look first. So we learn to check these rules of thumb when time and circumstance permit.

This brings me to the three most important lessons I have learned from studying the brain and the nervous system.

First, a lot of the wiring in our nervous system that influences us on a continuous and often profound basis, we are either born with or develop long before our brains are fully matured in adulthood. For example, the autonomic system is largely hard-wired. The binary fight-or-flight reflex is hard-wired in our lower brain at birth and is powerful and near instantaneous in its actions. Our genes affect the development of our brains and its wiring. We have all observed how differently the structures of the limbic system manifest in families. Some families are very laid-back; some are more high-strung. We know that genes play a predisposing role in conditions such as anxiety and depression, for example.

Our experiences as we grow up can affect the wiring of our brains. Chronic stress and trauma can have adverse effects on our hippocampus and its ability for memory storage and retrieval. We see this in cases of post-traumatic stress disorder.

In the last several decades we have come to appreciate the profound effect child-rearing can have on development of our brains. Families that are chaotic and disorganized produce children with poorer emotional control who struggle in relationships. Neuronal maturation and functioning in the amygdala and hypothalamus, critical parts of the limbic system with respect to emotion and meaning, are adversely affected if children are not raised in a secure household.

If children are not nurtured so as to establish a coherent sense of who they are, they are at increased risk of developing what is referred to as a "narcissistic personal disorder." They cannot see other people as separate from themselves, with their own views and desires, and this can profoundly affect their ability for deep and satisfying interpersonal relationships. At the extreme, it can deteriorate into a borderline personality disorder. People with this disorder cannot draw a distinction between themselves and the uncontrollable, relentless, and complex universe in which they reside. They feel constantly threatened by the outside world. Because they feel invaded by it, they are terrified, and they behave accordingly.

The second lesson I have learned is that despite the fact that a lot of this wiring is well established by the time we hit adulthood, we do have the ability, through neuroplasticity, to change our neurons and their networks. Just as we can learn to play guitar and play goalie in hockey, we can rewire our heuristics, our perspectives, our attitudes, our values, and even our moods. That is an incredibly powerful concept, one that can truly be transformative in our lives.

This brings me to the third lesson: how we make this transformation happen.

Thinking

On a daily basis, we rely heavily on our automatic lower brain functions. We also utilize the heuristics we developed in the more primitive parts of our upper brain during childhood when our ability to formulate complex and abstract thoughts was still somewhat limited.

In childhood, we still have a sense of naive realism; we are more easily influenced into making inaccurate rules of thumb. Many of the heuristics that we construct quite consciously when we are young, with repetition become subconscious as part of our implicit memory. We stop thinking about them and simply assume that they are unassailably true and apply them in an unquestioning, almost reflex manner. We say or do things "without thinking."

For example, linear patterns are easier to see and process, so we are more likely to see everything as linear, even though a huge percentage of the processes that surround us are *not* linear. For that reason, if we see two events occur one after the other, we assume correlation and perhaps even causation. Because binary thinking makes things so simple (something is either good or bad), we prefer to see all problems as binary because it limits fear and keeps us safe by making decisions easier.

We do not like ambiguity because that leaves us feeling vulnerable; we do not always understand the nuances of reality, so we don't know what to do. We want clear, decisive rules to follow, so we invent and then follow rules of thumb. We feel threatened, at a level deep in our brains, by criticism or by confronting our errors, so we avoid admitting to blunders or wrongdoings.

We don't want to have to rethink all of our ways of doing things or all of our heuristics. It's scary, and it is a lot of work. Our deepest selves are designed to keep things simple and to be frugal. For that reason, from an evolutionary perspective animals learned never to pass up an easy meal because they never knew when the next one would come around. They learned to gorge when the food was available, just in case. It is not surprising that even though our fridge may be full and we are at no risk of starvation, we often still eat too much.

In the lower parts of our upper brains, we are highly motivated by pleasant sensations and stimuli. We crave new experiences, always wanting to push the limits. So we love bargains and are suckers for a sale. If we can get quantitatively or qualitatively more with little sacrifice, we are all in. We experience childlike delight whenever we sense a deal in the making; we brag to our friends about it. We are hard-wired to want something for nothing. We'll spend ten dollars in gas to drive for a five-dollar saving.

In other words, a lot of our faulty thinking and behaviours arise from, or are heavily influenced by, the lower levels of our brain, below the cerebral cortices. This is where fear and denial reside. It is where our desires for sensory stimulation and pleasure reside.

So given these innate tendencies that we all share, how do we make neuroplasticity happen?

We think.

Consciousness

Let's be really clear: as with all other vertebrates, we cannot survive without our lower brain, and we need heuristics in order to function on a daily basis in the world. We make generalizations all of the time and use them constantly. In a fast-paced complex world, we have to. We are programmed to fear, or at least be wary, of anything that is unfamiliar, irrespective of its actual danger. Our fear is protective and necessary. Our enjoyment of pleasurable sensations is a tremendous gift we have inherited, and it adds untold depth to our lives. We should not deny any of this, nor be ashamed of it. In fact, we should relish it. But what distinguishes *Homo sapiens* from other animals is the size of our upper brain, especially the cerebral cortices.

The left hemisphere, or left cerebral cortex, is the one associated (usually) with the more logical, concrete side of ourselves. The right is more associated with our creative, abstract aspects, with our autobiographical self. The two are connected by the corpus callosum and work intimately together (and with all other parts of our entire nervous system). We function best when both sides are healthy and operating well, especially when we can balance the two sides.

Many people would insist that our consciousness resides in our cerebral hemispheres and is purely a function of the physiology of our neurons. Is that so?

It is important to recall two things about our nervous system vis-à-vis our entire person. Firstly, neurons from our brain, either directly or indirectly through connections with neurons outside of the brain, extend to the farthest reaches of our bodies. This allows for two-way transfer of electric signals—that is, information—between the brain and the body. Secondly, various hormones in our body bathe our brains constantly through the rich blood supply to the brain. So in fact, sentience is not limited to only our cerebral hemispheres; it is contributed to by our entire being. I have read that patients who receive an organ transplant, like the heart, commonly will enjoy foods they never liked before but foods the donor had enjoyed!

But all of us know that consciousness is an experience of our complete being. We feel emotions in our bodies: our heart "aches" when we miss someone, and we feel "sick" when we hear of something unpleasant happening to someone close to us.

So consciousness, I think, cannot be simply defined as existing solely in the hemispheres. Beyond that, we are all well aware that it can vary over time. We experience this ourselves every day: sometimes we feel groggy and not at our best, other times we feel very sharp. Drugs, licit or otherwise, can affect it. A wide variety of insults to our brains, including trauma, can affect our level of consciousness. When we sleep, our consciousness is largely shut down, but fortunately our subconscious, lower brain continues to function for us.

More importantly, we can easily observe the growth of consciousness from infancy to adulthood. For example, in later childhood, we progress from concrete thinking, seeing an actual dog as a thing to be played with, to abstract thinking, the idea of a dog as a being with its own, albeit more limited, consciousness. We come to realize that it has feelings and, hence, can experience pain and pleasure too. We gradually learn to care for it in a manner different from caring for our inanimate toys. Our consciousness grows from being self-absorbed to caring for others.

Although animals, no doubt, have *some* level of consciousness, the fullest level of consciousness, which includes the abilities for self-recognition and self-reflection, introspection (self-awareness), altruism, and abstract thought, seems to reside solely in human beings.

This transition from the consciousness of animals to that of humans is profound. No other animal over the hundreds of millions of years that vertebrates have been on planet earth has evolved its consciousness as *Homo sapiens* have. Only we human beings have evolved to enact laws to guide our behaviour, written books to communicate with one another, and built hospitals to care for the most vulnerable among us.

This difference is not just a matter of degree.

The instant that life evolved from inorganic molecules billions of years ago, it was not simply a matter of degree either. Once the physiosphere reached a certain level of complexity, it mysteriously transformed into something unique: *life*. Life, the biosphere, though it included all of the realities of the physiosphere, transcended it to something the physiosphere could not describe nor explain.

And once our brains became sufficiently complex, something mysterious happened: the development of full consciousness—the noosphere. This cannot be described or explained by the biosphere any more than the laws of the physiosphere can do so of the biosphere.

Not everyone agrees with this, however. Many very bright people are convinced that we are simply the physiology of our neurons. But if that is so, what implication does that hold for thinking, for true consciousness and, particularly, for free will?

Of course, there are also many bright and insightful people over the millennia who disagree with this atomistic, mechanical view of the universe, and I am tempted to side with them. Why?

In part because I am aware of our tendency to simplify things, to see patterns with which we are familiar and thus make us feel more comfortable. We see and comprehend linear more easily than logarithmic or exponential. We have come to understand the physiosphere *far* better than the biosphere, so we like to make nice, neat laws for the biosphere that we make for the physiosphere. We can predict the orbits of the planets with far more accuracy than we can predict the behaviours of complex ecosystems. Sadly, we have had a difficult time admitting that, hence the destruction we have wreaked on poor planet earth!

A more important reason I side with those who disagree with the mechanical view of consciousness is this: we humans have become enthralled with our intelligence, with what our cerebral hemispheres can do. Some of what we have done is impressive, and we should be justifiably proud. However, this has led to a large degree of arrogance. We are not humble about how little we know or understand of the universe. Human history is rife with examples. We want to pretend that we are very wise because it makes us feel good; it makes us feel safe because we understand the world so well. I don't blame people for wanting to do this; it's in our nature.

This brings me back to the idea of consciousness. The great sages over the years have come to realize, often through meditation or prayer, that the thoughts that arise in our nervous system—the electric impulses running through our neurons—are just the beginning. When we are humble and allow ourselves to slow down our brains and try to step outside of them, so to speak, we realize that there is a thinker of those thoughts, the "I" of ourselves. If we continue to work at it, we can then observe that we are more than just our thoughts because we can actually observe ourselves thinking those thoughts.

In other words, there are thoughts, the thinker of those thoughts, and beyond that, the observer self. We have all experienced this to some degree, even if we do not meditate or pray. We look back at something we did and can actually observe our thinking process. For example, we may find ourselves saying, "Yes, I remember when I was sixteen; I was so insecure and I wanted so badly to fit in. I went to that party, and even though I had had a lot to drink, I knew that I should not have done X, but I did it anyway. Even though I bragged about it after, deep down I felt remorse."

The observer self could see it all unfold, and at some level could see and understand what he was doing and why. He could see the lower part of his brain wanting to fit in and have some fun. He could see the cerebral cortex thinking through how to do X. And he could also feel that something wasn't quite right, even though at one level it felt good. That was his consciousness, his internal observer, his *mind* looking more objectively at his self as a whole. But it is tough to engage the observer self when the music is pounding, the adrenaline is pumping, the hormones are raging, the alcohol is flowing, and deep inside we are worrying that we are not quite good enough.

The neurochemicals of our subconscious are powerful, and some of our neuronal networks were programmed years or even eons ago. They can override our higher brain and observer self very quickly. It is not difficult to lose your mind, even if only temporarily.

This is important to realize because it is the mind that we use to change our neuronal networks, to rewire our nervous systems. By analogy, it is life within a single-celled organism that organizes the use of chemicals and structures within the cell to maintain the living organism. It is hard to define exactly what this thing called "life" is. You cannot see it, per se. You see evidence of it. When my elderly patient with seizures died, life left her. I did not see it leave directly. I remember thinking to myself, "Okay, Barry, you have pronounced her dead. But what does that mean? Even though her heart and lungs have stopped working and she no longer exhibits consciousness, not every cell in her body has ceased all metabolic activity simultaneously, or died, at this very moment. Where did her life go? And what was it, anyway?"

Equally, we cannot see the mind. But we can all recognize what it does. In the Western world, we have been very influenced by the ancient Greeks and their logical, rational approach to understanding the nature of existence. However, the mind is not a thing we can grasp through a purely rational approach, with the left side of the cerebrum alone. Like values, there is a nonrational aspect to mind. We perhaps need both hemispheres to begin to comprehend it. Together they help us to focus our attention, to enter into our observer self where the mind seems to exist.

But I suspect that a full understanding of the mind, like a full understanding of life, may elude us. In order to confirm their existence, we can describe how they manifest and what tools they use to manifest. But we may have a hard time seeing what it is we call life or mind.

This brings me to the final, and perhaps most important, reason to believe that the mind is not simply a physiologic structure of the physiospheric or even biospheric domains: humility and awe.

As I have said many times in these musings, and will continue to say, the universe is both a complicated and complex system. Something is complicated if it is convoluted; for example, the forms governments have you fill out every tax season (don't get me started!). A complex system is one with deep interdependencies between components of a system. In other words, changing one thing changes everything else. With a tax form, changing my donations does not change my medical expenses. In the universe at large, that is not true, and it is particularly not true in living systems.

Life and mind are manifestations of an intense complexity, of which we fathom scarcely little. There appears to be a teleology to the universe—it appears to be constantly changing, from simple to complex, in a very specific direction with a very specific purpose. When we stand back and look at the really big picture, we ought to be in awe. It would be wise for us to be more humble.

We can use our mind to change the neuronal patterns of our brain. We do so by slowing down and quieting the cacophony of activity in our brain and focusing, from the perspective of the observer self. When we do so, we allow ourselves to be in awe of the tremendous power of the mind that evolution has provided for us. Then our mind can guide the structure and function of our brains and, thus, how we manifest ourselves in this world.

PART III: WHERE WE ARE GOING

Change: The Universe's Only Constant

Chapter 12

Change and Growth

DO YOU BELIEVE in evolution? I mean, really believe in evolution? I bet you don't. I don't think most people do, at least not fully. What do I mean by that?

I think many people see evolution as a process in nature that primarily happened long ago and whose ultimate goal was to produce human beings. Now that we are here, the process is essentially done.

Others perhaps believe that evolution is still continuing, but it no longer affects us. Nature produced the ultimate species, *Homo sapiens*, and as a final product, we are no longer part of nature. Nature is still constantly tinkering, of course, but now we have two separate realities: there is nature and there is humanity. Everything that nature does is, obviously, natural, and everything that we do is not natural; it is artificial. Creatures in nature continue to evolve, but we are out of that process since we are no longer part of nature.

A rough analogy would be a new automobile company that has

slowly grown from an idea in someone's head into an actual complex facility that produces a novel line of cars. Those cars, once they leave the factory, are no longer part of the company, no longer part of the process; they belong to the owners who buy them, so they become separate from the factory. The factory may continue to evolve many of its internal processes for producing the cars, but every car that it produces continues to be identical to all others and will remain so for the remainder of their existence. The cars, of course, slowly decay until all are eventually discarded one way or another years later.

So what do you really believe? Are we the final, perfect product of nature and like the cars leaving the showroom our evolution is done? We are what we are?

I hope you don't because the evidence against that is overwhelming.

One may argue that as a species we still do a lot of not-so-good things in the world, but hopefully we can agree that we have evolved over the last several thousand years. The Magna Carta, the English charter that put limits on the authority of the king, is one good example. The near abolition of formal slavery is another.

Every day at work I see evolution. No visit gives me more pleasure than a well-baby visit. The baby's parents and I celebrate the growth of their child; we know in our bones that we are meant to evolve. Few things give parents more angst than the possibility that their child is not growing and developing, not evolving. I see it, too, in the university students who consult me; I see their growth from their first years in academia through to their Ph.Ds. They, like my fellow medical students way back when, worry that their evolution won't continue to its desired conclusion.

We see growth in our own lives; we document it with photo albums. We reflect upon the maturation of our thinking and behaviours (and wonder how we ever made it this far!).

But somehow we miss the point, I think. Let me explain.

I remember one particular day when I was about twelve years old. It was late afternoon on a beautiful summer day. The twenty-five-year-old daughter of a couple who were good friends of my parents was just coming home from work. She was gorgeous, and as she climbed out of her shiny new green Mustang, the sun seemed to sparkle off of her as she kissed her waiting boyfriend. I thought to myself, "Man, I can hardly wait until I'm twenty-five! Life will be perfect. I'll have a job, money, a car, a girlfriend and then life really begins. I'll be free to do as I please. No more stress of going to school and people bossing me around. I'll be at the pinnacle of life, and it will be just smooth sailing from there on in. Just sit back, kick my feet up, and enjoy the fruits of all of my labours!"

Man, was I stupid. Or in love/lust? Or to be fair, just naive.

Most of us realize when we reach adulthood in our twenties that our journey of life is usually (but sadly not always) far from done. However, I often get the sense that we forget that our own personal *evolution* within that journey is far from done as well. There are still a lot of lessons to learn; lots of neurons to develop and modify. We still have a lot of growing to do, and it's hard work. This means that just like in evolution, parts of us need to change, parts of us have to whither and die, to be replaced by better parts, better ways of thinking, better values and priorities, and better behaviours. Neuroplasticity is a large part of this.

It is easy to make the same mistake that I did when I was twelve, that life is simply a race to accumulate as much sensory experience as possible, like a new car putting more miles on the odometer.

But evolution is intrinsic to the universe. Ken Wilber captures it in his four levels of growth: the physiosphere, the biosphere, the noosphere, and the theosphere. Evolution means the gradual, or not so gradual, development of something, implying that that something starts simple and becomes more complex. It is a constant process of *transcendence* and *inclusion*.

By definition, evolution means change and change, by definition, means that something loses aspects of what it had or was in becoming something different, something more complex. And as we have seen earlier, change can be painful and scary because it *always involves loss*.

Do you see yourself in a process of evolution? Do you welcome change? Or are you clinging desperately to the same heuristics you had years ago? Perhaps the ones your parents taught you? Are you like the children the parents at my daughter's school dreamed of—you have been loaded up with all of the necessary programs on your hard drive, and now it's just a matter of putting on the autopilot of avoiding pain and pursuing pleasure?

It seems to me we often want to believe we are at such a pinnacle that there is no more climbing to do. Like the Everest of age twenty-five I was dreaming to stand atop of when I was twelve, we want to think that we have finally made it, and there will be no longer be any need for change and loss.

But for a human being, what does it mean to evolve and grow? What does it mean for us as a species?

Well, to start with, it means expanding past our lower brain to utilize the full capabilities of our entire nervous system. Although we will never outgrow the need for our brainstem and limbic systems, for example, we must transcend them while being inclusive of them. That requires us to first acknowledge what they supply for us and, therefore, why we want them still.

As we have seen, they provide for us the ability to experience pain and fear, to fight-or-flight, and to deny, as well as to appreciate pleasure. However, in many respects, they provide them in a very raw, undisciplined form. Unsupervised, it is easy to let the instincts and desires to avoid pain and seek pleasure drive us places we might regret.

Thomas Aquinas said that there are four types of temptations in the world to which we are drawn: wealth, pleasure, power, and honour. All of the things that entice us on any level, particularly the level of our limbic systems, fall into one or more of these categories.

A tasty meal, a kiss, an orgasm, a beautiful sunset, and our favourite music all fall into the category of things we are willing to make sacrifices for because they feel good. We want to be happy, and we quite rightly believe that we deserve to be happy. Pleasure is an important part of our happiness.

As all organisms have done for millennia, we are drawn to abundance because it allays fear and feels good. Many creatures store food or water, either in an external location or even in their own bodies, for example as fat, for the lean times. More is better; our instinct is to hoard, to have wealth. It makes us feel safe. That's why we love a deal. It's why we can be so easily tricked by so-called sales and promotions.

We also want to belong; we want to feel needed. We don't want to be the weakest deer in the herd—we know what happens to them. So we crave honour. If we are important, certainly we will be protected, right?

Or we crave power in order to protect our fortress of safety and pleasure. I will be in control of others and, therefore, have more control of my life and my destiny, and be less controlled by external forces. Leave less to chance.

It's not hard to see, as Aquinas did, that things can go quickly off the rails if these drives go unchecked. Pursuit of any of these four temptations can become addictive. The wiring in our brains provides positive feedback when we obtain them, to the point where we can become completely consumed by them and lose ourselves.

We can become slaves to pleasure, like the lab rats that will forego fluids and nutrition and opt for cocaine to the point of self-harm. Making sure we have enough is important, but having a lot more than enough and not caring about how we get it becomes greed. We like the feeling of being centre of attention, but if it means that we ignore others, we can drift into sociopathic behaviour. Having control of our lives is laudable, but when that extends beyond controlling our own behaviour into controlling the behaviour of other humans, it degenerates into slavery.

The supervision we need to control our lower brain arises from our minds and manifests through the activities of our cerebral hemispheres. Our evolution, therefore, involves developing our mind and thus our brain; that's how we "conquer" ourselves. We don't eliminate parts of our nervous system; we learn to control them by focusing our thoughts and quite literally building our brain through neuroplasticity to its fullest potential.

We try, as much as possible, to avoid irrational behaviour—activities that run counter to both the logical and creative sides of our brain. We avoid thinking, speaking, and acting from our lower brain without reflecting first with our minds, utilizing the tools of our hemispheres. We take that extra time to be mindful, to let the observer self guide us. On occasion, fear and anger need to be expressed and acted upon as quickly as they can arise. But for modern humans, those occasions should be rare. The more we practise slowing things down, introspecting and reflecting, the better we get at recognizing when our lower brains are sending powerful signals that need to be vetted through higher levels of our brain before being acted upon.

All of this, of course, takes time, energy, and most of all courage. As we do so, we find that evolution is sending us an important message about its *telos*—its goal.

Growth for humans is fundamentally different than it is for all other species. We see it in evolution. Species higher up on the developmental ladder become progressively more social. Humans are head and shoulders above every other species in this regard.

In the smaller sense of evolution, we see that the same holds true for each one of us: our growth from infancy bears witness to increased sociality and interconnectedness. We evolve from the intense narcissism of reptiles to potentially the highest levels of altruism and self-sacrifice.

For billions of years, our evolutionary universe has been leading the way in this process of transcendence and inclusion, increasing complexity and interdependency, and it is calling us to do the same.

We would be wise to listen. And if we do, we will find that the message is a simple one, but one that can change everything.

Chapter 13

Jane

PERHAPS THE BEST way to introduce Jane is to first tell you briefly about her grandmother, Mae, a patient of mine.

I had known Mae for several years. She struck me as the quintessential grandmother, her eyes brightening when showing me photos of her grandchildren, delighting in their journeys through life and wanting very much to be part of them.

She had a sweet spot for Jane, or Janey as she referred to her. Jane's mother had been a rebellious teenager, and Mae admitted that she had had a tough time dealing with her. She was disappointed in herself for not having done a better job. I suspect it may have been that guilt that prompted Mae to consider Jane her "pet."

Mae hadn't been completely pleased with her daughter's choice of husband, Bill. It wasn't that Mae disliked Bill; in fact, she was quite fond of him. But Bill liked whiskey a little more than Mae thought was prudent, much like her own late husband. Sadly, Bill could become violent when under the influence.

Jane was born a few months after the wedding, a reality neither young parent was prepared for. When the second daughter came along, she was quietly shunted to Jane's aunt. After that, Jane's father wasn't around much, which wasn't altogether a bad thing. His violence had escalated, and the police had been called on more than one occasion.

Mae described Jane as a tomboy, a term no longer politically correct but one she found fitting nonetheless. When she showed me a picture of Jane, I knew what she meant: Jane was dressed like her idol, Pippi Longstocking—also a redhead—wearing her hair in two pigtails leaping out from the sides of her head. She was covered in dirt and, posed with flexed biceps, gave the impression of fearlessness. Even from a still photograph, I could tell that Jane had boundless energy. Mae's voice would hush in a sad kind of way as she described how independent Janey could be, using her lively imagination to keep herself entertained.

This was perhaps fortunate for Jane. After her father, Bill, had left, Johnnie Walker became her mother's closest companion, which meant little time for her children.

Needless to say, Jane became fairly self-reliant. She figured that life was just like that. You get plunged into the universe as an insignificant little speck, and you do the best you can. Mae would have liked to have seen more of her, but between the strained relations with her daughter and son-in-law and living six hours away, she had to be supportive from a distance.

Mae described Jane as a very bright young lady who should have done better in school. If only there weren't so many distractions: butterflies landing on the windowsill saying hello, clouds playing charades in the sky, kids dancing in the hallway.

According to Mae, although Jane wasn't terribly interested in boys, they were certainly interested in her. Without necessarily meaning to, Jane projected an image of wildness, and a lot of guys found that appealing. She was athletic and could hold her own when competing with her male classmates. For that reason, she probably got along better with them than her female peers, who in her opinion just wanted to talk and giggle a lot.

I would find out later that when the hormones of adolescence began flowing, Jane had felt uncomfortable. Given her family situation, she had been a bit of a loner. Consequently, she found it hard to read people. She wanted to fit in but was socially awkward. Alcohol and pot helped to a degree. But when combined with her innocence and gullibility, it led to some associations, and actions, that she would come to regret.

At sixteen she had an abortion. She hadn't planned on becoming pregnant nor was it a subconscious desire to have something to love. She simply believed guys when they said they would pull out in time, but, oops, things happen. Fortunately, she clued in when she missed her second period and felt horrible. Shocked and scared, she didn't know whom to turn to. She didn't have any close girlfriends, and she wasn't exactly sure who the father was because there had been a few partners. Despite her embarrassment, and with not much time to spare, she confided in her grandmother.

Her parents never found out; Grannie Mae made sure of that. Mae stood with her throughout the ordeal and helped her to get contraception and, hopefully, prevent another mishap.

For a while Jane swore off guys, but loneliness got the better of her. Despite Mae's pleadings, Jane got in with the wrong crowd. She seemed to have the habit of dating tough guys; guys who she knew deep down were sweet and lovable if you could break through the rough exterior. Unfortunately, trying to do that made Jane a target of their violence, and her life continued to spiral in an unhappy direction.

She cut off what little contact she had been having with her parents and managed to call Grannie Mae only when she needed money. She would tell Mae that this would be the last time because she was cleaning up her act. She may even have meant it occasionally. Sobbing in my office, Mae would confess that Jane's increased lying and conniving at times caused her to lose hope in her darling granddaughter. But then one day, after much cajoling, Jane agreed to live with her grandmother for a while. Mae was ecstatic. I happily agreed to take her on as a patient.

By the time I met Jane, she was in her early twenties, battling several addictions and struggling to hold down part-time jobs. But with Mae's help, she was already starting to bounce back. Mae introduced structure into her life. Simple things like three good meals per day, some fresh air and exercise, and helping out around the house and the neighbourhood. She could be a taskmaster at times, but always a gentle and loving one. She saw her granddaughter's potential and never let Jane forget it. Mae even got her to help at the church bazaar!

Our first visit was what I expected it to be. Mae accompanied her for the first few minutes and then tactfully left the two of us alone to chat. Despite the fact she had not taken very good care of herself, Jane was quite pretty with striking, angular features. Her once red hair was now a rainbow of colours, and she sported several tattoos and piercings. She established little eye contact and projected a sense of indifference to the point of boredom. It was like she was in the high-school principal's office.

I thanked Jane for coming in and told her how fond I was of her grandmother and how special Jane was to her. Here eyes rolled. I heard her mumble that she had plans and wasn't intending to stay long with Grannie Mae. We talked a little about her childhood, which she curtly described as okay. I performed a cursory physical exam, listening to her heart and lungs, not expecting to find anything in particular. It was the human touch I was interested in establishing. We humans need that.

At the end of the visit, she agreed to do some blood tests and grunted in agreement to come back and see me to review the results. Mae took Jane's hand as she exited the exam room and gave me a wink as they left.

Our second visit was a difficult one. Jane's blood tests revealed hepatitis C. It wasn't entirely clear how or when she had acquired it, which isn't uncommon. She presented a brave front when I told her the news, but the trembling she exhibited when I examined her abdomen confirmed her hidden terror.

I explained to her the options for treatment. At the time, medication regimens were less successful and had more side effects than the ones today. Nevertheless, she agreed to a referral to a specialist and seemed to understand that I was going to be seeing her fairly often to monitor her progress. I don't think she was all that excited about the likely frequency of our visits, but I was looking forward to them.

Like many of us, I have always had a soft spot for the underdog, the person who continues to battle against the odds when fate has dealt them a less than stellar hand. I had a great respect for Jane for that reason. She squirmed in her seat a little when I told her that during one of our visits.

One of the reasons she had managed to get by as well as she had, given her upbringing, was her sharp wit and intelligence. As Mae had said, Jane was, indeed, very bright, but she had a tough time focusing her thoughts. Jane told me that for her, life was like going into a store where there were a hundred televisions on at the same time, each showing a different and exciting program: it was hard to choose which one to watch. Her life reflected that. She would jump from one activity to another, one boyfriend to another, one illicit drug to another, without stopping to reflect very long on her decisions. When she did take time to introspect a little, however, she often got better results, like the decision to live with Mae, at least temporarily.

Somewhat counterintuitively, Jane did not cope well with externally derived change. If something unexpected or unwanted happened, she became easily overwhelmed. Her limited ability to cope with disappointment, in fact with change of any kind, left her progressively more paranoid and distrustful of people. For example, she became very defensive and felt that I was looking down on her when I had asked her if she knew how she might have contracted the hepatitis, listing the most common activities such as intravenous drug use or sexual relations without condoms. She calmed down a little when I explained to her that I was simply trying to figure out how long she might have had the disease, not making a moral judgment.

When she saw the liver specialist, she was angry that there was more testing to do before treatment could start. Although I had outlined the likely timelines for treatment before that appointment, Jane thought that she would simply be given a prescription for a week or two and that would be it. She had a tendency to be very concrete in her thinking and dramatic in her reactions to the world. Everything had to happen right now, exactly as she wanted it, or else the world was being mean to her.

On the other hand, Jane was honest, almost to a fault. She genuinely appreciated any kindness that you offered. And she really did want her life to be better, although she couldn't enunciate what that meant exactly.

Jane was a good person, but truth be known, in many ways she was still a child. She had a difficult time seeing other people's perspectives. During one of her visits, she complained bitterly about Mae's house rules, particularly that there was a curfew. Jane felt she was being treated like a little girl. Although I didn't say it, to some degree Jane needed to be treated that way because her judgment at times was like that of a little girl, and Mae knew it. It was difficult for Jane to understand that her grandmother, who was in her seventies, worried a lot about Jane and slept poorly if she was out too late.

Overall I enjoyed her visits, although I never knew which Jane was going to show up, as her moods could be quite labile. She stormed out of my office on more than one occasion but at the subsequent visit would bring cookies she and Mae had baked as a kind of peace offering.

A frequent source of her perceived instability was her binary thinking, seeing the world as only black and white. On her third visit, we talked about her use of alcohol, given her hepatitis and her impending treatment for it. She understood my suggestion that she abstain from alcohol as much as possible, but she had a minor meltdown when I suggested that she might want to curtail her use of pot as well. She accused me of implying that she was an out-of-control loser, that she was a bad person for using the stuff. I assured her that addictions don't mark people as bad or losers. People may do bad things in their quest to satisfy their addictions, but addictions are signs of internal pain needing to be soothed. I wanted to explore with her why she used it, to understand and help with what was going on inside of her head that instigated its use.

I suggested to her, as I do for many patients wanting to make any life changes like controlling addictions, that beating up on oneself seldom works. Guilt and shame are poor motivators because they don't dive deeply enough into the reasons for the behaviours.

We explored the difference between the brain and the mind. I explained to her that the brain is the organ we use to get things done; our mind is what tells the brain what to do. We can get a glimpse of the difference when we do things "without thinking": our brain just takes over, and we mindlessly do it. Sometimes that's a good thing, like when we remove our hand from a hot stove before we have time to think about it. Other times, it's not so good, like unconsciously lighting up a cigarette when we are trying to quit.

The mind is like the general deciding on the strategies for our lives, utilizing various areas of our brains—the privates and corporals—to accomplish them. Of course the brain does have lots of input coming from its privates and corporals, especially in the brainstem and midbrain. We can listen to them, but they often don't have a handle on the big picture. Letting the general, which engages the cerebral hemispheres, mull it over and decide upon the ultimate strategy tends to give better results than purely reflexive behaviour alone.

Initially she wasn't all that enthused, but over time she came to appreciate the analogy. We spoke at length about instances in her life when she had listened to the privates and corporals and hadn't been happy with the outcomes. I suggested that she work on becoming more mindful, by putting time and space between her reflex feelings and impulses, and her more thoughtful responses to them. Try to be more an observer and contemplator of her brain activity before becoming the actor.

One day, she came in the office and told me that I looked a little like Kenny Rogers. I joked that the pot and the booze had finally caught up with her! After a little hesitation, she quipped, "Don't get all serious on me, Doc; I just think you need a haircut; you're looking mangy like him." We both chuckled. She would never have been able to respond so adeptly a few months before. It was a pleasure seeing her mature to the point that she was comfortable enough accepting my playful teasing and be able to respond in kind.

But the most telling aspect of Jane's development was her devotion to Mae when her grandmother fell and broke her hip. Jane was working part time and made tremendous sacrifices by getting Mae to her medical appointments and nursing her at home. I don't know what Mae would have done without her.

After completing her rehab and treatment for the hepatitis, Jane was able to find more permanent work. Not surprisingly, she eventually moved out of Mae's home and began to make a life for herself. During our last visit, I mentioned that she had a lot to give the world, and she might want to go back to school or take some part-time courses. I think she might have blushed a little as she hugged me before leaving, simply muttering, "Thanks, Doc."

I lost touch with her when she left town, but Mae always kept me in the loop.

In retrospect, it is hard to identify *why* Jane pulled back from the brink exactly when she did. But there is no doubt in my mind as to *what* pulled her back.

I learned from Jane and Mae that, as is always the case in life, whenever we mature through our pain, the foundation for our growth is love. There were times when Mae had doubts about her granddaughter; the paradox of true faith is that it always embodies doubt. But Jane always knew, at a very deep level, that Grannie Mae truly loved her.

And when Jane was at her lowest ebb, that love is what brought her home.

Chapter 14

Love

What is hateful to you do not do to your neighbor: That is the whole Torah; the rest is commentary.

—Rabbi Hillel, Jewish sage

LET ME START this chapter by being completely honest with you: the story of Jane *is* a true story. But it is not the story of one person alone. It is a compilation of the many Janes, Maes, and Bills that I have met over the years. All are wonderful people, and all are deserving of happiness and love. And I have learned from all of them.

I wrote a compilation for two reasons. Firstly, I did not want to relate a story of one person in such detail that their confidentiality would be compromised. Secondly, the point of the story is to illustrate that we all share the same humanity as a starting point, even though we are all struggling with our own unique and deeply personal evolutions. I suspect that each of us can see ourselves somewhere in the story; I know that I can.

Perhaps as you read the story of Jane you had the feeling that in many ways she was very childlike. She could be gullible, approaching the world with an almost naive realism. You may have felt sorry for her when she was taken advantage of for that reason. You may have recognized that often her thoughts and actions arose from her lower brain and were not filtered by her higher brain as often as they could have been. In other words, she wasn't always mindful.

Her internal rules of thumb, her heuristics, did not always get her the results she wanted. The role model she had for what constituted a husband or father was one mired in addiction and violence, so these are the behaviours she learned and internalized. She loved her father and wanted desperately to 'fix' him so that she could have a happier family life. Her romantic pursuits later in life were repeated attempts to do the same thing with men who were similar to her father. Her concept of love was not a sophisticated adult one; it was one still rooted in her early childhood. Her faulty rubric told her that men who love you beat you up.

We may wonder how we come to adopt such seemingly self-contradictory, irrational heuristics. How could anyone ever come to believe that being violent is being loving?

It is not difficult to understand if you look carefully at where we start our evolution.

Remember that as infants we are born with an intense, naive realism because we lack the cognitive abilities of a fully formed nervous system, particularly the cerebral hemispheres. We see that people who say they love you hit you, so you deduce in your simplistic way that people who love you hit you. And because our thinking is initially only binary, like our reptile cousins, we figure that there are only two choices: either I am not loved or I am loved and beaten. Our deep-seated fear of being abandoned, like solitary confinement, is powerful and often wins out.

The other deduction is even more tragic: I cannot be loved. So we incorporate whichever rule of thumb we choose very early on in our lives, when our brain is like a blank slate with little to challenge new input. Intrinsic memories and heuristics from our childhood can exert great control over us well into adulthood for that reason. And it can take a lifetime to undo them.

Understandably, then, our relationships with our parents play a pivotal role in our evolution. When we are six years old, we believe that our parents can completely protect us from boogey monsters underneath our beds and burglars who might break into our homes under the cover of night. If not, we would never be able to fall asleep. Sensing our own vulnerability, we need to believe that our parents are invincible and, therefore, that we are utterly safe. Naive realism, binary thinking, denial, and deep reptilian fear combine to elevate our parents to near godlike status. No wonder their role modelling is so critical in our early development.

Entering adolescence, as our abilities to reason and engage in abstract thinking begin to flourish, we appreciate that life is not so simple, and we start to glimpse the fragility of life. Not only can our parents not protect us completely, but mommy and daddy aren't going to live forever either. It can be terrifying.

And to make matters worse, not only are mommy and daddy not godlike, they are hopelessly flawed. Please don't tell me I'm like them! We are all embarrassed to some degree by our parents because, by seeing them so close-up, we are convinced that they are the dorkiest things on the planet (which means we might be, too). It can be a tall pedestal they fall from.

From grade school through well into adulthood, our life is a litany of struggles to break away from these horribly imperfect, former godlike creatures to a life of complete independence. Sometimes the process is relatively smooth but is rarely without some degree of awkwardness and pain.

A good friend of mine years ago told me that the majority of people never separate from their parents, and the minority who do don't do so until sometime between thirty-five and forty-five years of age. I thought he was kidding, and I laughed. I don't laugh anymore.

Maybe you are as skeptical as I was. To convince you, let me tell you about Pat.

I had known Pat for several years. Pat had diabetes and popped in every few months for it to be checked. On one such visit, I noticed that his blood sugars were significantly higher than usual, and I enquired as to the possible causes. Pat admitted to feeling very stressed recently and suspected that was the origin. What was the stress, I enquired?

Pat was going to visit his eight-five-year-old father. Normally that would be no big deal. But this visit was going to be different.

You see, Pat's spouse had died five years earlier after more than thirty years together. They had raised three children, all now adults, one of whom had children of her own. Pat had retired from a successful career and was financially comfortable. But loneliness had caught up with Pat. Having been dating someone new for the last two years, he felt the urge to settle down again in a long-term relationship. So what was the problem?

Pat's new partner wanted to meet her father-in-law before finalizing wedding plans. Pat understood and agreed with the request. The problem was, Pat was not at all sure that his father would approve of either his choice of partner or the idea of remarrying. Hence the raised blood sugars.

So despite having lived almost six decades of a very full, satisfying, and productive life, Pat still needed dad's approval. Pat had not yet completely "separated."

Does that surprise you?

It's a lot commoner than you think, and it is completely understandable. Our parents, because they help form so many of our first impressions of the world, are responsible for many of our implicit memories and provide many of our internal heuristics, which hold a special place in our psyche. Separating from them is like disavowing our innermost selves. Such fundamental change is painful, and it scares us because then, to some degree, we have to start all over again. Venture into the great unknown where nothing is guaranteed to be safe. It's so much easier just to stay the course, avoid change, and not evolve.

And it terrifies parents, too. It was fear that parents at my daughter's school meeting were expressing. "Look, as long as I just load up their hard drives with all of the tried-and-true heuristics I have, some from my parents, some I have learned on my own, then my kids will do as well as I have. They will be safe, and I can rest easy knowing that everything will be all right." In other words, don't let them venture out on their own and take unnecessary chances creating their own heuristics. It's too stressful for me, the parent. I couldn't cope if anything bad happened to them. It's primal.

It's the same fear, and reaction to that fear, that mother bears express when someone is messing around with their cubs. Teenagers are correct when they accuse their parents of irrational worry about events that are highly unlikely to occur. They fail to recognize, however, that a horrible event, no matter how improbable, will be devastating for their parents. And no one knows what that feels like until you're a parent. There is simply no life experience prior to parenthood that approximates it. It's part of being a mammal, a social creature, compounded by a fully conscious human mind.

So, can we separate from our parents, and if so, how do we do it?

Separate does not mean physical separation, living somewhere else; you can live in the same house and still separate. It does not mean getting married and having children such that your family becomes your primary obligation and focus of your life; you can separate and still be devoted to your parents. It does not mean that you separate simply because your parents die; you can separate before they die or even after.

To separate from your parents means that you mature to the point where you no longer see them, nor need to see them, as demigods. You are allowed to see them as imperfect and flawed beings and still love them. You no longer cringe at their foibles and idiosyncrasies, or at least no more than you do with the other people in your life that you love (or even yourself). You understand their humanity and forgive them for that. You respect them and their perspectives, but you don't live and die with their opinions and approval. You have evolved to the point that you have your own worldview and feel comfortable being responsible for your own values.

You are always interested in what they say because you trust that it is being said with the best of intentions. But you will reflect upon it before incorporating it into your belief system. Much as you would do with anyone else's opinion, you will not let pressure or guilt force you into believing or doing something with which you do not agree.

This inability to separate from our parents can produce no end of problems in our lives. In our long-term romantic relationships, both parties can fall into the trap of thinking that only their own family of origin has all of the answers.

But we all know that no person or family has all of the answers. I am always surprised at how little faith parents have in their children. They forget that they, themselves, ventured out into the world once upon a time, and the heuristics their parents gave them weren't all flawless. They had to modify a lot of their rules of thumb along the way, and some they frankly ditched long before they ever left home. And yet they survived. So will their children.

It is easy to continually shirk responsibility for our actions and expect our parents to constantly bail us out, and it is tempting for parents to continue to rescue us, thinking that that is love. However, maturity requires that authority and responsibility be parallel; the umbilical cord must be let out appropriately so as not to feel overwhelmed. We can't learn and grow if we continually deny and fail to face the consequences of our behaviours.

Once you have truly separated from your parents, you are prepared to take on the full responsibility of adulthood: you not only make your own decisions and have authority over your life, but you are also prepared to face the consequences, both pleasurable and painful, and to learn from both.

Growth, as we have seen, is one the hallmarks of life: something that is alive independently utilizes nutrients to sustain itself and increasing in its complexity. The seed we plant in the garden will grow to a complex plant, and all it needs is soil, water, and sun to do so. It will spontaneously organize itself to become more interconnected with the world around it, using roots and branches. We do not need to construct and then affix roots or branches or leaves for it. Just give the seed the requisite nutritional elements and life will take care of the rest.

We can add programs to computers, and they can be programmed to improve the sophistication of their functioning. But they cannot grow as living things do. Human beings are living things, not computers. We do not need to affix arms and legs to our children or manually connect the circuitry in their brain. Provided we supply the appropriate nutrients, they will grow in complexity: physically, emotionally, intellectually, psychologically, and spiritually. Like all living things, of course, they will have limitations. No amount of nurturing can make an acorn mature into a maple tree.

Unlike reptiles and amphibians, that nurturing necessitates more than just the simple fertilization of an egg. It also involves more than feeding and protecting them when young and vulnerable, like other mammals. It even requires more than being taught ways to fend for oneself and defend oneself. It demands the nurturing of the full gamut of human experience—speech, higher cognitive functioning, emotional continence, et cetera.

As parents, we often forget that. We are there to nurture, not create from scratch. We are there to role model, not to force-feed. Every one of us resists force-feeding because we don't need to be force-fed; we are not computers. We are there to cultivate all aspects of human existence, including, and perhaps particularly, those aspects we find deficient in ourselves. We do so by evolving through the entirety of our own lives, role modelling such lifelong growth for our children.

This means that we must remain humble. Our parents did not have all of the answers for our lives. We don't have all of the answers for our children's lives either. Even if all of our parents' rules had been perfect, many might only have been applicable in their particular circumstances—their location, their time, their context. Ditto for us. Evolution is a dynamic process in a complex world that is constantly changing. Buddhism refers to it as "impermanence." When one thing changes, it forces everything else with which it interacts to change as well. How many beliefs or rules that you had as a youth have you long since abandoned?

We trust that we have some timeless truths that our children will incorporate into their worldview and value system. But the best way to ensure that that unfolds is to model that behaviour consistently. Walk the walk, don't just talk the talk. And admit when you stumble and fall. Provided that they will not incur major or lethal trauma, let your children stumble and fall too. Let them conjure up some of their own heuristics and learn resiliency. Show that you are introspective and self-reflective and are prepared to face your fears and grow so that they learn how to do that as well. Teach them to evolve by evolving yourself.

In other words, share your mind with them. In many ways, I guess that is the most important reason for me writing this book: I want to share my mind with my children. And I want to help myself. As a good friend of mine Robert Burns (not *the* Robert Burns) said, "Barry, this is a true self-help book—you are doing it to help yourself." We both laughed, knowing how true it is.

Some of the most important rules and tools we can give our children (or anyone, for that reason, including patients) involve the use of our mind through the upper brain. These include facing our fears. Given that our lower brains are powerful and work nearly instantaneously, the more carefully we monitor and control them, the better people we will be and the better our lives well be.

That involves taking time to become more mindful, learning the self-discipline not to act on impulsive thoughts, and to delay gratification. As we talked about earlier in practising medicine, sometimes the hardest thing to do is sit with our fear and do nothing until we know the right thing to do, which may be little more than supportive care. Occasionally, the best thing to do in life, even when raising kids, is to get out of the way.

We can teach them to think well. Sometimes we need to improve our own thinking, first. For example, few things in life are truly binary; most things lie along a spectrum. Any time you are in a situation that appears to have only two possible choices, beware! It may be your inner reptile at work. Our right hemisphere in particular is the creative side of our brain, and it can help us to look for those grey areas if we take the time and let it. But we have to want it, first.

We can learn the difference between an argument and an opinion. An *argument* (not in the sense of a fight but in the philosophical sense of something used in a discussion) is a statement that uses reason to justify a conclusion drawn from a premise. For example, "The Ottawa Senators are a *winning* hockey team because they have won more games this season than they have lost." The strength of the justification used for an argument can lie anywhere along a spectrum from very weak to very strong, and it behooves us to analyze the potency of the argument before we simply agree with it.

An *opinion* is a statement without a justification. "I think the Toronto Maple Leafs are a good hockey team." There is no justification in that statement. (Some Senators' fans would argue that no such justification exists, period, but we won't get into that here and offend Maple Leaf fans!).

We can learn to respect and value other people and their thoughts by using dialogue, not debate. Debate involves binary thinking: one person takes the position *x*, and another takes the position *anti-x*. One person wins; the other person loses. It's a zero-sum game, and nothing new evolves from it. Dialogue, however, opens up the possibility of other positions. One person proposes *a*, another *b*, and yet another *c*. Together they take the best of each to form a new and better proposal *d*, transcending (and including) what they started with. We do so by listening carefully to one another's arguments, weighing the justifications and reasoning. We don't always have to agree, but we would be wise to at least listen with an open mind.

It is said that the scariest thing in the world is a closed mind. It is not a humble or wise mind; it is a stubborn mind born from fear and resistant to evolution. It is a mind capable of great harm because it clings desperately to what are referred to as "the killing certainties." The universe is a very complex place. Anytime you are absolutely certain of something, pause for a moment to ponder it a little further. Ask yourself, Am I so sure of this that I would die for it? If not, then do not kill for it either. This won't always keep you out of trouble, but it is a good start.

It would be helpful to acknowledge and accept that we are motivated by fear, avoidance of pain, and the pursuit of pleasure. It is our starting point, but not our destination. Our evolutionary universe has used fear, pain, and pleasure as part of a teleological journey for us. The journey is not yet done; we are still evolving.

The journey is one transcending our primitive narcissism. Just as the universe is becoming more complex and interconnected, with our large brains capable of intense sociality and communication, so are we. We are evolving past the point of being obsessed solely with *our* own fears, pain, and pleasures. We are capable of caring about others, and *their* fears, pains, and pleasures. With our mirror neurons, we are capable of empathy, actually *feeling*, to some degree, *their* fear, pain, and pleasure. We cringe when we watch horror movies and see the protagonist in peril. We wince when we see a stranger wounded and want to help. We share in the delight of our children opening our birthday gifts to them.

In other words, we are not only *capable* of self-sacrifice and altruism; we are *drawn* to them. How can that be?

We need only look at Mae and Jane. Our purpose as human beings is to grow closer to one another, more interconnected. We care desperately about being accepted by others. Nothing will prompt suicidal thoughts the way abandonment will. We all crave intimacy. Our brains have been evolving toward this for millions of years. That's what makes us so unique.

We want good for ourselves, but we also want good for others, even people on the other side of the planet. We seldom feel content when our inner reptile speaks and acts for us unchecked. We want to grow, and we want others to grow too. Not just our children, but everyone.

If you don't believe that love is about growth, then imagine the following scenario. Your friend says to you repeatedly that she loves her dog. One day, you visit and you find the dog tied by a short leash to a rigid post in the ground that allows for little movement. The doggy is scrawny and filthy; it clearly has not been fed or washed for quite some time. It is far smaller than it should be for its age. Instead of excitedly trying to jump up and lick you, it recoils in fear or lies placidly ignoring you. Your immediate impression is that this dog is not growing because it has not been nurtured in any way—with food, with attention, with exercise. Would you still believe your friend when she says that she "loves" her dog? Ditto if you found the garden she "loves" in total disrepair—unwatered, unpruned, and unfertilized with plants drooping because of lack of supports.

A mature mind yearns for a world full of individuals who are less narcissistic and more altruistic. We may deny this, but look at our disappointment and cynicism when someone in a privileged position, especially one of power in whom we trust, behaves selfishly. We want to live in a world where people care about each other more generously, without ulterior motives; not a world where fear drives us only to look out for number one and, subsequently, not care about hurting others. We conquer ourselves by moving beyond ourselves in a symbiotic, not parasitic, fashion.

Willing the good and growth of the other, as other.*

That's the best definition of love I know. And love is our destiny. Evolution tells us so.

Mae and Janey knew that too.

*This definition is a modification of one by Bishop Robert Barron. I have added, and I think it is crucial, the element "growth." We will explore why that it so important in the following chapters as well.

Chapter 15

Motive and Mind

For him who is not self-mastered, the self is the cruelest foe.

—The Bhagavad Gita

I SUSPECT THAT many of you are doubtful that evolution has a purpose—teleology—and that it is to give rise to love. Perhaps you feel that it is far too simple a concept, to the point of being simplistic. Or that it is dangerous to cling to such naïveté, given the nature of humanity, as witnessed in our past and present behaviours. Maybe you sense that it is just far too difficult to accomplish. I fully understand your pessimism. I disagree, nonetheless, but *not* because I differ with you about the simplicity, naïveté, or tremendous challenge of love given our history. I disagree with you because I don't think we have any choice *but* to believe it.

What do I mean by that?

Let's go back to the mythical days of the caveman. I call them mythical because, like G. K. Chesterton, I am not sure that we can ever really know what it was like way back then because it is *pre*historical. By definition, we have no record of how people lived; we can only make inferences from artifacts we find and take our best guesses.

However, we are pretty sure that they did not live in large and complex cities, but rather small tribes. Before we had invented the wheel and tools, our ability to inflict damage, either on each other or on the environment, was limited.

Now, let's imagine a hypothetical caveman. We'll call him Fred after Fred Flintstone. Suppose Fred had occasion to be in a foul and ornery mood. Perhaps he was genetically predisposed to it or had incurred some illness that affected his brain functioning (like trauma, physical or otherwise) or he, like us, was just having a bad hair day.

If he decided, consciously or subconsciously, to lay a beating on a fellow tribesman because of his foul mood, his other tribesmen would likely step in very quickly to curtail it (unless, perhaps, the group agreed that the person being beaten really deserved it for the sake of protection of the group). A small group living in such vulnerable times could not tolerate such anarchy. People had to get along fairly well together merely for survival. Collectively, they faced enough external threats on a daily basis that they could ill afford to have such endemic dissension if they wanted to survive the rigours of such a harsh milieu. More practically, you had to get along with your fellow tribesmen because you could not possibly defend yourself if they all turned against you.

However, with a burgeoning cerebrum, primitive man mastered the construction of tools, and that opened the door to using them, of course, as weapons. In addition, social structures became more complex, so subgroups formed within tribes. These two developments allowed for a very different dynamic. Firstly, one person behaving badly (for whatever reason) could, with the use of a club or a sword, kill, not just injure, *many* people before they could be stopped. Secondly, if that person had elicited the assistance of several tribesmen within their subgroup, they could inflict considerably more damage before being subdued.

Over time, the upper brain of humans continued to grow but, of course, the lower brain did not disappear. Fear and other powerful emotions continued to exert a tremendous influence on our behaviours. However, the unrelenting development of our cerebral hemispheres facilitated the invention of even more sophisticated weapons. These were not only more lethal but could act from a distance: guns and their variations like cannon.

Our social structures became even more complex as well. As we began to live in larger groupings, we organized ourselves hierarchically. Naturally some people acquired greater power and influence than others. With better weapons and a pyramidal infrastructure, one individual could control the lives of many others, including inflicting harm. The situation magnified as we also ventured out to explore other groupings of people in faraway places, people who were often very different from us.

Fast forward to today. A person with narcissistic or borderline tendencies, sometimes referred to as "sociopaths," can inflict tremendous harm in the world. They can obtain weapons that can kill or maim potentially thousands of people half a world away. They can, if they are clever, come to control large organizations, even countries, and utilize huge infrastructures to inflict no end of harm if they do not learn to control their lower brains with their minds. In other words, if they do not learn how to love.

So please do not believe that my premise that evolution's goal for us to love is based on some Pollyannaish naïveté. Nor do I look at the world through childish, rose-coloured glasses. I know exactly how flawed we are; exactly how driven we are by fear and anger. I am fully aware of how reptilian we can be and how difficult it is to control such powerful, deep-seated, and instantaneous behaviours. I appreciate how complex the universe is, how many factors influence human development, and how many things can go awry along the way. I have studied human beings for almost forty years and lived for almost sixty. I have read history. I continue to read the news.

But I believe that evolution is leading us to love out of necessity: with such powerful intellects, we can create no end of powerful weapons to hurt one another and the planet. And I do not mean just physical weapons. Weapons of the mind are the most dangerous of all: coercion, humiliation, and disrespect. The most dangerous people on the planet often wear suits or elegant uniforms. When they run organizations of great influence using their lower brain and not love, they use people like pawns to acquire power, honour, pleasure, or wealth in a highly narcissistic fashion. Destruction frequently lies in their wake.

I firmly believe the only thing that lies between Armageddon and us is love, so I desperately hope that evolution is leading us, and continues to lead us, in that direction or else we are doomed. Period.

I am often reminded of Martin Luther King Jr.'s solemn observation:
We have guided missiles but misguided men.

For years I had wondered how we came to be so misguided until I heard a statement that has stuck with me. I do not know its origin, but it has been of great value to me in my own life. It speaks to the importance of the *mind*.

There are no pure motives this side of heaven.

This should not surprise us. Our mind operates through our brain; *all* of our brain. Our cerebral hemispheres may transcend our brainstem and powerful, emotional limbic systems. But our brain does not; it includes these necessary lower structures. Nothing we do is ever *completely* devoid of their influence, at least not this side of heaven. Ever since Fred we have been this way.

The sooner we acknowledge this bitter truth, the better our world will be. We urgently need to recognize that none of us is ever completely selfless and altruistic and *accept* that as part of our being human. We need to forgive one another for this while still holding ourselves, and each other, accountable to do better, to becoming more mindful. We need to love each other—*will* the good and growth of the other as other. Not just hope for it or pray for it, but *will* it. That means action. Grow out of our fear, grow beyond our own pain and pleasure toward the only thing that can save us—wanting the best for each other.

Immanuel Kant, a German philosopher of the 1700s, has had a tremendous influence on Western society and present-day medical ethics in particular. His philosophy was one based on duty, referred to as "deontology" (from the Greek word *deon*, meaning "duty"). He developed what he referred to as "categorical imperatives," or formulae; rules to guide us. His second one goes something like this:

Act with reference to every rational being (whether yourself or another) so that it is an end in itself in your maxim.

He recognized that we never act with only one motive; it is an inescapable fact. People must be treated primarily as an end in themselves, not primarily as a means to an end of another person's choosing. In other words, treated as a person not as a thing. This means that we must always acknowledge our hidden motives and be sure that we act first and foremost in such a way that *we* do not use other people for our gains *primarily*.

Kant was clear that we should behave this way not because we necessarily *want* to treat people this way, but rather that we *ought* to; it is *our duty* to do so as human beings. In fact, he was almost disappointed if you enjoyed doing your duty since that was not the point—it was not about your feelings but about ethical behaviour. The same is true of love. It feels wonderful when you have affection for someone you love, but it is not necessary to feel affection for someone in order to love them. Why? Because love is not about you and your feelings; it is about the *good and growth of the other as other*. In fact, the most difficult love is love for someone for whom you have no affection or even detest—your enemy.

As a physician, the implication for me is this: I recognize my desire to help others, but I also concede that there is always something in it for me as well. I may get paid (wealth). I may enjoy performing surgery or being thanked (pleasure). I may be granted special privileges (power). I may be respected more (honour). And there is nothing wrong, per se, with me getting something in return; I am human, after all. But Kant says that my duty is not primarily for these things. My duty, first and foremost, is *to the other as other.*

I must never let my personal gains become more important to me than helping the other and particularly not to adversely affect my treatment of the other as an equally valued individual. First I must always do what is best for the patient; anything else that I receive is subsequent and secondary to that. Don't use patients as things, as a means to my end. Ring any bells?

Equally, I do not have to *like* a patient or feel affection for him. My duty is to care for him; my feelings are not part of the equation.

So despite what the love songs on the radio say, love is *not* a warm and fuzzy *feeling*. It is *willing* the good and growth of the other as other. You may not even like someone, but you can still desire that this person should grow to goodness and happiness, to greater maturity and *selflessness*. Why selflessness? Because we know deep down that no one can be truly happy being completely disconnected from the rest of humanity. John Donne wrote:

> *No man is an Island, entire of itself; every man is a piece of the Continent, a part of the main....; any man's death diminishes me, because I am involved in Mankind.*

We are designed to be in relationship with one another, and that implies relinquishing some of our narcissistic tendencies. That's why solitary confinement is the worst torture of all. Shouldering the burden of another's pain, sharing our pleasures with the person and, perhaps most importantly, mentoring him to grow so that he will do the same to others (pay it forward) is in the very fabric of what it means to be human. Evolution designed us this way; it's why so much of our brain is involved in communication and why we have mirror neurons.

Growth is crucial. Our goal is not, as the old expression goes, "to *give* the other *a* fish" but to "*teach* the other *to* fish" (and I would add, to teach the other how to teach fishing). We *will* that the other person should grow and become an even better fisherman than we are. It's why we take such pride when we mentor a protege to greatness. That's why so many of us are drawn to raise children. It's intrinsic to evolution; the universe is about growth.

Loving parents wants their children to be even happier, more mature, and more loving than they are. That's why parents who conquer their fears don't look at their children as just computers to be loaded up with *only* their old, potentially corrupt, programs. They know the potential for their children to grow beyond them with the right nurturing. Loving parents know that they will always have their own fears and selfish desires. But they listen to Kant as best they can and mentor, not download; encourage, not obsessively control; and criticize constructively, not destructively.

I cringe when I hear the term "tough love." I worry that the supposed purely altruistic love mentioned is little more than an opportunity to vent deep anger when something hasn't turned out as hoped. I suspect that tough love is a good example of "there is no pure motive this side of heaven."

> *Love is patient, love is kind. It does not envy, it does not boast, it is not proud. It does not dishonor others, it is not self-seeking, it is not easily angered, it keeps no record of wrongs. Love does not delight in evil but rejoices with the truth. It always protects, always trusts, always hopes, always perseveres.*
>
> —Corinthians 1:13

Unconditional love is willing the good and growth of the other as other without the contamination of other motives. Perhaps on this side of heaven, it is an unattainable goal, but it is our ultimate aspiration.

We must never forget that all of our acts of kindness, no matter how noble, almost always have an element of selfishness. The wonderful book *The White Man's Burden* by William Easterly (based on Rudyard Kipling's poem of the same name) explores the harm done over the last many decades by well-meaning people who felt that huge problems can be solved by having outsiders come with big plans to "save" the downtrodden. We constantly provide fish (and sometimes the wrong fish) to developing countries, for example, rather than teach them to fish or, better still, humbly provide the resources for them to improve their own fishing techniques.

It's easy to define good only in our terms, failing to take into account the perspective of the other. We must be willing to recognize when our solutions become more about our own ego needs than about helping others. More importantly, if we only do good for others with no intention of helping them grow, then we reinforce their continued inferiority and dependence on us. We run the risk of infantilizing them with a demeaning and disrespectful hierarchical structure from which they cannot extricate themselves. That is not love; that is using others for our own self-aggrandizement.

So learning to love is difficult because our primal and self-centred desires and tendencies have a habit of tainting our efforts: there are no pure motives this side of heaven. It is very difficult to put others first and not use them in order to satisfy our own temptations (i.e., wealth, pleasure, honour, power).

Fortunately, our minds engage neuroplasticity so that we can learn to control and thus balance our own fears and desires by wiring new attitudes, values, and behaviours that can transcend our narcissism. We grow to our full humanity by engaging more altruistically with one another even when it may hurt. Ask any parent.

So now it is time for me to lay my cards on the table, to fess up. To what, you may be asking?

I have written this book primarily because I have enjoyed doing so. I do not want to profit from it from it financially (so I am donating the profits) because I have enough money; more money would not help me to grow or make me happier. I don't know why, but I have never had any interest in power. So my only other ulterior motive is relatively simple: I am at the tail end of a wonderful and satisfying career, and I am feeling a lot less useful than I used to. In part, that's because the things that I used to be good at, I am no longer so good at; it's hard to tame the ego, isn't it? But in part, it's because I am interested less in the mechanical things of medical practice, and life, and more in the abstract aspects. I enjoy my contacts with family, friends, and patients, but I yearn to connect with people at a deeper level. I have failed in my attempts to do so during the last decade, and I am hoping that this book will correct that. I don't want fame, but I do want to expand my horizons, make new connections, and continue to grow. I told you it was a self-help book, didn't I?

Many years ago I read a book, on the advice of a good friend of mine, David McQuarrie, called *The Road Less Traveled*, by M. Scott Peck. In many ways, that book began the journey that I am still on, part of which is sharing my book with you.

In his book, Scott Peck said something I had never heard or read before, something that sounded almost outrageous to me.

He said that as a physician, his job was to love his patients. I knew that he did not mean romantic love, but beyond that I didn't understand what he meant, really. But having now explored with me what love actually is, I suspect that you do understand what he meant. That he, and I, should "will the good and growth of our patients as other."

But it is not a one-way street. My patients can love me; they can will my good and growth as well. And they have, for which I am forever grateful; so much of this book I owe to them. Without their influence, I would not have learned as much as I have about maturity.

Chapter 16

Maturity

Who is wise? One who learns from every man. Who is strong? One who overpowers his inclinations.
Who is rich? One who is satisfied with his lot.

—Ben Zoma

SEVERAL YEARS AGO, I took a course designed to assist adults in helping youth. I have to admit that I was skeptical, but it was a wonderful experience from which I grew in many ways.

In retrospect, one of the most important truths I learned in the course is incredibly obvious now that someone wiser than me has pointed it out:

By definition, the path to maturity consists of immature steps.

I know what you are thinking: "Duh." *Mea culpa.*

But the truth is, we forget this fact on a regular basis. We get upset at ourselves when we err, forgetting that we all can do dumb things no matter how far along we are in our journey. Often, we are irritated when our children act like, well, children. We abhor mistakes and errors, but they are part of life and we learn and grow from them.

Evolution, maturation, can be a slow, nonlinear process. As parents, we have to learn to let out the umbilical cord at the right speed, a speed that is always changing because every child (and adult), on a regular basis, is going to slip into subconscious behaviours, triggered by deep neural networks in their brains. The process of letting out the umbilical cord involves allowing our children to have authority for decision making in their lives to the degree that they can take responsibility. In other words, their ability to face up to and deal with the consequences of their behaviours.

It's a difficult process because all of us have inherited from our primitive ancestors myriad eons-old pathways that are running constantly in the background, below our conscious radar. In addition, we have all been heavily influenced by cultural memes, and all of us engage heuristics without reevaluating them on a routine basis to see if they are still (or ever were) accurate and useful. It's the unavoidable wiring of millions of years of evolution and thousands of years of socialization, so we may as well get used to it. It isn't going to change any time soon.

I am convinced that most of the things that we do that we come to regret or that don't make the world a better place arise from the less altruistic thoughts and behaviours of a less mature mind. Socrates meant this when he said that if we fully understood, we would not do bad things. When we take the time, and courage, to reflect upon our lives, we often recognize that our "bad" behaviours were more likely selfish ones motivated more by deep-seated fear, pain, and insecurity than by a fundamental inner "badness."

We need to put time and space between the workings of our brain, particularly the lower more primitive levels, and the observer. Otherwise, our lives can devolve into a mindless merry-go-round, obsessively chasing after ever more grandiose sensory stimulation (i.e., wealth, pleasure, honour, power) in order to avoid pain and existential angst. These behaviours stunt our growth, hurting others and ourselves in the process.

I do not want to minimize the very real possibility of true evil in the world, but rather point out that most of what the majority of us do that is considered "bad" I don't think arises from evil per se. It arises from ancient narcissism and selfishness triggered by the fundamental and inescapable fragility of existence, the fear we have spoken of in earlier chapters. Perhaps this is akin to the concept of "original sin" and the Genesis myth: the immutable reality that when we left Eden as fully conscious beings, we still retained all of the primitive neuronal networks of our cousins. Our journey became a perpetual challenge of taming, but likely never eliminating, these networks with our newly acquired consciousness—our mind.

For this reason, I think it is important that we be gentle with ourselves. We do bad things not so much because we are inherently bad, but because to get to this point in evolution we had to be narcissistic: survival of the fittest. Nature is amoral, not immoral. Its duty is to its own preservation and advancement. A wolf is not being selfish when it kills the weakest deer in the heard to feed its young. It does not have morality because it does not have full consciousness. For this reason, it is narcissistic but not selfish: unlike us, it does not know any better. It cannot be mindful.

At times I am very mindful, at other times less so. I suspect you are the same. So this business of maturity is a tough one because it is not binary: you are not either mature or immature. We need to free ourselves from dualistic thinking; think instead "both-and" not "either-or."

In order to do so, there are three important aspects of this concept of maturity I want to explore.

Maturity as a Process

Let's start with a definition of maturity or, maybe more accurately, an examination. Consider the tree genus *Quercus*. When very immature, it is an acorn; when more mature, it is a sapling; and when fully mature, it is a mighty oak. Maturity for plants translates into *structural* changes—taller and thicker trunk, many branches, an extensive root system, and lots of leaves; as well as *functional* changes—photosynthesis, reproduction, and primitive (relatively) communication with its environment. It's a more or less steady process, although as we all know, growth is not consistently linear: trees grow more in the summer, less in the winter.

For lower animals, maturation includes similar structural and functional elements, but also includes mobility aspects as well. Reptiles develop their ability to find and procure sustenance as well as defend themselves. Higher animals include these components but transcend them in their maturation process with the progressive acquisition of social behaviours, including more sophisticated communication.

Homo sapiens add to this repertoire aspects of full consciousness, slowly attaining capacities for introspection, self-reflection, abstract thinking, sentience, and profound levels of communication.

What does evolution say the final product, a mature adult, looks like? Most of us are aware of the *structural* aspects that differentiate adults from children, and we have already explored in a little detail some aspects of brain development. From a *functional* perspective, maturity for humans begins, of course, with developing our powerful cerebral hemispheres. This involves nurturing our intellectual and creative faculties.

But far more important is developing our mind, the observer self, which can focus actively on not only the brain as a whole, but also on the entire, integrated self from whence consciousness arises. We learn to slow down our thoughts long enough to reflect upon sensory and other input before making decisions or undertaking some course of action. We learn to question our heuristics and, when necessary, devise better ones. We do so through neuroplasticity, the ability to alter neural connections at the level of neurons and their axons and dendrites by mindfully focusing our attention—our consciousness.

Consequently, we retain our base emotion of fear and the fight-or-flight response, but we learn to temper it, utilizing it only when we are truly threatened. We enjoy the pursuit of various kinds of pleasure, but we do not let them control us. As we cultivate self-discipline, we improve our capacity to delay gratification, minimizing our tendency to wallow in narcissistic behaviour. We grow from concrete to more abstract thinking, relishing not just sensual stimuli but intellectual and creative ones as well. We see ourselves as a member of the world around us and reflect upon our place in it and our contribution to it. We nurture our mirror neurons so as to cultivate compassion and empathy for others. We begin to contemplate the concept of morality, understanding that we are now capable of selfish behaviour because with our full consciousness we can know right from wrong.

We learn to love. And a crucial part of that is to transcend our own personal desires and ask ourselves the critical question: what kind of person do I want to be for this world? In order to do this, we need to quiet the noise of our lives, both internally and externally. We gradually resist the adrenaline rushes and overstimulation we sought in our youth to simply be the observer self. The observer self tries to get to know us better, what "makes us tick." We learn more about our subterranean selves: archetypal perceptions, thinking and behaviours imprinted from eons of evolution; memes inherited from our families and societies in which we grew; and our own internally derived heuristics and self-narratives that we formulated in our youth.

We often find that we become more comfortable in our own skin in the process. We become more thoughtful. This process of rewiring our brain requires humility, honesty, patience, and courage. Letting ourselves sense awe in even the simple things of life is likely a prerequisite as well. Only when we do so can we fully appreciate the enormous complexity of the universe and develop an appropriate humility regarding our place in it.

It is no accident that our brains had to develop to a certain level of complexity for full consciousness to arise. As we discussed earlier, denial may have been a necessary prerequisite for the development of full consciousness. Equally, until we had the capabilities of protecting ourselves from our environment utilizing our powerful cerebral hemispheres, we did not have the luxury of the time and space necessary for the ascension of the observer mind. When you live in a dangerous and convoluted world over which you have little control, all of your energy has to be directed to shear survival. It's hard to relax and ponder life's mysteries when a hungry wolf is chasing you!

I want to be clear that maturity is *not* about intellect alone. It is not primarily about other manifestations of our cerebral hemispheres like creativity either. It is about the mind growing its ability to develop, integrate, and then utilize the complete self—the whole brain and body. It involves all aspects of what makes us human, physical and nonphysical.

So when I speak of human maturation, these are some of the elements to which I refer. It is not an exhaustive list, just a beginning. All are within the reach of each of us, at least to some degree; they are part of being human. But it is a slow process, one punctuated by occasional aha moments—epiphanies. Accepting the invariably circuitous and plodding reality of maturation is critical. We frequently take one step forward and two steps back. It takes a lot of focus and work to rewire old networks. After all, we are naturally somewhat averse to change because it entails the pain of loss. But with repeated practise, we can learn new ways of thinking and behaving, ones more reflective of our full, loving potential.

Maturity as a Spectrum

Maturation is perhaps the quintessential example of the concept of spectrum. Most things in the universe lie along a spectrum. But as we have learned, our default lower brain position is designed to think binary. So, any time we find ourselves thinking binary, we would be wise to step back for a few moments and allow our observer self to ask: Am I engaging my full self, including my full brain, here? In other words, am I being *mindful?*

When we are young, we want simple, black-and-white answers because we need to feel safe. As we mature, we realize that life is full of grey zones. We come to accept that context matters, like when you have a sore throat. Few things irritate me more then when individuals or organizations mindlessly opt for zero-tolerance policies. They want to absolve themselves of their humanity and become robots or lizards. Searching for the "right" thing to do is always going to be a challenge when you are a fully conscious and sentient being. We left the Garden of Eden a very long time ago. Love means willing the good and growth of the other as other, not treating people like things to assuage our own fears or foster our careers and other hidden agendas.

When people behave badly, including ourselves, we need to understand why they do so. Why are they behaving selfishly? Why are they not following the rules? Why is it that they are not engaging like more mature adults? What is missing in their evolution? If we choose not to ask and, subsequently, answer these questions, then we limit any chance for them to grow. This means that their behaviours will likely not change, and they will continue to behave badly, and we will continue to be the recipients of their bad behaviour. Such a choice is born of fear and anger, not of wisdom and love.

Since maturity is a process, by definition at any given time, each one of us lies at a particular point on the maturity spectrum. Mindless busyness aimed at satisfying all desires for wealth, pleasure, power, and honour so as to relentlessly feel ahead of the pack, safe from the hungry wolf, cannot advance us along the spectrum. It is critical to take time to reflect upon where we are and what we need to think and do in order to continue to evolve.

A crucial insight is the realization that we are all insecure. We have evolved from simple creatures that have lived, and continue to live, in a complex universe that is immensely powerful and beyond their comprehension and, thus, their control. They had every right to feel insignificant. But it was the humility that arose from that realization that fostered many of the behaviours that assured their survival and flourishing. All of us, wealthy and poor, handsome and homely, famous and unknown, have inherited that self-doubt as a starting point.

Further, we begin our lives totally dependent on the care of those who love us, and we require nearly two decades of nurturing before we can survive well on our own. So every one of us—no matter what advantages of health, talent, or treasures have blessed us—is insecure. The struggle of maturation is *not*, I repeat *not*, one of overcoming this insecurity, this low self-esteem. Maturation is coming to the realization that you (and everyone else on the planet) can't escape it and, therefore, it doesn't matter. *You are insignificant, so get used to it.* There are seven billion people on the planet today. There have lived more than sixty billion people.

I am but a speck of sand on a very large beach; so are you.

You can spend your entire life trying to convince yourself otherwise. Deny your fears or run away from them. Cram your life full of more and better sensory stimuli. Attempt to satisfy all of your desires if you want. But at your core, you are insecure because ultimately the universe is more powerful than you are. You can forestall death, but you cannot avoid it. You can work hard to minimize pain, illness and disability, but you cannot eliminate them.

Once you accept this, you begin to free yourself from the neural networks that deal only with fear or other raw emotions that can make you feel that *you alone* are insignificant and vulnerable. You grant yourself the strength and courage to evaluate your old heuristics and build better ones. You free yourself from your narcissism to look beyond yourself and connect with those around you, sharing in the struggle of maturation. You learn to love more fully.

In practical terms, how do we overcome this innate insecurity?

Maturity as Forgiveness

Under threat, our immediate and sensible response is to fight-or-flight, and we are very good at it. For example, we push back when a bookcase topples toward us. Sometimes we do not act, of course, and fright takes control; we stand there paralyzed by fear because too many conflicting signals have been generated (and risk incontinence!).

Our ability to control our environment so well, relative to our animal cousins and ancient forefathers, should obviate the use of fight-or-flight for the most part; serious minute-by-minute threats are relatively rare at this point in our history. However, I suspect that many of us recognize that we utilize the flight, fight, or fright reflex far more often than we really need to. Our adrenaline pumps in situations out of proportion to the actual level of threat we are facing. Perhaps we get a flat tire and are going to be late for a meeting and freak out; but no one's life is likely at stake.

Or someone criticizes us, perhaps for no good reason, and we retreat into a reclusive self-nihilism building up resentment, or we adopt an offensive ready-to-fight posture. In other words, we behave in a binary, passive-aggressive fashion, not a mindful, assertive one.

Equally, compared to our cousins and forebears, most of us have a large array of pleasant sensations available to us in conditions safe enough to enjoy. Most of us seldom have to worry about not having enough of the essentials, at least in North America. In fact, most of us have access to no end of luxuries that most people on the planet have never had.

Despite that, we continually seek more. We crave pleasurable stimulation of all types. We often eat more than we need to. Becoming bored with our usual surroundings, we seek exotic travel to enjoy new visual or other stimuli. We turn to mind-altering drugs, licit and otherwise. We want a bigger house, a faster car, a more prestigious job, and more recognition for our accomplishments; the list is near endless.

But human maturation involves leaving our narcissism and entails caring for others. It hinges on respect and starts with self-respect. That means you have to deal with your own insecurity first. Not by denying it or trying to outrun it, but by sitting with it and accepting it as a fundamental part of you—your foundation. Then doing the same for others.

And that is not easy. When others behave badly, especially toward us, it can trigger immediate and primal neural pathways. Ones filled with resentment, disappointment, confusion, anger, and revenge. Those feelings may blind us to the realization that they, too, are on a journey of maturation that is comprised of immature steps. It can be especially frustrating when they are very early in their process and still thinking in very binary terms, not open to the vast spectrum of possibilities.

So far we have talked a lot about the influence our lower brain can have with respect to holding back our ability to grow given its lightning-fast and primal neural networks. However, as much as our cerebral hemispheres allow us the opportunity to think deep thoughts and be creative, our autobiographical self seems to reside on the right side, and the networks residing here can produce their own kind of problem for us.

As we examined earlier, children raised in chaotic environments can be deprived of the opportunity to develop an integrated sense of self. All of us, to some degree or another, have aspects of our autobiographical self that are inaccurate and often self-punishing. That's because none of us had perfect childhoods, and none of us could possibly have interpreted all events of our childhoods perfectly well anyway. Almost invariably we carry with us, as part of our internal narrative, some negativity about ourselves. Given how directly our right brain is wired to our limbic structures, the more extreme that negativity, the more painful that insecurity can feel.

All of us, owing to the basic insecurity of being human, and perhaps compounded by the addition of a self-deprecating internal narrative, reflexively resist further assaults to our sense of self by avoiding criticism, whether internal or external. We all have witnessed a two-year-old responding no to every suggestion made by a caring parent.

We often want to believe that we are at the pinnacle of our maturation far earlier than we really are. Remember me at twelve dreaming of nirvana at twenty-five? We feel that way in part because we resist change, and in part because we feel threatened—on many levels—when we find out that the heuristics we have laboured so hard to acquire continue to be a work in progress. It can be embarrassing to realize how immaturely we have been in both our thoughts and behaviour.

But a third aspect of this resistance relates to the fact that criticism is often not given well; it is not constructive. Why is that? We may think that we are offering purely selfless criticism. But hidden in the message is often another agenda, one that subtly (or not so subtly) is about us being better than the other person. The advice itself may be useful, but the less obvious impact is that it reinforces to the other that they are bad or unworthy. That's destructive criticism. It's a little like the idea of tough love; it's really more about aggrandizing *us* (propping up our ego) than helping *them* grow.

When we love another, we want them to grow, and we use constructive criticism. When we do so as unconditionally and as humbly as possible, the message is "I care about you and respect you. Maybe I am further along my journey of maturity than you and maybe I am not. But regardless, we can help each other grow because we both are fully capable of it. It is our destiny. So let's not let our insecurities resist this growth. For what it is worth, here is my take on the situation and the justification for it. I don't have all of the answers, but this is an insight I have at the moment; it may change as I continue to learn more and grow. So ignore it if you want; I will not think less of you. But realize that I offer it respectfully with no strings attached in order that you may grow."

I think that's how we grow best. We learn to become more mindful because we have loving role models who mentor us, not bully us. But it is a two-way street. We have to be open to correction. We have to be willing to change. We have to be humble enough to admit when we are wrong, and in a very complex universe that may occur more often than we would like. Despite our tendency to believe that we have figured it all out, we need to accept the fact that this business of maturation is a lifelong process of immature steps. And sometimes the toughest steps are the first steps, especially if we only start to take them when we are adults.

One concept that is often confused with constructive criticism is that of judging. Part of it relates, of course, to the fact that we don't criticize constructively or humbly. So we interpret any analysis aimed in our direction as an attack on our very being, on our integrity as a moral agent.

But much of the confusion arises because we conflate judgment of an *action* as a judgment upon *us*. If I *do* something bad, then I must *be* bad. That simply does not follow, although historically people have often made that error. Behaviours lie along a spectrum of good to bad, with pure to impure motives. Our level of maturity lies along a spectrum: supremely selfish to supremely altruistic.

We can move along these spectra in a good direction, a more loving direction, if we choose to be more mindful. In order to do so, though, we must of necessity monitor where we are and seek assistance in moving along. That means, at least in part, welcoming constructive criticism, perhaps most importantly from our observer self. If we do not analyze (another word for that is "judge") our own behaviours, we cannot grow.

I think the biggest challenge to that process is forgiveness. Can we forgive ourselves for messing up? For acting selfishly? For being relatively immature and narcissistic? In other words, for being human?

Once we learn to forgive ourselves, we can learn to forgive others. Only by doing that can we learn to criticize constructively and help others mature. We ensure the continued integrity of the other as an individual worthy of respect and capable of growth. We love.

There is nothing harder than forgiveness, especially if someone has been hurt. The anger we experience when another has hurt us can be terrifying and can be a tremendous obstacle in any attempt to forgive.

Equally, when we realize that we have erred and hurt another and contemplate asking for forgiveness, the threat we feel to our own existence is almost palpable; shame is deeply uncomfortable. So our tendencies at one extreme are to simply deny our error or at the other to beat ourselves up excessively. Often we are angry at that person inside of ourselves who acted so badly.

But as the Great Buddha said, "Revenge is like drinking poison and expecting the other person to die." Poisoning ourselves (or others) will not make the immature part of us die. We can overcome having it act unchecked by being more mindful, but we cannot kill it, and to try to do so is literally self-destructive.

There are two potentials for growth when we forgive. The first is for the person doing the forgiving. The "forgiver" empties herself of the anger she is holding. That anger blocks her ability to see the one who has hurt her as a fragile and insecure human being like herself. It reminds her that she, too, has likely harmed others in much the same way for much the same reasons. In other words, it humbles the forgiver. And that does not require that the one being forgiven admits to the harm, takes responsibility for it, or even feels remorse. The forgiver benefits regardless; she grows in her ability to love unconditionally through her self-imposed humility.

The second potential for growth is for the person being forgiven. He is allowed to confront his wrongdoings in a way that humbles but does not humiliate. In other words, the forgiver acknowledges to the person being forgiven that we are all human, we all err, so that we are all on equal footing, so to speak. The person being forgiven may have done something bad, but *that does not make him bad*. It does not mean that he must always do bad; he can grow to be more loving.

The forgiver does not lord it over him with an air of superiority, objectifying the one being forgiven. That would be a form of humiliation. Instead, through forgiveness, both are offered the opportunity to reflect on the painful reality that all of us can behave selfishly and hurt others; that life is a constant struggle to grow from childish narcissism to adult altruism. The goal of the mature person who forgives is for the growth of the other so that they will not harm again. It is not about the forgiver's feelings of hurt or need for attention, compensation, or pity.

But what about when someone demands an apology? What is it this person is asking for? That the words "I'm sorry" be said to her, irrespective of how sincere they may be? For a public acknowledgement that she has suffered harm? Does it have anything to do with humility? Forgiveness? Growth?

Or is it just a way to garner self-pity? Or to let the person being told to apologize know that he is bad and inferior to the person demanding the apology, as though the person harmed has never harmed anyone? The forgiver may say she forgives the other once he apologizes, but does she really? Or is it all about establishing a clear moral hierarchy between the two?

Often some person or some group seeks an apology from another person or group for wrongs committed by a third party. For example, a group who was wronged by a government years ago demands that the present-day government apologize on behalf of that government whose members are long since dead.

First of all, I am not sure how a government, which is only an abstract concept, can apologize. A person can apologize; I am not sure an organization can. An organization has no conscience or soul of its own; only its constituent members do. I certainly understand that a group or individual wants to have a public acknowledgement by one government that something bad was done to them by another government. And I certainly understand why they may want some compensation, as well as promises, perhaps in the form of legislation, that it will never happen again. A government can do that.

Members of the present government can and should be feel badly that harm was done, but if none of their number was actually involved in the perpetration of that harm, I do not think their members can apologize for something they did not do, no matter how much they regret that it was done. They may be sorry that it happened, but they cannot apologize for something they did not do.

In a similar way, if a parent lets her five-year-old run rampant in a friend's home wreaking destruction, she ought not apologize for harm done by her five-year-old. The child is simply acting like a child. If the parent is going to apologize at all, she should at least have the courage to apologize for her own behaviour—for not supervising the child appropriately—and not cop out by blaming a child for her parental lapse. No one can apologize for the behaviour of someone else.

This brings me back to the question—why do people demand an apology? There may be many good reasons for doing so. But it strikes me that often it is not about forgiveness, not about humility, and not about growth. It's about putting people in their place, an inferior place. It's about humiliation and one-upmanship.

What about accepting an apology? What does that mean? It strikes me that there are at least three requirements for an apology to be sincere and meaningful. First, the person doing the apologizing acknowledges that he did something inappropriate. Second, that person has remorse for having done so. Third, that person is going to try not to do that again. In other words, he is going to learn and grow from the experience, become a better person. An apology that lacks these components is not much of an apology.

So, just like forgiveness, one can apologize and grow in the process irrespective of whether the other person accepts it. That's because the primary objective in apologizing is for the person apologizing to grow. If he doesn't, then it's a phony apology and a waste of time. If the person continues to behave exactly the same way, it would be hard to believe that his apology was sincere. The person being apologized to may very well be interested in having her hurt recognized and offered the opportunity to forgive, but she can forgive without an apology ever being offered. And a mature person is most interested not in her own pain but in the growth and maturing of the person doing the apologizing. Accepting an apology is noble only if that means that the person has sincerely forgiven, and it need not, and should not, be on condition of an apology being offered first.

Apologizing, sincerely asking to be forgiven, is one thing. Demanding an apology with a view to a conditional forgiveness is quite another.

One involves maturity and humility; the other involves childish feelings of hurt and revenge. Don't mistake the two.

Equally, mature forgiveness should not be conditional on an apology first, any more than a mature apology should be conditional on being forgiven. Both are done primarily for personal growth with a desire for growth of the other as other. Both are about love.

Addiction

Nowhere is this idea of forgiveness more necessary than with respect to addictions. A friend of mine was going through an addiction program and related to me some of what his counsellors had been telling him in order to help in recovery. He explained that people with his type of addiction had been shown, through blood tests and brain MRIs, to have different genes and brain structure than people without his addiction. Somehow that was supposed to help him, I guess. Maybe make him feel okay about himself because he had been saddled with these particular "defects" that people without his particular dependence don't have.

But I said to him that such a perspective misses the essence of addiction. Addictions are part of the normal human condition. He seemed shocked.

I explained to him that everyone, not just addicts, has a huge amount of their nervous system that is devoted to processing both pain *and pleasure*. There are countless sensory neurons that transmit signals to our brains from all over our bodies and within the brain itself. There is a very wide array of signals that are sent—smell, taste, touch, et cetera. These sensory stimuli affect our cerebral hemispheres directly and also indirectly as they are intimately wired through the emotional parts of our brain, for example the amygdala and other parts of our limbic systems. So we enjoy and desire pleasant sensory stimulation on many levels. In fact, we have been programmed over millennia to seek out and even hoard these pleasures. Why? Because in a harsh world designed for the survival of the fittest, we never know if and when the next meal may arrive, for example. Consequently, we have been hard-wired never to pass up a free lunch.

We come to realize that painful stimuli tend to warn of danger and pleasant stimuli tend to promise safety and abundance. The problem is, some of these pleasures stimulate us at very deep levels in our brains, levels whose neural networks are intense, powerful, and run at lightning-fast speeds. Rats will preferentially opt for cocaine to the exclusion of food and water, even to the point of death. The same can happen to us.

Everyone, including you and me, has genes, brain structures, and life experiences that can lead to getting hooked on something(s). There are no exceptions. This is why there are so many addictions out there, and very few of us can avoid all of them for a lifetime.

We often have a very narrow concept of addictions. We don't recognize a lot of them because some are socially acceptable (even desirable), so we don't think of them as addictions. But think for a moment of all of the addictions one can succumb to.

Recall Aquinas's four temptations. They can all become problems—wealth, pleasure, power, honour.

If you are addicted to some of these, like wealth or power, you can become very successful in our society. People will respect you and want to be with you. If you become obsessed with a certain activity, based perhaps on a musical or athletic aptitude, you can be worshipped in our society and receive no end of attention should you excel at it. It is not difficult to fall prey to the idea that you *are* your talent and crave the continued adoration that comes with that. That's because others believe, or want to believe, that when you excel at this one activity, you excel at everything; that you are special. Then you start to believe that you are better than other people because of it and treat them accordingly. Descend into greater narcissism.

There are a plethora of addictions—food, sex, power, money, sensory pleasures, weight loss, gambling, drugs, alcohol, smoking, fame, adrenaline rushes, power and control, gaming, work, television, technology—the list is near endless. Activities which in and of themselves are *not bad per se,* but when engaged in nonmindfully, can lead to obsessive, self-centred behaviours. The fallout from that is a lack of balance in our lives, in which we do not take care of our whole self. Like the cocaine addicted lab rat, we *disintegrate,* because our addictions control us. Worse still, we lose our interest in connecting and helping others. Our ability to love atrophies, and our ability to be loved, to want to grow, does so as well.

None of us should feel that we are exempt from addiction; *I am certainly not.* Why? Because none of these basic desires are abnormal—we are designed to enjoy pleasure and to avoid pain and death. We are hard-wired not to be the weakest deer in the herd, so we seek safety in power and honour and wealth. We are motivated to seek that which is enjoyable, so we seek pleasure. But we need to monitor and engage them mindfully as nature planned when it imbued us with full consciousness. Otherwise, we will fall into mindless, low-level cravings that will be our downfall. We *can* have too much of a good thing.

When I walk downtown, I know to my very core that the individuals panhandling for my donations are hooked on something and that I could easily be among them if I am not careful. Equally, I know that I could be like those with socially acceptable addictions—the wealthy and powerful—who lord it over their fellow humans. As I said earlier, that is why I am donating any proceeds from this book—I fear having too much and becoming addicted. I have enough and having more will not help me grow and evolve. When we reflect at a mindful level, we come to recognize when we have enough and lay down better neural pathways that supersede the reflex desires for more and more and more.

Part of this mindfulness is forgiveness. Any of us, under the right circumstances, is perfectly capable of becoming addicted to something, and we would be wise to always remember that. We must be humble, both to avoid dependencies ourselves and to help others who are in the chokehold of addictions. People do not yield to addictions out of *badness,* but out of *sadness.* They are people who have succumbed to eons-old temptations—partly born of pain, partly born of desire—and they need our love to help them grow beyond them.

Making someone feel bad is never going to help. I become more convinced that the problem with addictions is as much about how we beat up on ourselves about our addictions as it is about the addictions themselves. How we have to find some excuse, some gene or structural abnormality on an MRI, to make us feel that we are not bad and inferior to everyone else on the planet who is good. Forget about it! Welcome to humanity! We are all in the same boat, and we are all seasick! (The last line I think was from G. K. Chesterton.)

Of course, it is important to deal with the very real and very unpleasant aspects of withdrawal. But letting individuals with addictions know that they are not inferior to us and that they are just as deserving of happiness as the rest of us are important messages. Convincing them that they can rise above their addictions is critical. With help, they can come to appreciate that our shared ancestry and shared memes, as well as our personal genetics and life stories, greatly influence all of the choices we make. Maturity involves the triad of accepting the reality of change in the universe, the depth and creativity to explore change that helps us to grow and the self-discipline to bring it about. Together they constitute what we refer to as resiliency, something evolution has provided and we can nurture in others and ourselves.

Some of our choices guide us toward behaviours at the altruistic end of the spectrum, and others toward the narcissistic end. The more mindful we are, the better *integrated* we become, and the more able we are to tame, without having to eliminate, our desires to avoid pain and death and to seek pleasure and joy. To know when we have *enough*.

The hallmark of a more mature person is that he has learned to forgive another (or himself) for behaving immaturely, selfishly, or narcissistically, and by doing so encourage his growth.

In many respects, forgiveness is the theme for the rest of this book. But forgiveness involves an element of paradox, and to understand it, we must delve into the heart of paradox.

Chapter 17

Paradox

The opposite of a correct statement is a false statement. The opposite of a profound truth may be another profound truth.

—Niels Bohr, theoretical physicist

FIRST, LET'S CLARIFY how paradox differs from contradiction.

A contradiction is a statement that falsifies itself. For example: "I don't want to get hurt, so I am going to play goalie in ice hockey with very good players using a puck and not wear any equipment." Sound familiar? Yes, contradictions involve irrational thought. They are statements that involve reason but are logically flawed. I have certainly played goalie with miniature hockey sticks and a small ball, so you don't need equipment because you really can't get hurt. Hence, it is possible to play some types of hockey without equipment and not get hurt. But it is irrational to think that one can play goalie in ice hockey without equipment with good players using a puck and expect not to get hurt.

Either you wear equipment and likely don't get hurt, *or* you don't wear it and likely do get hurt. They are mutually exclusive of each other; you can't have both of them at the same time.

Paradox is a little different. It can seem irrational, like a contradiction, but on closer inspection, it is clear that although it may not be completely rational, neither is it irrational.

Paradox challenges our full brain—the logical left hemisphere and the more creative right hemisphere. As Mr. Spock, the Vulcan archetype of supreme logic, once said, "Logic is just the beginning of wisdom." The Greeks, Socrates in particular, may not have fully understood that statement, and we have inherited that legacy from them. In recent years, however, we have come to recognize the idea of emotional intelligence, the ability for our brain to understand in ways other than logic. It is not, as we used to believe, *irrational* but rather *nonrational.* "We often know before we understand" is a truism I read somewhere. We have *gut feelings*, instincts. Mathematician Henri Poincaré stated, "It is by logic that we prove, but by intuition that we discover."

If you look back on your life, you will probably come to realize that most of the really big decisions you made were not based primarily on logic. Logic may have prevented you from doing something really dumb, and likely logic did not disagree with any decision you made that turned out really well. But nonrational thinking often informs us about the right thing to do. Marrying my wife, having children, moving to Ottawa, and taking up goaltending and countless other of my best choices in life were not irrational and did pass the logic test. But I could not justify any of them on purely logical, rational grounds. They were highly influenced by the nonrational part of me.

I am reminded of Blaise Pascal's dictum: "The heart has its reasons for which reason knows nothing." A mature mind knows how to balance all parts of our self, how to deal with the tensions inherent in the multiple spectra of which our world, and our lives, are composed.

Let me give you a concrete example. In goaltending, I don't want to get hurt, and I want to play well. That means I have to wear equipment but not so much equipment that I can't move sufficiently to play well. One spectrum is about avoiding injury (rational—self-preservation); the other is about stopping the puck (nonrational—having fun). But minimizing one may maximize the other, and the optimal situation involves balancing the tension of the two of them.

Paradox is a "both/and" scenario, not "either/or." It involves a certain tension of what appear to be opposites (getting hurt and playing well), but in fact they are not because they are not mutually exclusive (not either/or). In other words, there is a sweet spot, and it likely varies from goalie to goalie.

For example, it is more fun to make a great save against a great player than a mediocre save against an average player. However, playing against great players increases the likelihood of me letting a goal in, something I do not like to do.

Pleasure has its own paradox. We seek pleasurable sensory stimuli: we taste novel foods, try new activities, travel to exotic places, and pursue new adrenaline rushes and other forms of entertainment. But the great Buddhist monks can meditate for hours on a single flower they see daily in their own backyard and still never plumb the full depths of its mysteries. We miss most of the pleasure, and magic, of the universe because it is too close for us to see.

This innate desire for pleasure is a challenge for us. Just as we cannot and should not eliminate all of our primal fear and pain, we should not eliminate all pleasurable sensations in our lives either. Would there be much point in living if we did? But we don't want fear, pain, or pleasure to control us, to become addictions. There is a certain tension in all of this.

As I said in my preface to the book, although we want to avoid pain, we also know that all growth involves loss, and in turn all loss involves pain. So we cannot grow without pain, but we have to manage growth because we cannot handle constant, overwhelming pain.

Humans do much better with acute stress than with chronic stress. Equally, we seek pleasure, but if we do so mindlessly, then it becomes an addiction: we devolve into such a profound narcissism that it prevents us from growing, from learning to love and integrating with others. Our lives are a journey of balancing the tension of our desires to grow and love others with our desires to avoid pain and to seek our own pleasure. That's why the path to maturity involves many immature steps.

Intimacy has elements of paradox. We are hard-wired for intimacy; we crave it. We can die (the hopelessness of solitary confinement), or make ourselves die (suicide), without it. Yet at the same time, it terrifies us because intimacy leaves us exposed and vulnerable. When we let our guard down and share our innermost selves, we risk rejection, ridicule, and shame. The negative feelings these generate can feel like death for us, too.

Growth itself has elements of paradox. We transcend but include what we have learned from those who have gone before us. As much as we want to become more complex and interact more intensely with the world and each other, we do not renounce our primal selves nor do we lose ourselves in the other. We learn to tame and integrate our lower brains as we commune with others, and yet we retain our own uniqueness.

The same goes for love. Love is not a sentiment but a willing the good and growth of the other as other. In marriage, we remain two separate individuals within the intimacy of being one in union. We will the other to grow—to change, mature, and reach their full potential—even though we want to remain with one another as a couple.

But there is also unrequited love. You may desire for someone to grow, perhaps transcend an addiction, but she may not be open or ready to do so. This means your love may not be effective or returned. When you don't get the results you want, it is easy to feel frustrated or hurt. But love in its purest form, without other motives, is unconditional—it is given freely with no strings attached. When we love, we do not focus on our feelings; we focus on those of the other. Love requires a mature mind, one more interested in giving than getting.

Our most intimate loving relationships, particularly ones with romance, have a visceral component that affects us deep in ourselves. We *feel* physical sensations, including ones controlled by our autonomic nervous systems and ones generated in our limbic systems. It is easy to confuse lust with love. True love, lasting love, will encompass these primal desires but also tempers and regulates them—transcends them—with our mind, utilizing our entire being to will the good and growth of the other as other.

As romantic relationships progress, occasionally people worry that the spark has left their relationship, that they have fallen out of love and that something is wrong. But a maturing relationship requires the ascendance of the higher centres of our being and, ultimately, the primacy not of physical satisfaction but of mindfulness.

When we first fall in love, we are drawn to one another because of mutual visceral attraction, shared pleasures, similar interests, and common goals. Much of this relates to avoidance of pain and seeking of pleasure. However, as we evolve, we develop a deeper understanding of each other's autobiographical selves, each other's internal narratives and heuristics, each other's deeply held values and beliefs, all stuff influenced by our cerebral hemispheres. We find a safe place in which to be ourselves and share our deepest fears and joys. In such a context, we can begin to grow.

Our job as parents is to love our children so much that we want them to eventually separate from us. If we have loved them well, they will *want* to leave, but they will also *want* to return, not as needy or guilt-ridden children, but as mature adults seeking union in mutual love.

Nowhere is this more beautifully expressed than in Kahlil Gibran's *The Prophet*:

> *And a woman who held a babe against her bosom said, Speak to us of Children.*

And he said:

Your children are not your children.

They are the sons and daughters of Life's longing for itself.

They come through you but not from you,

And though they are with you yet they belong not to you.

You may give them your love but not your thoughts,

For they have their own thoughts.

You may house their bodies but not their souls,

For their souls dwell in the house of tomorrow, which you cannot visit, not even in your dreams.

You may strive to be like them, but seek not to make them like you.

For life goes not backward nor tarries with yesterday.

You are the bows from which your children as living arrows are sent forth.

The archer sees the mark upon the path of the infinite, and He bends you with His might that His arrows may go swift and far.

Let your bending in the archer's hand be for gladness;

For even as He loves the arrow that flies, so He loves also the bow that is stable.

This piece of what I would refer to as "wisdom literature" is atypical because Khalil directly addresses the unique challenges of parenthood. In my experience, individuals who have not been parents have written much of the wisdom literature. Perhaps it's because only they had the free time necessary to write!

However, even in instances where the writer is a parent, seldom is parenthood a focus of their insights. I find this both surprising and disturbing because the overwhelming majority of us are parents, so insights on parenthood are highly relevant for most readers. Also, I do not think there is a more difficult vocation than parenthood, one that would benefit more from wisdom. Finally, there is no more important vocation than parenthood. Wisdom literature that does not explore the special challenges, and importance, of raising children may be theoretically interesting but practically irrelevant.

Virtually every parent knows that the journey of children separating from parents hits speed bumps; parents and children can be out of sync for a while. Sometimes, because they do not have to separate as intensely from grandparents as from their parents, children may turn to their grandparents for advice and guidance instead. That's what Jane did with Mae. At times the extreme proximity and emotion of a parent-child relationship can paradoxically interfere with the honesty and intimacy needed for authentic separation.

Authentic separation requires mindful releasing of the "umbilical cord." Maturation takes time, and although both child and parent want and need the cord to be loosened, if it is let out too quickly, it can be scary for children (and parents!). The process is very much a push-pull one, and it can generate much emotion, not all of which is pleasant. The wise and loving parent assesses her child's level of integration, of mindfulness, and provides the appropriate freedom that allows for growth but not destabilization and potential disaster.

Although children perceive that the freedom they are seeking is from their parents, the paradox is that it is freedom from the tyranny of their own unmonitored and unchecked lower brains—their fears, their desires, their faulty heuristics and analyses—that they are truly searching for. In truth, their ultimate mission is to conquer themselves, not to separate from their parents.

At one end of the spectrum, the unduly anxious parent fears easing the grip on the cord, and so the child rebels in an immature way. At the other end, the overly liberal parent, perhaps more concerned with his image of being cool and therefore liked by his children (and his children's friends), releases the cord far too readily, and children flounder in the context of too little wisdom, guidance, and structure.

In truth, the most liberating and enjoyable things in life have rules and structure. We attach rules to the things we most value to protect them. No one pays money to watch professional athletes engage in a sport that has no boundaries whatsoever. No one enjoys a musician playing his instrument incoherently. When you learn a new language, there are rules to follow if you want to be understood. Because love is willing the good and growth of the other, it requires a progressive integration and coherence of the self, and boundaries are a necessary part of that reality. Without them, we can devolve into serious mental illness, into disintegration.

The most important thing we do as a parent is teach our children how to love—how to rise above their narcissism and care about others. Intimacy requires the maturity to love. Without it, our children will live a lonely existence because few people want to spend much time with individuals who are only consumed with themselves. When people do spend time with narcissists, it is often primarily to gain from the wealth, pleasure, power, or honour that the self-absorbed person may have accumulated. Relationships like these contradict Kant's second categorical imperative (i.e., treat others as ends in themselves); everyone ends up getting used as a means to an end, as a thing. That's not love.

Our journey as human beings is to become more integrated within ourselves and within our society. It is fascinating to me that as we mature, as we change in so many ways on a daily basis, we nevertheless continue as the same ontological self. (Ontology, from the Greek *ont*, meaning "being," and *logos*, meaning "study," is the philosophical study of being, becoming, existence, or reality itself.) In other words, even though your body, including your entire nervous system, has changed tremendously since you were first conceived, you are still you. Every morning you wake up knowing that you are the same person you were the previous morning (barring serious illness or disintegration). Even though you may have grown a lot from the previous day, perhaps even experienced an epiphany of some type, you don't feel like you have become someone else *entirely* foreign.

It is one of life's great mysteries: how, when I look back at pictures of myself as a youth, can I still feel like the same guy in the photo when so many of the atoms and cells that comprise me have changed, so many of my attitudes and perspectives have changed, so much of me has changed. I suspect the answer is that my consciousness, my mind, is what has persevered and constituted what I refer to as "me."

We can even change the past and still be us if we want. Don't believe me?

Think of some event in the past, in particular think of an unpleasant one, maybe a time when someone did something mean to you, and you felt hurt. Further, pick an example in which you still have strong emotion, perhaps lingering frustration or anger. Now, as we all know, you can't change the details of the encounter—what was said or done or the fallout of it. But suppose I provided you with more information about the encounter than you had before, information that greatly changed the context of the event. I supplied data that offered a deeper understanding of the behaviours of the person who hurt you. And once you knew this, your perspective of the event, and the person involved, altered radically. You understood why they did what they did, and maybe even acknowledge that you might have done the same thing as they did, given those particular circumstances.

Now, do you feel differently about the event? About them? Would you treat them differently now if you were to see them again? Do you feel differently about the past? In other words, in your mind, have you essentially changed the past?

That's the essence of forgiveness. The paradox of forgiveness is that it changes the past for us. It is the mindful rewiring of circuitry in our brain that results in our ability, even desire, to help ourselves and others grow rather than wallow in narcissistic self-pity or the desire for revenge. Pity is a normal compassionate reaction, even when directed toward oneself. But when it interferes with growth of the self or the other, it becomes problematic. That's why the great Buddha said, "Revenge is like drinking poison and expecting the other person to die."

To better understand this paradox called forgiveness, watch the movie *The Railway Man* with Colin Firth. It is based on a true story with a remarkable ending that reveals not just the mystery and power of forgiveness, but the necessity of it if we are to grow. Often the hardest person to forgive is us—it is too painful to admit our wrongdoings to ourselves. But learning to forgive ourselves helps us to forgive others, and vice versa. Forgiving, like most activities, improves with repeated practice. We learn to rewire our brain through neuroplasticity. It requires mindful, courageous, and continuous introspection and self-reflection. It is how we grow.

It is likely clear that paradox is intimately associated with the concept of spectrum. Rather then resorting reflexively to binary thinking, we can mindfully immerse ourselves in spectra whose tensions are anchored in those opposites. We leave the concrete land of simply either/or and journey to a more abstract place of both/and.

As we mature, we begin to grasp and become more comfortable with the reality that most elements of the universe lie along some kind of spectrum. When we only see the world as either x or anti-x, then there are no in-betweens. If you believe that only x is correct, then everything else, any other shade of grey between, is anti-x. Consequently, we fail to appreciate the importance of context, and that makes forgiving a lot more difficult and loving someone, including ourselves, considerably more challenging as well.

Nowhere is this truer than with respect to our own self-narratives. Our starting point in life is one of insecurity—both from an evolutionary perspective and a developmental one. We fear death, we dread loneliness and abandonment, and we seek lasting pleasure that seems constantly just beyond our reach. Bombarded by the complexity of the universe, we feel insignificant in the world, even impotent. We bounce between feelings of worthlessness and desire to be special to compensate for those feelings. We grab onto anything that will confirm our specialness and make us feel safe and loved. Wanting to feel special is a normal and understandable attempt to compensate for our innate insecurities. However, it arises from the narcissism of our lower brains and needs to be overcome if we want to conquer ourselves.

Parents love their children so much that they tell them that they are special. Parents and children alike can confuse that idea of specialness. A child should always be special to their parents and vice versa. But if that is conflated with being special in the world *in general*, it can lead, as we have seen, to difficulty with separation as well as connectedness with others. A child who cannot see and accept his parents as imperfect humans will have a tough time ever feeling like an equal adult with them. Similarly, a child who comes to believe that he is special in the world will have a difficult time when he faces the inevitable reality that others in the world do not agree with his specialness. Narcissism is an impediment to growth and love.

Sometimes children will be told, particularly by their parents, that they are so special that they can do anything if they work hard enough at it. They can't, of course, because they are finite creatures; by definition they have limitations and boundaries. Leading anyone to believe otherwise puts incredible pressure on people to pretend to be gods or demigods. That kind of overconfidence and, frankly, arrogance, will not help them to conquer themselves. It will simply feed their innate narcissism.

Nonetheless, you may still feel that there are special people in the world, and perhaps that you are one of them. The first question I would ask you is, Why do you feel a need to believe that there are special people in the world? And if you believe that you are one of them, why do you need to believe that you are special? What's wrong with being ordinary? Does that thought scare you too much?

The second question I would ask is, What is it about these special people that makes them special? Is it their talents? Their wealth? Their looks? Their wonderful or privileged lives? If that is the case, then you are mistaken. That is not who they are. They may have been born into wealth or a life of privilege, *but that is not who they are.* They may have been blessed with neural pathways that have been nurtured to allow them to manifest a musical talent or athletic ability, *but that is not who they are either*.

How we start at birth is pure luck (for us), and much of what we accomplish during our lives, notwithstanding the requirement of hard work and perseverance, is luck too. Don't believe me? If Bill Gates had been born 100 years earlier, or in a different country to a different family, would he still be the same Bill Gates today? In one respect, yes, he would be. The unique essence (ontological being) of Bill Gates would still be Bill Gates. However, the details of his life would be very, very different. Would that make *him* less special? Or would it just make the *details of his life* less special?

We are far more than just our bodies or neural pathways or cerebral hemispheres. We are far more than just our social position, the stuff we own, or the letters after our name. We all have minds, and all minds are unique and special. Some people may be fortunate enough to be born and live in circumstances (e.g., time, place, family of origin, health) where their talents and other gifts are highly valued. But talents are not always appreciated appropriately. How many great artists did not have their work valued during their lifetimes but only long after they left us?

Again, *that is not who they are*. You are you, and what you do in the world is under your control. If I asked you to name the individual who placed second in a specific event during a specific Olympic Games, chances are you would not be able to do so. But if I asked you to name your favourite teachers and why, I bet you easily could. They likely were not famous or accomplished, and yet you remember them, and likely with fondness. Why? *Because you remember who they were*, not what they accomplished. Their deep selves, their minds, manifested to you in such a way that they helped you grow. In other words, they loved you. And that was a choice they made; they willed the good and growth of the other (you) as other.

All of us are capable of love, so all of us are equally special in the only way that really matters. We are a balance of being and doing. We often forget in our busy world that we refer to ourselves as human "beings," not human "doings."

We may seek relationships with people who tell us that we are special. They tell us that they need us, that they cannot live without us, or that we complete them. It is easy to believe that that is love. However, such sentiments, as romantic as they may sound, are about *our feelings* of dependency, of fearful neediness, not about willing the good and growth of the other as other. They stem from our insecurities and desire for pleasure, not from a mature and mindful willingness to sacrifice for the other.

So the issue is not whether we are insecure—all of us are. The issue is how do we deal with it? Do we plunge into one or more of Aquinas's four temptations to convince ourselves that we are all right, that we belong, that we are special and therefore not the last, lonely deer in the herd? Do we accumulate more wealth, pleasure, power, and honour to assure ourselves a safe, privileged, and special life? Do we fall into addictions to escape our pain?

So often our insecurity leads to jealousy. We try to tear down other people simply because they have something we do not have, especially if we want it and feel we deserve it as much or more. We raise ourselves up by putting others down.

One of the subtle ways we do so is by pretending that we all have identical talents and gifts, aptitudes and abilities. News flash: we don't! We are all ontologically equal, but that does not translate into being identical in *every* way. Our insecurity does not allow us to be different but valued. We can stunt the growth of others by forcing everyone to the same level, insisting that everyone receive a gold star. It's one thing to speak and act against someone's behaviour on moral grounds. It's quite another to diminish someone's accomplishment or talent because you are insecure and jealous that they are better at something than you are.

If we learn to conquer ourselves, we will encourage rather than deny the opportunity for others to develop their skill sets, knowing that if they do so and use them in a moral fashion, the collective, which includes us, will benefit. Life is full of hierarchies of talents and gifts; it is not the aesthetics of them but how we use them that matters.

Another common way we deal with our insecurity is to associate ourselves or immerse ourselves in a tribe. It may be a tribe based on citizenship, on a certain culture or religion, on a certain talent we have, on a profession, or on an area of interest. There is no end to the tribes we belong to and in and of itself this is not a problem. In fact, it can bring us much pleasure and can help us to grow and love others.

I must admit that I am not very tribal, and I am not entirely sure why. Perhaps it relates to the fact that I have a very mixed ancestry—I am a bit of a mutt. Maybe it stems from the fact that I have no particular skill sets that qualify me for any elite tribe. I have conceded to being a generalist, a jack of all trades but master of none.

However, I think it mostly stems from the fact that tribal thinking scares me. There is a certain tension in being a member of a tribe, any tribe. One the one hand, we feel connected and benefit from the safety in numbers embodied in membership. We can be nurtured by the tribe and inherit useful memes and heuristics that can advance our growth.

But membership in the tribe can also limit or even interfere with our growth. Not all tribes value creativity to the same degree. Many tribes expect conformity because there is a collective fear of change, the pain of losing what is familiar and known. Uniqueness may not be appreciated; blending in is highly valued. It has been said that culture is "our way of hiding our hatred of change."

We fall prey to social fads to fit in. As I said earlier, in many ways, we like what we are told to like. The herd mentality is powerful. Radicals and people who "think outside the box" can scare us.

That's why playing by the rules is often of supreme importance for tribes. Questioning those rules, exploring grey zones, and acknowledging elephants in the room can be frowned upon. To keep the social order, binary thinking is often engaged: you are either with us or against us. Robert Milgram's various experiments in the 1960s confirmed the social pressures we feel in this regard and goes a long way in explaining the atrocities committed throughout human history. When members don't play by the rules or when things aren't going well for the group, tribes often look for scapegoats to blame, either within the tribe or outside of it.

This is the basis for the concept of sinfulness and the burden of shame. The problem is not so much that we label bad actions as bad or sinful but that we want to label individuals as bad or sinful once we have caught them doing something of which we, or our tribe, don't approve. Then they are no longer part of "us," the good people, but "them," the bad people.

Conscientious objectors are a classic example; they are not always treated fairly. The shame and guilt we encourage them to feel allows us to separate them from us and make us feel safe again. After all, as long as us good people stick together and get rid of the bad ones, we'll be okay, and they'll get what's coming to them, right? They will be the ones eaten by the wolf, not me, thank heavens. As long as I'm safe with my tribe, that's all that matters.

That's why bullying behaviour can be successful. The bully picks a whipping boy, and the rest of us stick together, run and hide, and leave the unfortunate victim to fend for himself. We're safe; but it sucks to be the weakest deer in the herd, doesn't it?

The wolves and bullies prey on our black-and-white thinking. That's why they get away with what they get away with. Evil flourishes because good people do nothing. Instead of standing up to the bully, we take flight. We would seldom have to fight the bully if we confronted him; paradoxically the bully is usually as scared as we are because we are all insecure. The bully simply counts on us blinking first. He counts on the neurons deep in our brain triggering the rushes of adrenaline that produce so many terrifying feelings—heart pounding, dizziness, weakness, nausea, near incontinence—that prompt us to run and hide.

So we find many ways to deal with our innate insecurity. We join a tribe and give into our own fear by mindlessly following the rules, avoiding becoming a pariah at all costs. Or we capitalize on the fear of the collective and become bullies or wolves. Some of us try to convince ourselves, and anyone else who will listen, that we are special. Others do the opposite and recoil into a self-narrative of inferiority and hopelessness. All of these are completely understandable, but they are not mature or mindful.

Think of the tribes that you belong to. Perhaps they are based on a shared culture, religion, hobby, or other interest. Tribes often compare themselves to other tribes, just as individuals do. That can lead to fear and jealousy and the desire to feel special or superior. And, of course, the need to prove it, one way or another, often follows.

The word "compete" comes from two Latin words: the "pete" part is from the word *petire*, which means "to seek." The "com" part is from *cum* meaning "with." Therefore, compete means to "seek with"; in other words, work with each other to find something better, along the lines of dialogue. However, many individuals and tribes commonly misinterpret competition as being adversarial, like debate, when in fact it is meant to be cooperative.

Sadly, tribal thinking can be the starting point for hatred of any tribe that is different from ours. It starts from the primal fear of anything new or foreign. It's in our DNA; every culture on the planet has an inherent unease and fear of unknown tribes. How much misery have we inflicted on one another because one tribe fears another simply because they are different? All forms of racism and bigotry are manifestations of this need to feel special in the face of fear, jealousy, and envy. We like to believe that we are exempt, but none of us is.

We may be mindful of our prejudices and prevent them from manifesting or from influencing us excessively, but they are always there, *no exceptions*. In fact, often people who have been the victims of such prejudice have the most difficult time suppressing their own prejudicial tendencies.

Perhaps the tribes we belong to don't hate other tribes or act aggressively toward them. However, all tribes have their own narratives, rules, and rituals, which can be internalized and followed mindfully, encouraging members to meditate on deep truths in the process of making the world a better place. Or they can be followed mindlessly, from a primitive part of our selves full of fear and insecurity. In such instances, the rules and rituals are not about openness to others but about exclusivity, segregating us from the rest of humanity who are not members of our tribe. Beware any tribe that does not value inclusivity. It can be the start of the "us and them" mentality that has led to so much suffering in the world.

Exclusivity, the unwavering belief that your tribe is better than another, is the breeding ground for what is referred to as "the killing certainties." The tribe is so certain of its specialness that its members will kill to protect it. When we are young and more easily influenced, we can fall prey to this mentality. Our insecurity and need to belong drive us to be part of a tribe that is special. I wonder how many wars would have been averted had we disallowed those less than thirty years of age from entering military service?

None of these modes of thinking and behaving are surprising—tribes consist of humans at varying levels of maturity, so they are not going to behave better than their constituents. We want to believe that our various tribes and institutions will represent the best of us, but that is not always so. Each one of us must come to realize that no matter what tribe we think we belong to, there is one tribe we all belong to that matters most: the tribe called *Homo sapiens*, the only tribe with minds. We must utilize the wonderful gift of full consciousness mindfully because if we don't, our species risks disintegration and so does our planet.

Mindfulness involves two components. The first is taking the time to be the observer self to see and understand how our brains and bodies are working—our reflex behaviours, our feelings and desires, our perceptions, our internal heuristics, and our higher thinking. It requires us to slow down and be courageous. By doing so, we can see ourselves as we are, without guilt or despairing negative judgment, with an attitude of forgiveness. Yes, we do crave things and engage in behaviours that can be narcissistic or selfish; that's a given. We may be able to understand why that is so, and we may not. What is most important, however, is to simply grant that *it is so*. This is the starting point for psychotherapy.

The second part of mindfulness is using our complete and true self, our mind, to then rewire ourselves. Focus less on things we want to be rid of—neural networks that are hindering our growth—and focus more on things we want to adopt—creating new neural networks that foster greater connectedness with one another. This requires engaging our hemispheres more fully—the emotional intelligence of our right hemisphere (nonrational) and the logical intelligence of our left hemisphere (rational).

Using our mirror neurons, we learn to respect the other, have compassion and empathy for the other, and emote with the other. Very often people stress the importance of good communication as a starting point for good relationships. However, before we communicate our thoughts, we must develop our thoughts, and that takes time and practice. After all, well-communicated gibberish is still gibberish.

We can learn to develop our thoughts more clearly and effectively by

- avoiding binary thinking and becoming more comfortable with the concept of spectrum;
- understanding the use of reason in supplying justification for an argument rather than just dealing in opinions;
- engaging in dialogue not debate;
- accepting the reality and importance of paradox;
- avoiding fallacious reasoning (of which there are many examples); and
- avoiding assumptions by being explicit.

These are all skills that we can and must nurture. Simply being good observers is not enough; we must learn to manage change and growth. Simply being good communicators is not enough; we need to learn to think better, rationally and nonrationally, and avoid irrational, contradictory thought.

The path to maturity involves many immature steps. We can do so individually as well as collectively, within our various tribes.

Chapter 18

The Medical Tribe

Humility is the only lens though which great things can be seen—and once we have seen them, humility is the only posture possible.

—Parker Palmer

I HAD A wonderful experience in the office recently, one that inspired me.

A middle-aged man (which at my age makes him a young man!) was following up with me after a very eventful visit to one of our local hospitals. He had been awoken in the early part of the night with a terrible pain that would not abate. After several hours he had had enough, and he proceeded to the emerg, where he was eventually seen by a surgeon who suggested, quite wisely, to undergo urgent surgery to correct the problem. He spent a couple of days recovering in hospital before discharge, and when he saw me he was almost back to normal. Doesn't really sound very inspiring, does it? Well, there's more.

First of all, it took a while for the medical team to make the diagnosis because his case was a little atypical, and it was in the middle of the night when services were less available. Because the hospital was so full, he spent a considerable amount of time on a stretcher in emerg, even after the surgery. During that time, he slept very little because the emerg is a busy, and noisy, place pretty much twenty-four hours a day. In fact, in the middle of the night, it is often the noisiest because people get themselves into all kinds of trouble after midnight (and often there are alcohol or other mind-altering substances involved).

To add to his stress, the patient in the stretcher next to him was dying of cancer.

Even after he got out of emerg into his hospital room, he did not sleep well because of commotion in his shared room.

I know what you are thinking: "What a horrible story" or "Man, is our health-care system ever broken" or "I would be writing to the CEO to complain about that experience if it were me."

But this man did not see things that way. Remember what I said in an earlier chapter about perception? This man's eyes were opened to a world he did not really know existed. He allowed his observer self to simply witness the lives of the emerg nurses, doctors, ambulance attendants, police officers, orderlies, cleaning staff, lab and X-ray technicians, et cetera. who had to deal with no end of human suffering day in and day out, at all hours of the day and night. He saw the people who came into emerg on their own or with family or friends or by ambulance or with police. He saw people with minor problems and people dying. He saw people with problems that could be fixed and problems that could only be managed.

Rather than complain, he introspected and reflected about his own life. About how lucky he was not to have a more serious problem. That he lived in a country with good hospitals that are open 24/7 in a health-care system that is publicly funded. He sadly realized that the dying man beside him had probably been urged to stop smoking many times. Then he realized that one day he, too, was going to die, and he wanted that to be later than sooner. This meant that he was going to have to get more serious about his own health before it was too late.

Talk about mindfulness! I have rarely had a patient speak so eloquently or move me as he did, which is why I am relating it to you.

I don't do hospital work any longer, and my patient's story reminded me how much I miss it. I have spent considerable time in operating rooms as both an anaesthetist and an assistant, and although it can be stressful and involve odd hours, it can also be very satisfying work. Ditto for emerg shifts.

Taking care of patients in hospital was also part of my practice for about twenty-five years. At one end of life's spectrum I delivered babies, and at the other end I did palliative care. There were some very happy moments and, of course, some very sad moments as well. In all of those years, involving thousands of patients, there was one thing I found rather disappointing. Seldom did anyone ever reflect upon their time in hospital the way my patient above did.

Except for the life-changing experience of childbirth, most times when a person is admitted to hospital, it is because of a significant negative medical event and, thus, not a pleasant one. As with my friend above, the hospital environment offers individuals an opportunity to step outside of their usual lives to realize that they are mortal and that life, and health, are but fleeting gifts. I would have thought that patients would take advantage of this time to meditate on that, to become more mindful, to make some significant life changes.

I have seen a few people experience epiphanies in their lives, but not as many as I could have. Seldom did I see people confront their own mortality. People did slow down and catch up on their golf magazines or read a good whodunit. But I don't recall seeing many patients read anything deeply philosophical or spiritual. Occasionally, especially if it appeared that death could be imminent, they would invite a visit from someone representing their religious affiliation. Otherwise, their focus was primarily about getting out of hospital and getting back to their usual routine as much as possible. It was not common for patients to reevaluate their life focus or routines, to see if this illness they had was telling them something about their lives that they needed to change.

Several years ago I was a patient. I had a heart problem—paroxysmal atrial fibrillation—the commonest arrhythmia we see. Generally, it is not serious, but it is annoying. Having said that, it is, nevertheless, a problem with my heart, which is unsettling. I went to our local hospital, and because I did not know how long I would be there, I brought along a book I was reading, Ken Wilber's *A Theory of Everything*. I was treated very well and was converted easily back to a normal rhythm, and after a night in the emerg on a stretcher I was released home, tired but otherwise normal and healthy. And thankful.

Lying there on the stretcher, I knew that my life would never be the same. I now had a chronic medical problem, albeit rather minor in the big picture, but more importantly, I was mortal and I was getting old. For the first time in my adult life, I experienced medicine from the other side of the stethoscope and it humbled me. I reflected upon the many joys and blessings of my life, and I also started to introspect about the source of my problem—what was this atrial fibrillation telling me about myself?

During our medical training, we are led to believe that our job as doctors is to fix patients' problems. Early on in medical school that provokes naive visions, garnered largely from television shows, of brilliant diagnoses followed by dazzling cures. I suspect that patients are as influenced by the same television shows as we are.

But as our education continues, we come to realize that cures are not that common. When I used to teach family medicine residents, I would ask them what we, as doctors, can hope to accomplish when patients visit us. I would give them a clue: all of the things we can do for them fall into one of four categories. No group of residents I did this exercise with ever got it right. It's harder than you think. Do you know?

As far as I can tell, everything we can offer patients falls into these four categories: educate, prevent, cure, or palliate.

The residents, after some discussion, would agree.

Hopefully, we always educate patients with every encounter; they should always leave our visit knowing more than they did before.

There are some diseases and conditions the medical profession can prevent, but not as many as you think. There are lots that you, the patient, can prevent, with a healthy lifestyle, but not that many that doctors can do for you on their own.

There are, in fact, two kinds of prevention. There is true prevention (less common), and there is postponement (more common). In true prevention, for example a tetanus immunization, you actually do not get tetanus *at all, ever*. As I said earlier, immunizations are the one prevention doctors can offer you that really work. Nothing else even comes close.

However, much of what we call prevention is not really prevention in the same sense, but rather postponement. For example, if you take blood pressure medications or cholesterol-lowering drugs, no one is going to guarantee that you won't *ever* have a heart attack or a stroke. You will always be at risk for them if you live long enough. The best we could hope for is that we can postpone it for many years, in your eighties as opposed to your fifties if you are *really* lucky. And that's only if the medications work for you—more on that later (most people do not benefit from these drugs).

When I asked the residents how often they effect a cure, they chuckled; they knew it was infrequent. Infectious diseases are perhaps the commonest, but as we discussed earlier, a lot of those are viral for which we often have no cure per se.

After education, the most likely way we can help patients is by palliating their disease or condition. "Palliate" comes from the Latin word *palliare*, to cloak, which means that we cannot make it go away, but we can hide it, so to speak, and make it less of a burden.

I taught this seminar to residents in the context of a palliative care course, but the lesson for the residents, as it is for the population at large, is perhaps shocking. Palliation is not just about helping people with serious disease in the process of dying. It is about the overwhelming majority of all the work we do for patients who have conditions or diseases because we cannot prevent or cure very many.

I am sorry if you find this disturbing. It's a bit of a letdown for us, too, both during our formal education and the rest of our careers. I am not sure that we are very well trained to deal with this reality either. It's tough coming to peace with the fact that bad things happen, even when we take good care of ourselves, and we are often powerless to make them go away. Most often all we can do is cloak them.

On the other hand, there is an upside. What, you ask, could possibly be the upside?

The upside is that there is, in fact, a fifth thing we can do for patients that can ease their pain, and by now I bet you know what that is: we can help patients grow.

This would seem like an obvious thing to do and that we must certainly attempt it, if not accomplish it, during every encounter. However, I would suspect that it is a relatively rare phenomenon. Don't believe me?

Growth requires a few things in order for it to occur. A person has to understand the idea of growth. If someone believes that she is already at the pinnacle of her life and that there is no longer any need or room to grow, then growth is less likely.

At one end of the spectrum, there are times when disease or illness befalls us, and it was completely unpredictable and beyond our control: a driver falls asleep, veers off the road onto the sidewalk, and hits us. It's just really bad luck. At the other end of the spectrum are situations in which bad luck has much less to do with it. We make some very irrational choices and an inevitable and undesirable result ensues: we get drunk and, without using condoms or asking a few questions first, have sex with someone we don't know well and get herpes.

Of course, most disorders that affect our health, physical or mental, lie somewhere between the two ends of the spectrum. This means that in the majority of instances, we *own* at least some responsibility for how things turned out.

Now that may seem rather obvious when looked at objectively as we are now, but in the midst of unpleasant symptomatology, it can be hard to see, and acknowledge, that bitter reality.

Patients, myself included, want quick, painless fixes generated "out there," not slower, more ponderous palliation involving introspection with a goal of personal change. Remember my shift in the walk-in clinic?

It's always more satisfying to please than to displease someone. It's less risky and less threatening; confrontation is not something most of us enjoy. It's not fun giving bad news when you're a member of the medical tribe. I have had to let staff go when I ran a clinic, and I have personally had investment disasters, but none of those compare to telling someone that she or her loved one is seriously ill and may not survive. Only someone with sociopathic tendencies wouldn't feel the same way.

Given what we have learned during our exploration of how we humans work, it's perfectly understandable that there is a lot of pressure on the medical tribe to erase people's pain. We generally don't like pain. As creatures that appear to have the fullest consciousness of any species on the planet, this aversion to pain applies not just for us but also for our loved ones and even strangers. So we all want it gone. But is that realistic or even desirable?

Sometimes there are opportunities for growth hidden in our pain, life lessons to reflect upon as my patient in emerg recognized. I learned a lot about myself—and grew—from my experience with my heart. It told me a lot about how I handled stress and that my life was too busy. I was not being mindful enough. It continues to be an ongoing process of self-discovery and self-conquering.

As patients, we often just want a quick fix. As I have said many times, the universe is a complex place, and at a deep level we know that that is true, which is why so many of us are attracted to experiences that awe us, like standing at the edge of the Niagara Falls. It is also why we are drawn to magic: we relish the feeling of wonderment when something unexpected, and seemingly impossible, happens.

Often, we have the same approach to medicine. We really do believe that these fellow *Homo sapiens* called doctors have, through reading books too complicated for us to understand (or so we think) and having experiences we have not had, acquired special if not magical powers to rid us of our pains and problems.

There was a time when physicians were far more educated than most of the population, but that is no longer true. Yet the mystique to some degree persists. Why is that?

As with any tribe, we have our own lingo, our unique terms and language. Much of it is in Latin, or Latin in origin, and thus it seems almost incomprehensible. To be honest, this excessive use of Latin is a bit of a farce—conditions that sound so impressive in Latin when translated often offer little or no insight into the nature of the illness. Often the vernacular translation simply *describes* features of the illness, and often rather esoteric ones at that, which add minimal insights into either etiology (cause) or potential cure.

Let's look at the word "dermatitis." Whenever you see *itis*, it means "inflammation"; *derm* refers to "skin." So dermatitis means inflammation of the skin. It does not explain the pathophysiology (the development of disease) at all, just the end product, so it is somewhat helpful, but it is primarily descriptive. Interestingly, it sounds so much more sophisticated when you tell your friend that you have dermatitis rather than just say your skin is inflamed (which they probably already knew just from looking at it!). Multiple sclerosis is another good example. *Sclerosis* means "hardening," and when they performed autopsies on patients suffering from this disease, they found multiple plaques of neural tissue that looked hardened, hence the name. It tells you nothing of the origins or cause of the disease, just what it looked like. Equally, it gives you no clue as to the cure.

Like most tribes, there are special ceremonies and qualifications that must be satisfied for admission to the medical tribe. Somewhat unique to the tribe is the fact that one acquires a special appellation, "Doctor," that is used not just within the tribe but also by everyone outside the tribe as well. The mystique grows more.

Frequently, when we interact with the health-care system, we are either in pain or afraid of impending pain, so we feel vulnerable. Our judgment may be clouded by these feelings or by the medical condition itself. The extreme is in the case of altered levels of consciousness, for example a coma, in which we are completely at the mercy of the profession. Another example is when one deteriorates into a psychosis. In such cases, there is little one can do to control the power differential inherent in the physician-patient relationship.

However, those extremes are fortunately rather uncommon. In most cases, we can minimize this differential, and doing so would make for a much better encounter. Why? Because the practice of medicine, as Scott Peck indicated, should be about the good and growth of the other as other. But how do we effect this growth? It starts with understanding the nature of the patient-physician relationship.

A number of years ago, a couple, Ezekiel Emanuel and Linda Emanuel, developed a concept referred to as "the four models of the physician-patient relationship."

At one end of the spectrum is the paternalistic model (I refer to is as the "parentalistic model") that was common through much of medical history. Doctors acted much like well-meaning parents and patients like well-behaved children: doctors spoke and patients listened and did as they were told. As people became better educated this model fell into disfavour. It is still a useful model, but *only* in situations in which patients are incapable of making a decision, for example, when they are in a coma or psychotic. In such situations, the physician must make decisions in the best interest of the patient (particularly if the patient has already indicated their preferences, for example, in a living will) and only act only insofar as to bring the patient back to a condition in which they can resume their own decision making as soon as possible. In other words, physicians should not overstep their mandate and address all kinds of other issues beyond the immediate condition resulting in loss of decision-making ability.

The second model is the informative model. In such a model, the role of the physician is at the other end of the spectrum. She is simply there to provide relatively raw data for the patient to contemplate. For example, ordering a blood test to assess cholesterol and presenting the results and generally accepted guidelines to the patient. This model is becoming more commonly used but has its limitations. Patients are left to understand the information on their own, and so the quality of decision making is highly dependent on the level of understanding of the patients or the sources they refer to (like the internet!).

The third model is the interpretive model. In this scenario, the patient engages with the physician in a more interactive way, seeking the doctor's interpretation of the raw data in the context of the patient's present condition and past medical history. So, for example, although the patient using the second model may feel that his cholesterol is at a reasonable level, the physician may point out that the patient has a very significant family history of heart disease, already smokes, and has high blood pressure and diabetes. Using a calculation tool based on the Framingham study, the physician may help the patient realize that, in fact, his risk for heart disease is very high (more than 35 percent in the next five years, potentially). Sometimes this kind of interaction can be more helpful than consulting Dr. Google, who does not know you very well and, therefore, cannot contextualize the data.

The final model is the deliberative model. Much like the third model, it involves a mutual engagement. However, added to the dialogue is a mutual reflection upon the *values* of the patient. The patient may have a natural aversion to taking medication, and that is perfectly understandable. In fact, this model welcomes skepticism because it wants both parties to reflect upon the data as mature adults. The patient and physician together examine and critique the evidence in the context of the patient's other risk factors and values.

Not taking medications may be a very important value to the patient. He will have to weigh this value with the value of maintaining good cardiac health. If he perceives that his likelihood of living long enough to benefit from the drugs is too low, he may opt not to take the drugs. Or if he would prefer to die of a sudden cardiac event instead of some other more lingering and painful condition, he may opt against the drugs as well. Or maybe he is just comfortable taking risks. What matters is that the physician assists the patient in weighing and balancing all of his values in the context of medical decision making.

Often, information is all that need be exchanged. However, there are a couple of important points to consider.

Firstly, we often assume that because we are educated in general, or very knowledgeable in one area of life in particular, that that level of sophistication or expertise translates directly into our understanding of medicine. These assumptions are often quite erroneous. For most of us who have not completed medical school, the sum total understanding of the human body comes from grade ten health class and our own, potentially flawed, interpretations of our own body's functioning.

In addition, knowing a lot about playing piano, for example, does not equate to an equal proficiency in medicine. As I have said earlier, although I took a lot of biology courses in high school and university prior to medical school, I would know little of human functioning if I had not gone to medical school. Our intuitions about how complicated things, like human beings, work is seldom completely accurate. I would suggest that most of us would benefit from listening to our physician's interpretation of data with an open mind. As I said about strep throat, it is surprising how few patients ask me what I do when I have a sore throat.

I am always surprised when patients express disappointment when they visit a surgeon who counsels against surgery. Look, surgeons love doing surgery; that's why they went into their discipline, just like how a car salesperson loves selling cars. If they don't think they can make you better with surgery, pay heed. They are not trying to be mean; they likely have your best interests at heart. You may well be disappointed that your problem cannot be fixed by them, but don't be disappointed that the fix may come from something nonsurgical. Avoid the scalpel as much as you can.

In fact, one of the problems these days is that because anaesthesia is so good and surgical techniques are so much safer and less invasive, there is a tendency to occasionally have the threshold for surgery set too low. As we have said earlier, we all feel a tremendous pressure to always act simply because we can, but sometimes the best thing is to do nothing (or at least nothing surgical) and let nature do its thing.

As much as I would implore patients to ask for more education from their physicians, I would also remind physicians that the one thing we can always provide to patients every visit is education.

This brings me to the second issue around information: context matters. So although raw data is useful, it most often needs to be interpreted within the context of the life of the unique patient in front of you. This is not something Dr. Google can do for you. I remember once finishing off a morning office and the staff asking me to see one more patient before noon, a young lady experiencing cystitis, a benign bladder infection. Thinking this would be a short visit and I could still cram in my lunch, I agreed.

The analysis of her urine and her symptoms all pointed to a simple lower urinary tract infection (cystitis) for which a short prescription of an antibiotic might help. Much to my surprise, she broke into tears! She had Googled her symptoms and was convinced that she had bladder cancer. It took a while to convince her that such was unlikely the case. So much for a leisurely lunch break.

This is an extreme case, I admit. However, I am finding that patients often have their agendas set by the time they see me. Their neighbour has counselled, or they have read, or their gut tells them that they need an MRI, for example. I am simply there to provide for them what they want. They cannot recognize that fear or pain may be motivating them to investigate further. Equally, their sources of information may not be appropriate in their particular set of circumstances. Patients often don't have a plan, just a blind stabbing in the dark to find answers. An awful lot of investigations are done today whose results are normal for that reason. And in retrospect, those normal (or even abnormal) results could well have been known prior to the test had patient and physician taken the time to interpret information, not just react reflexively to it.

The third and final point is that all decisions are ethical ones. By that I mean all decisions in medicine involve asking what *should* be done, not what *can* be done. Sometimes the "should" is very obvious: you are young and healthy and have bacterial pneumonia, so we treat with the appropriate antibiotic. But sometimes it is not so clear: you suffer from moderately severe dementia and you have suffered a number of complications recently that have hastened your decline. Perhaps the wise decision, the "should," is simply to keep you comfortable, even though we "can" do more.

This is where the discussion of values enters into the picture. We answer the "should" questions based on our values. Years ago I had a wonderful patient who was retired and was probably the handiest guy I had ever known. He could fix anything and was always busy helping out his kids and grandkids with home renovations and work around the house. He loved to cut grass. He came to see me one day because he was getting terrible leg pains cutting his grass. He had circulatory issues in his legs that caused the pain, referred to as "claudication." Although he was a heavy smoker, he was otherwise healthy. He was terrified of having the surgery (and I don't blame him), but given the severe narrowing in his arteries, there were few other choices.

Medications and smoking cessation had helped minimally. We spent a lot of time trying to balance his different values—enjoying activity versus his distaste for surgery—trying to figure a way out of his conundrum. He eventually opted for the surgery and did very well.

We hear a lot about values these days—every business seems to have them. Although we recognize that they are important, I am not sure that we completely understand them. So before we go any further we should take a look at values and how they relate to the practice of medicine.

As a springboard to exploring values, let's start with special kind of experiment.

PART III: WHERE WE ARE GOING

Endless Possibilities

Chapter 19

Thought Experiment 1

You don't become completely free by just avoiding to be a slave; you also need to avoid becoming a master.

—Nassim Taleb, *The Bed of Procrustes*

YOU ARE PROBABLY wondering what kind of experiment we can do together and how could it help to understand values. Well, have you ever done a thought experiment?

Chances are you have without knowing it. Philosophers use them a lot. As mental games, they are often contrived and artificial. By design, they are not meant to be applied in real life. Rather, their purpose is to tease out particular aspects of an issue in order to better comprehend both the issue itself and how we reason it out.

For example, someone poses a hypothetical situation to you: If you knew that this is your last day alive on earth, how would you spend it? The person is not implying that you are actually going to die tomorrow. They pose the thought experiment as a way to get to know you better, to understand how you think about the world. By pretending to put you in such an extreme and unlikely scenario, they are asking you to reflect upon and share your values with them.

So I am going to present to you a thought experiment. Now remember, this is *not real*! Don't get all heated up about it as though it could really happen; it can't. Ready? Here we go.

I have developed a medical program that I will offer to you completely free of charge. You can opt out at any point.

This program, if followed to the letter, will offer you many rewards. Specifically, I absolutely guarantee that if you cooperate, you will live to be two hundred years old and be perfectly healthy every day of your life. (Remember—this is just a thought experiment!)

During your two hundred years, you will not suffer from any disease or illness. For example, if you fall and break your leg, it will be instantly healed without sequelae. You will incur no physical pain of any kind. You will be as hale and hardy on your two-hundredth birthday as you were every other day. And the evening of that momentous birthday, you will go peacefully to bed and die suddenly, and without discomfort, in your sleep.

Sound interesting? Want to hear more?

To further entice you, I assure that you will never have to endure anything unwanted. For instance, if you can't stomach opera, you will never be subjected to opera. The same will be true if you can't stomach rock 'n' roll.

If you hate vegetables, you will never have to eat them. Same if you hate tofu. If you detest reading, you will never have to do so. Furthermore, if you detest exercise, you will be under no obligation to do that either.

And so on. Get my drift?

Remember, this is all free and guaranteed. Want to sign up?

Wait, you are wondering if there is a catch?

Ah, good question! Because there is always a catch when it comes to thought experiments (so get used to it). That's what makes them so useful.

Yes, I admit there is one small catch. Well, maybe not so small.

For the entire duration of your two-hundred-year lifespan, you will not be allowed to do anything you really enjoy.

If you love chocolate ice cream, you can't have it, but of course we will never force you to eat vanilla if you hate it. If you are neutral about banana ice cream, then there will be lots of that for the taking.

If you abhor playing soccer, then no soccer for you. However, if hockey is your game, there will be none of it either. Indifferent to tiddlywinks? Then play as much as you want.

If you treasure living in the country but loathe life in the downtown, we'll stick you in the suburbs.

Should you come to enjoy something you didn't enjoy before, it will then become off-limits. Conversely, if you find yourself despising something you once felt neutral about, it, too, will cease.

If you...need I go on? I'm sure you get the picture.

Okay, excited to sign up? What, you are having second thoughts? How come?

What fun is there in living if all of the things you love doing you can't do, you are asking?

If all of the people you like doing things with can't do those things with you, then what will give your life meaning, you wonder?

If you are not allowed to use your talents to accomplish things you desire, then what is the purpose of your existence, you implore?

Come on now! I am guaranteeing you safety and health for two hundred years! Moreover, it's all free! You seem a little unappreciative.

Well, for what it's worth, I agree with you. I haven't signed up either. In fact, having presented this program to many, many people, I have yet to have anyone sign up.

Why is that?

The answer takes us to a discussion of axiology—the study of values.

Chapter 20

Values

We are more likely to make ethical mistakes trying to reconcile the irreconcilable than living with the irreconcilable and acknowledging that we are doing so.

—Margaret Somerville, *The Ethical Imagination*

VALUES: IDEAS, IMAGES, notions we use to explain why various realities matter to us; values attract us, and we aspire after the good they articulate; things that are valued are referred to as "the good"

Axiology: the study of the origin of values and types of values

Whether you realize it or not, you have values. In fact, you probably have lots of them. Like most of us, you likely treasure your family, friends, and community. People generally desire a home and steady employment. We are willing to spend energy and money on hobbies, entertainment, and pastimes. We consider these to be good things in our lives; we value them.

That's why you were not interested in my medical program. It was devoid of many of the things that give your life pleasure and meaning.

There are two aspects of values that are worth exploring. The first is that there are different categories of values. The second is that not all of our values have equal weight. Both of these concepts probably make intuitive sense to you, but we often forget them when we are making decisions in our lives.

Let's start by exploring how we categorize values. One way to catalogue values is by examining *how* they are valuable to us. Another is to explore *why* they are valuable to us. Let's look at the *how* question first.

Some values we refer to as "intrinsic." They provide value to us *directly*. In a straightforward fashion, they help us to realize our full potential as human beings. For example, we value freedom in principle because it reflects and respects our individuality as conscious and sentient beings. It is a desirable foundation for our lives. We value education for the same reason. We may value the arts or athletics in a similar fashion; we enjoy them.

Health, which for the sake of simplicity I will define as at minimum the absence of any disease or illness that interferes with our self-actualization, can be seen as an intrinsic good. All things considered, we would prefer to be free of disease or illness as a starting point from which to launch our lives.

On the other hand, some values are *instrumental*. How do they operate compared to intrinsic values? Instrumental values benefit us not so much by what they offer us directly as by what they facilitate for us *in*directly.

For example, political institutions have an instrumental value to us because they enable and safeguard (hopefully) our freedom, which is an intrinsic value as we have seen above. The same is true of schools, art galleries, and sports arenas; they facilitate the acquisition of the intrinsic goods of education, the arts, and athletics. You can probably see that many values can be both intrinsic and instrumental at the same time.

What about health care? Is it an intrinsic value or an instrumental value or both?

If you think back to our thought experiment, you are probably starting to realize that, indeed, health has instrumental value as well as intrinsic value. True, in and of itself, being healthy is a good thing—who wants to be in pain, for example? Who would choose to be blind? But being healthy also facilitates our attainment of so many of the other intrinsic goods we savour. It's harder to enjoy music if we are deaf. It can be significantly more challenging to enjoy sports if we are physically incapacitated. It may be incredibly difficult to become more learned if we have incurred a serious brain injury.

Is it possible, in fact, that the instrumental value of health care is more precious to us than its intrinsic value?

I think that our thought experiment might be telling us just that. And if that is true, then we have some sobering repercussions to face.

Firstly, we need to acknowledge that health is not the only intrinsic value in our lives. We also value freedom, education, the arts, athletics, et cetera. Health without all of these leads to a rather shallow, meaningless life as we have seen in our thought experiment. So we need a balance among all of the various intrinsic goods.

Secondly, health *may not be the most important intrinsic value*. We don't need to be perfectly healthy, nor do we need a guarantee of a two-hundred-year lifespan to be happy and content. A modicum of good health will allow for a reasonably full life. In fact, on a regular basis all of us risk our health to engage in experiences we consider valuable. We leave our homes and cross streets, drive cars, fly in planes, downhill ski, and try new foods. This means, ultimately, that compromising all other goods to the high altar of perfect health cannot give us what we really desire from our lives: a smorgasbord of experiences, challenges, and depth.

Thirdly, we need to see health care as a *means* to an end

(instrumental) as well as an *end* in itself (intrinsic). We do not want people to suffer from poor health, but we must be cognizant that they can suffer lots of other ways, through political persecution, through deprivation of personal fulfillment, and through economic strife. We need to manage health care such that all other aspects of people's lives receive the appropriate attention to allow for the development and protection of the complete person.

So health is not the only value we have. It will not always trump all other values, and its greatest applicability in our lives may reside more in its instrumental value than its intrinsic value.

Finally, this implies the necessity of boundaries to health care. We cannot let fear run rampant and allow health-care concerns to bulldoze over all of the other values and types of suffering. We may have to make decisions about health care based not on an isolated desire to have perfect health, but in the context of whether certain choices facilitate the acquisition or maintenance of other intrinsic values. For example, we cannot afford to compromise the integrity of our political or judicial systems by putting all of our attention and resources into attaining perfect health to the detriment of personal or communal freedom. Health-care decisions will of necessity have to be made using, to some degree, a utilitarian calculus that respects and upholds our other values. Health is more a facilitator of a full and balanced life than the sole constituent of a one-dimensional life.

So we have explored the cataloguing of values on the basis of *how* they are valuable to us. Now let's investigate the *why*.

If you think about the various aspects of your life that you value, you may notice that they fall into two groupings. We have explored this before, but it is worth a second look because of its importance.

The first group is composed of things that primarily give you pleasure. I play hockey, and I am willing to take time out of my life, pay money, and take risks to engage in this behaviour. You may well wonder what one could possibly enjoy about having people fire a hard rubber disc at you (remember I am a goalie), and to be honest, I can't explain it to you. I don't understand why players like to make me look bad by launching the puck into the net behind me either. Be that as it may, we all enjoy certain experiences because they resonate within us; it is highly personal. Some people like rock 'n' roll, others like opera.

More important about this group, however, is that we do not feel that everyone ought to prefer what we prefer. I like stopping pucks; others enjoy shooting pucks. We might *like* others to enjoy the same music we do, but we do not see any need for them to *have* to feel the same way we do.

The second group is quite different, however. It is composed not of things we like to experience but rather of attitudes and behaviours that we feel we should exhibit toward others. Critical to this group is a sense of universalizability of these values. We can accept that not everyone fancies impressionist paintings, but we would like to have everyone agree not to inflict unwanted pain on others.

The first group of values is referred to as "aesthetic." For aesthetics, the answer to the question "Why do you value it?" is that we find it personally pleasing in a sensual sense. The second group of values is referred to as "ethics." For ethics, the answer to the question "Why do you value it?" is that we think this is how all of us should treat one another in a moral sense, not in a sensual sense.

So we have covered the categories of values in both the *how* sense and the *why* sense.

As mentioned above, the second interesting aspect of values is that they are not all equally weighted. I would much sooner give up ice cream, as much as I enjoy it, than give up playing hockey. I believe that we should not lie to each other, but I feel extremely strongly that we should not kill each other.

Hopefully, we feel more strongly about the importance of ethical values than aesthetic values, but I am not sure that that is always the case. So, as we shall see, this prioritizing of values can get very complicated. And to make matters worse, our values, aesthetic and ethical, often change over time, and that has potential to be a very good thing.

It's important to realize that any lasting and loving relationships are always based on shared ethical values. Ethical values, not aesthetic values, are the glue that keep us together. Shallow relationships based on aesthetic values fade when times get tough; deeply mature and loving relationships don't because they are based on ethical values. Occasionally, as we get to know others better, we discover that their ethical values have changed, or we simply come to recognize and understand their values better. That may draw us closer together or push us further apart, irrespective of our aesthetic tastes.

I remember my grandmother saying, "Tell me your company [the people you hang around with], and I'll tell you your name." It is so true. We are often initially attracted to people who have similar likes and dislikes, but what keeps us together are shared ethical values. So we can tell a lot about you by seeing the ethical values of the people you hang around with. If you associate with people who cheat or lie or abuse others, we are going to assume that you share similar values. Either you don't value honesty and compassionate treatment of others very highly, or some other values outweigh them. If we really value honesty and compassionate behaviour, those other values better be pretty impressive or else we won't be impressed, at least in a good way, with you and your "associates."

This brings us to the topic of judging. It is curious these days how much we claim to be against judging—"live and let live" is part of the common parlance. I understand where it comes from. At a very deep level we are insecure, and anything that challenges our existing neural networks—particularly our internal heuristics—feels very threatening.

But how do we grow if we do not reflect upon our own thoughts and behaviours? For example, we often stress the importance of role models. But by definition, a role model is someone you have assessed to be worthy of emulating, which means that someone you do not consider a role model is someone not worthy of emulating. Isn't that judging? Who are we kidding?

So whether we want to admit it or not, in every aspect of our lives, consciously or subconsciously, we use others as a reference point for our own thoughts and behaviours. I assess the play of other goaltenders to see if anything they do would help my game. That's why I went to goalie school.

I do the same when it comes to ethical behaviours—how would people more advanced in their development handle a situation? What decisions would they make? How can I change, based on that, to become a better person? I want to compete with them, not in the sense of fighting them but in the sense of seeking with them to become more mature, more loving. It is not jealousy; I respect them and want to imitate them, not disparage them. As I have read, the only person you should be jealous of is the person you want to become.

Growing, maturing, requires that we admit to mistakes and even failure. Sadly, our culture sees mistakes as something negative. Even the Nobel Prize for scientific achievements tends overwhelmingly to be granted to discoveries that involve positive results rather than negative ones, even though both are equally scientific since they both add to our understanding of the universe.

People judge all of the time, *but they don't like to be judged*. Of course even that is simply *not* true. We *love* to be judged, as long as we are judged *positively*! We seldom tire of hearing that we're the best at x or are just amazing because of y. However, we are not nearly so enamoured by negative judgments, no matter how true, well intentioned, or helpful. As we explored earlier in the book, we can find introspection and self-reflection rather threatening at a very deep level and for good reason. However, growth requires us to do both of these processes.

Failure, like pain, is an unavoidable reality of life. We can try to minimize mistakes, but we cannot eliminate them. Nor, perhaps, should we aspire to do so. Innocent mistakes, ones not done intentionally to hurt oneself or others, are a necessary part of risk taking. And risk taking is a necessary element of living in a complex and incompletely understood world. We should do so mindfully as much as possible, but without risk taking, we would be paralyzed, living lives not dissimilar to my theoretical two-hundred-year program. We learn, grow, and build resiliency through making mistakes, provided that they are not serious.

Just like so many of our most important decisions in life, the process of determining values involves our entire person, including not just the logical left hemisphere but the creative right side as well. This means that values will have both rational and nonrational elements, but not contradictory, irrational ones. To a certain degree, how we develop our values is a bit mysterious, something I refer to as the "black box" inside of our heads—the mind.

Children do not have the capability of processing information and formulating the complex and abstract ideas and theories required for developing values. We need to mentor them, which means that we must assist them in developing the boundaries necessary in which to structure their creative thoughts. In truth, we never stop doing this throughout our entire lives, hopefully. We must constantly and mindfully reevaluate our internal heuristics, including our values, in our never-ending journey of personal growth.

We often think that our job is done as soon as we have developed the right values. But that is just the beginning. We need to be careful not to confuse or conflate aesthetic values with moral ones. Not everything has intrinsic moral content; moral content may be determined by how we use something instrumentally. One of the most challenging aspects of values is the fact that no matter how good your values may be, they will almost certainly come into conflict with one another on a regular basis. This means that in many decisions you make, you will have to carefully weigh different values against one another in order to reach a conclusion. Internal heuristics can't do it for you; you have to use your full mind to contemplate the solution, knowing that you must live with the discomfort of never being sure that you chose the best option. "Moral residue" is what the ethicists call it.

For example, in medicine we value truth telling, but sometimes patients are not ready to hear the truth, and we need to respect that as well. What do we do? How do we balance patients' rights to know critical information about their health and yet maintain our oath of *primum non nocere*, above all do no harm?

In the not so distant past, many individuals had few, if any, rights within their society. It is better today, thank goodness, but far from perfect. However, in the process of advocating for human rights, we have not realized a very critical element of the discussion: human obligations.

I spoke with a university student several years ago who was very excited about the human rights courses he was taking. I asked him if he was taking any courses on human obligations. He looked puzzled. Had his professors not mentioned them to him? I asked him how they can talk in an isolated fashion about human rights without speaking simultaneously about human obligations? He saw my point. You cannot have a right without me having a commensurate and parallel obligation to that right. The same holds true in reverse.

It's a lot easier to get people excited about human rights because it involves them *getting something*. It appeals to our primal narcissism. But people don't get nearly as excited about human obligations because that means they have to *give something*, perhaps even sacrifice something, which is much less fun. Politicians, for example, have learned long ago during election campaigns to promise rights to people, not obligations, if they want to get elected. How many of us are in favour of a policy that will *cost us* but benefit the collective? How many of us see paying taxes as a privilege earned by making enough money to warrant being taxed?

Because our health and even our very lives are at stake in health care, values play a critical role. So it's time for another thought experiment exploring values and health care.

But I have a funny feeling that a lot of you are not going to like this next experiment very much. Facing our deepest fears is seldom something we enjoy.

Chapter 21

Thought Experiment 2

We must safeguard each person's power to become fully themselves—when we do we are acting morally.

—Søren Kierkegaard

WE ARE NOT always consciously aware of our values; they often guide us from a deeply hidden place from which content and origin are not always clear. Often values conflict: we want to drive a fancier car, but we don't want to spend too much of our money on just a car.

Often we confuse values; a value we consider to be of the ethical realm may, in fact, be more aesthetic in nature. When that occurs, we can react as strongly to trivial breaches of protocol or etiquette in the same way we would respond to legitimate moral transgressions. Using the wrong fork at the table is not as heinous as stabbing somebody with a fork. We may see someone with a low pain threshold as a weak person morally even though one has nothing to do with the other. Often we base our likes or dislikes of others on fairly superficial aesthetic criteria.

Sometimes we think we understand our values, and we believe that they should be universal ones—values that everyone should agree with. We can be tempted to adopt a holier-than-thou attitude or react with righteous indignation rather than dialogue respectfully with others about their values and be open to change.

For example, many people think that age should not be a factor in medical decision making. They accuse people who disagree of being guilty of ageism, an unfair bias against the elderly akin to a bias against people on the basis of skin colour or gender. They consider ageism equally unethical. What do you think?

Before you decide, let's do another thought experiment.

Suppose we have one kidney available for transplantation, but we have two potential recipients. To keep it simple, let's call them Jim and Bart.

Jim is a twenty-two-year-old, quite healthy male. Bart is a fifty-nine-year-old male who has a minor health problem for which he takes medications. His life expectancy and quality of life are minimally compromised by this condition. Apart from this, Jim and Bart are identical in terms of all other factors that might influence medical decisions.

Now, both Jim and Bart develop kidney failure that can only be remedied with a kidney transplant. The one available kidney is an equally good match for both. The one who receives it will do very well, the one who doesn't will die. Again, except for Bart's trivial medical problem, which would in no way interfere with receiving a kidney, they are equally good candidates for the transplant. Who do we give the kidney to?

Assume that the doctors involved are convinced from a medical perspective that Bart's medical issue should not be counted against him in making the decision because it is so insignificant. For those of you who want to avoid being labelled ageists, do we then just flip a coin?

Suppose we do so, and Bart wins the coin toss and gets the kidney.

Bad luck for Jim, but since they were essentially equally good candidates, that's the luck of the draw, right?

Well, not quite. In this thought experiment, if you give Bart the kidney, not only does Jim die but Bart is dead as well. Confused?

Remember we talked earlier about making assumptions?

Well, you assumed that Jim and Bart were two *different* people. I never said they were. You see, Jim is the name this person went by when he was twenty-two, but as he grew up he developed the nickname Bart. They are the same guy; their stories are just separated by thirty-seven years. That's why if you let Jim die, then Bart will be dead as well. Jim won't be able to grow up and become Bart.

In case you didn't realize it, Jim and Bart are both me. My first name is James, which is where "Jim" comes from, and one of my many nicknames (thanks to my brothers, Frank and Steve) is Bart. I have a minor heart problem that I didn't have when I was twenty-two. The part about kidney failure is made up, of course. I have never had to have a transplant.

You are probably feeling like I tricked you, and in a way I did. But hopefully you also realized an important lesson.

Being old versus being young is *not at all the same* as being black versus being white or being male versus being female. You are the same ontological person when you are old as when you are young. We are not biasing against you—you are the same person, just older (or younger). A black person named Jim does not become a white person named Bart; they are two different people. Someone with XY chromosomes named Bart does not develop XX chromosomes and become Jamie; they are two different people.

I have been blessed with three grandchildren. Does anyone honestly think, all other things being equal, that they and I should have equal claim to a kidney for fear of ageism? I hope not. It would be profoundly narcissistic of me to feel that I have an equivalent claim. I have lived for fifty-nine years; they have the right to do the same before I should be blessed with any more.

Let's be honest: life is sweet, and we are all afraid of losing it. Just like the reptiles, we cling to life at all costs. We find acceptable facades for our fear, inventing pseudobiases like ageism to justify our behaviours.

We complain that the elderly are deprived of interventions and treatments simply because they are old. However, all interventions and treatments carry risks, and the bulk of the risk is usually upfront, for example with surgery. The most likely time to suffer a complication is either during the surgery or very soon after. And the older we are, the more likely are the complications, particularly because we often have accumulated other concomitant diseases. So we have to pay a bigger price (more complications) right away to obtain less benefit (because we have other medical issues to detract from the value of the intervention) for a shorter duration (because our life expectancy is less). When we advise against interventions and treatment in the elderly, it's not because we are biasing against them; it's because as we age, the ratio of benefit to risks and costs (e.g., longer recovery) declines substantially.

Okay, so you might disagree with me if it were between you and your grandchild. But would you feel the same way if it were someone else's grandchild we were talking about instead?

Now level with me: Did this little thought experiment annoy you? How mad are you at me for tricking you?

You see, values are tricky things, and they affect us deeply. I am pretty sure that people over sixty have a different perspective on this thought experiment than people under thirty. There is no view from nowhere.

This reinforces to us that often our values change throughout our lives because our worldview changes. Two of the great challenges of ethics and values are fairness and consistency. Do you apply your values and ethical rules no matter what side of the coin you are on? Or is there one set of rules for you and a very different set for other people? Is it okay when you cheat but not when they cheat? Or do your rules change willy-nilly depending on your particular circumstances? Are you as compassionate and reasonable with others as you would like them to be with you?

We have to remember that we do not just see the world, we interpret it: not merely with our senses and brain, but also through our mind and our values. We are biased by our values, and our values are biased by our experiences and the shared experiences of others (among other things). A big part of that involves feelings of many different kinds, not just logic. Objectivity is a myth—we do not develop our values in a vacuum devoid of emotion and personal motives. To some degree, we are always invested in our values.

This means that all of us can behave inconsistently and unfairly, especially when we are afraid, because we all have narcissistic tendencies. And the higher the stakes, the more likely we are to look out for number one.

But there is a more important message from this thought experiment. Every morning I wake up, and as I make my way to the shower, I am surprised by who I see in the bathroom mirror. I still feel the same as that twenty-something-year-old me, but I am clearly a grey, much more wrinkly and saggy Barry.

We are so influenced by appearances, by superficial perceptions and feelings, by aesthetics. We are so driven by fear, pain, and the pursuit of pleasure. We can come to believe that we are the dye in our hair, the ink tattooed into our skin, the spare tire around our middle, our age, our gender, the piercings dangling from our extremities, the perfectly faded and torn designer blue jeans we wear, the titles we have, the colour of our skin, the stuff we own, the places we have been, or the talents that we have. But those are not who we are; we are something deeper—our ontological selves. With mindful introspection and self-reflection, we can come to know who we really are and try to accept, and love, who we really are. But it can take a lifetime to do so.

And there is one time in our lives, in particular, when we are faced with that opportunity. It's a time that terrifies us the most, something even doctors don't like to talk about: death.

Chapter 22

Death

An ordinary man will work every day for a year shovelling dirt to support his body, or a family of bodies, but he is an extraordinary man who will work a whole day in a year for the support of his soul.

—Henry David Thoreau

LET'S BE HONEST with each other: this is not a chapter many people are going to want to read, nor one many will enjoying reading. But given its importance, it ought not be avoided. If we are going to grow, we need to deal with the really tough stuff too.

As I said earlier in the book, it is somewhat bizarre that few medical schools or residency programs have a course specifically on the topic of death, especially since there are few disciplines where death is not a possibility. Even specialists like dermatologists and ophthalmologists are going to interact with people who are dying even if they are not dying directly of a skin or ocular problem.

I will start this chapter with a rather uncomplimentary statement of our culture and our health-care system: we deal with death in a very binary fashion. In other words, our approach to death is immature. Before you freak out on me, let me explain.

Years ago, I read that two-thirds of all people dying do so without a will (intestate). It's as though they think they are never going to die. We don't even like using the D-word. Instead, we choose less painful euphemisms like "pass on" or "cross over." I fully appreciate why we do this; I do it sometimes too.

But there is a more important reason why I say that we are immature in our dealing with death. At one end of the binary spectrum, we avoid acknowledging the possibility of death and do everything we can to prevent it. As proof, the statistics reveal that somewhere between 50 and 80 percent of all the money spent on health care for an individual will be spent in the last six to twelve months of a person's life. It would not be an exaggeration to call our system a death-avoidance system not a health-care system. It wouldn't be so embarrassing if the money and resources were spent wisely and provided individuals and their families with wonderful palliative care experiences in their final days. But far too many individuals die in sterile hospital settings or in facilities that are unsuitable or underfunded.

Even more tragic, in many Western countries this approach often leads to the inevitable situation where life becomes unbearable, and now we are choosing to leap to the other end of the spectrum: physician-assisted death and euthanasia. Just about as binary as it gets: prolong your life for as long as possible using any means possible then essentially resort to killing you when we run out of options and you're in misery (and we are too).

Now I know that sounds rather harsh, but there was a time when we lived in smaller or more rural communities, and we saw death on a regular basis. We saw plants die. We witnessed, even engaged in, the death of animals on farms. We experienced the deaths of our pets, not in veterinary clinics but in our homes. We took care of ailing grandparents in our humble abodes, not in government or for-profit residences. Death was not necessarily always embraced but neither was it denied and avoided. We were thrown into the full spectrum of death, and we learned to deal with the tensions it presented.

By that I mean we came to realize that death could not be cheated indefinitely and that the goal was as much for a pleasant exit surrounded by loved ones as it was for a maximum duration of life. We lived the tension of balancing the two. Modern medical science has done a lot to prolong life and reduce needless pain, but it has also unwittingly helped us to avoid dealing with this tension.

Part of this is because we have come to worship science and logic. We have fallen in love with all things *quantitative*: age, tumour size, blood pressure, cholesterol level, et cetera. Studies on cancer treatments are judged almost exclusively on the quantitative measure of life prolongation (often only months). Qualitative things seem to elude medicine; we are ruled far more by our left hemisphere than our right. Our left hemisphere counts the trees; our right hemisphere recognizes the grandeur of the forest. Even when we deal with quality of life issues, we want to quantify them.

Now it is common for people to die of "a million little cuts." In other words, we continue to treat every possible cause of death, and so we die slow and lingering deaths in a state of perpetual angst. There was a time when we referred to pneumonia as "the old man's friend." No longer. We have forgotten that you actually have to die *of something*. For example, nobody really dies of cancer per se; they die of complications that cancer predisposes us to, like pneumonia. And those illnesses, of which there are many, are often ordinary *and treatable*. So we treat them because we cannot have an adult discussion about the many other possibilities that lie along the spectrum between continual avoidance of death at one end and killing on the other.

Physicians are not trained to talk about the dying process, and the public often prefers to avoid the discussion anyway. We choose not to dialogue about the many ways there are to die naturally along the spectrum. Illnesses that could lead to our final demise relatively comfortably if only we would let them.

Many years ago, when I took care of patients in nursing homes, I had under my care an elderly lady with moderately severe dementia. She developed pneumonia and was quite unwell. I presented the options to the family. At one end of the spectrum, we could simply keep her comfortable among the people who had cared for her for the last several years and comfortably let nature take its course, whatever that would be. The other end of the spectrum would be very aggressive treatment including transfer to an ICU and even intubation and ventilation.

The family struggled with the decision but eventually opted for transfer to the hospital with intravenous antibiotics, but without highly aggressive interventions like the ICU.

After a few days in hospital, she started to improve, but of course she became even more confused as she was still very sickly and in a facility that was completely foreign, among people she did not know. One day she tried to get out of bed and fell, breaking her hip. Now she had to go to the operating room to have that repaired. Not doing so was not an option as nursing her for the weeks it would take for her hip to heal on its own would be miserable for her.

During the surgery, she had a heart attack and postoperatively developed heart failure, so she was admitted to the coronary care unit. After a few days there, she was transferred to the regular hospital ward to recover from her surgery, heart attack, and heart failure.

I would strongly suggest that you spend as little time as a patient in hospital as you can. I say that because hospitals are loaded, not surprisingly, with lots of germs, and some of them can be quite resistant to even the best antimicrobials. Sadly, this lady developed another pneumonia. However, this time it was too much for her. In her now emaciated and immune-compromised state, she could not fend off the organism even with powerful intravenous antibiotics. The family did not want her in an ICU or on ventilators, and she peacefully succumbed to her illness a few days later.

One daughter sent me a letter some time later thanking me for my care but also reflecting about a conversation we had had when her mother had first developed pneumonia in the nursing home. She remembered me mentioning that we can treat a lot of medical illnesses, but our treatments are not always affective. Our treatments work in conjunction with the patient, not independently, so the patient's status is a large determinant of success. More importantly, she recalled that I had said that often we are offered an opportunity to choose how we might die. If we know that our time is near, it might be wise to reflect upon what mechanisms of dying we might want to accept, like pneumonia. When we don't opt for one of the less unpleasant and more manageable exits, the next one that comes along might not be so pleasant or manageable.

She saw the irony in rejecting what would have been a peaceful death in the nursing home among people who knew and loved her only to die of the same illness in a strange hospital many weeks later after having suffered through many complications in the interim. I encouraged her not to beat up on herself for the decisions they had made; the future is hard to predict. But I also suggested that like all painful experiences in life, this one offered an opportunity for growth because this would not be her last exposure to these kinds of decisions. Sooner or later we all die.

Look, I enjoy life as much as anyone, and I am not looking forward to being dead or to dying any more than you likely are. But we have to start talking about it a little more, have a respectful dialogue about the universal struggle of dying and death. For example, I am not at all sure that I want to get the flu shot when my time seems near. I would much rather die a few months too soon of the flu than have a long miserable demise while taking the chance of eking out every possible extra second of existence. That's just me, and you don't have to feel the same way, and I fully respect whatever sentiments you have on the matter. All I would ask is that you spend some time talking with your loved ones, mindfully reflecting on the various possibilities.

At the very least, have a will and ideally have a living will. My experience is that the details of the living will should be minimal. I say this because, as Yogi Berra once said, "It's hard making predictions, especially about the future." Studies have shown that often living wills are not followed very closely because they are overly prescriptive, trying to anticipate all possible eventualities, and that is simply not realistic. I think the most important thing is to talk honestly with your loved ones, the ones who will have to make the decisions when you can't. Make it clear to them what your priorities are *in general*: in other words, not what interventions you do or don't want so much as what quality of life you want to have and what likelihoods of success interventions should offer before opting for them.

A good example of this is the issue of sudden cardiac death. First of all, let me state clearly that I am all in favour of the widespread availability of automated external defibrillators (AEDs), as well as increased education of the public regarding CPR. However, having done many CPR courses (as well as more advanced resuscitation courses) over the years, I am well aware of how questionable the science behind the protocols has sometimes been. Beyond that, there are three other issues that are seldom discussed vis-à-vis sudden cardiac death.

Firstly, we have often ignored the fact that the people administering CPR and using AEDs are humans, not machines. That means they have feelings, and they get scared. The early protocols tried to make CPR very scientific and exact, forgetting that the biggest challenges are not the technical aspects but the emotional ones. Chest compressions are *not* difficult to do; practising on a dummy is easy. But most individuals using CPR in the real world have never seen anyone die, and there is a profound difference between that and the artificial environment of the course where they learned CPR (especially if you know the person you are working on).

When a real person suddenly and unexpectedly drops dead, it can be very challenging just to check for a pulse—your hands are sweaty, you are trembling, you can't tell if it's the person's pulse or yours you are feeling—let alone do simple chest compressions well. The goal should have been, and is to a greater degree now, to keep the protocol simple for that reason.

Secondly, I often found that there was little emphasis put on the low success rate of CPR and the significant likelihood that even if successful, the recipient's prognosis is often not good, particularly if their premorbid status was already compromised by other medical conditions. For example, AEDs are not good for all dysrhythmias, and the survival rate for combined CPR and AED is at best 20 percent in *witnessed* out-of-hospital cardiac arrests (unwitnessed are much worse). Furthermore, as many as half of all survivors do not return to their premorbid status (how they were before the arrest), and many never leave hospital.

More importantly, there is little discussion about feelings, especially if the attempts are not successful (as is usually the case). Sure, everyone is elated when there is complete success, but what about the guilt when it doesn't? Did I do compressions too quickly or not quickly enough? Were they good quality compressions? Is there something else I should have done?

Thirdly, there is the question of doing CPR at all. It is hard to imagine a more merciful way to leave this world when your time comes than a sudden cardiac arrest. We all have to die, and we all have to die of something. Yes, the discussion regarding the institution of CPR can be a difficult and awkward one, but sometimes it is also the mature and humane one.

You may believe that this business of dying is being dealt with well enough at the moment by the health-care system, so "if it ain't broke, don't fix it." However, the statistics regarding the higher amounts of money we spend at the end of life tell a different story. So do the studies indicating the relative scarcity of excellent palliative care (there could be a lot more). There is, as we have already explored, a finite amount of money available to health care, and we need to spend it wisely. In my opinion, we spend far too little money on good palliative care, including research, because we are spending far too much trying to avoid death quite literally at all costs.

Beyond the purely humane arguments for better palliative care and less aggressive prolongation of the dying process, there is a strong ethical argument as well. As our population ages, our present approach will simply become unsustainable. As we will explore later, sustainability is an ethical issue. Our children and grandchildren cannot be expected to pony up vast and ever-increasing sums of money for health care to the exclusion of all other social programs for which the collective provides.

I have no doubt that these financial issues will begin to influence our approach to medical assistance in dying. If we do not have the courage and maturity to explore the grey zones in the spectrum, as we run out of resources to provide the kind of intense care we have been providing, we will be forced to the other end of the spectrum to find solutions—medical assistance in death (MAID). I am concerned that MAID may devolve from a legitimate solicitation by the patient to a prescription forced upon them by impatient others with less than mercy-laden hidden agendas heavily influenced by crass economics.

Perhaps more importantly, the suggestion to discuss death and dying and reevaluate our approach to them is one encouraging us to greater mindfulness and maturity. The paradox is that by reflecting and talking about the finitude of life, we offer ourselves the possibility of enhancing our lives by slowing down and really appreciating this gift of life. The more we come to peace with death, the more liberated we are to deeply enjoy life. (Read the wonderful book *What Dying People Want* by Dr. David Kuhl.) I have often found it strange that once a friend or loved one dies, we often reflect upon the fullness, meaning, or purpose of the person's life, but we rarely speak of it while the person is alive.

If we are going to conquer ourselves and become the persons we want to be, we need to take time out of our busy routines and reflect upon the fact that life does not last forever. We may develop a greater sense of urgency and focus, rather than simply chasing mindlessly after more sensual pleasures while avoiding all pain, including the unwelcome realization of our eventual death.

If we are fortunate to survive into our sixties and beyond, we should come to recognize this as a great gift, one much more attributable to good luck than we would like to admit. It is an opportunity for us to reflect upon our lives and then to fine-tune them or even make wholesale changes. As I mentioned in my foreword, Søren Kierkegaard said that we "live life forward but understand it backward." In our final stages, we can try to make sense of our lives, prepare for death, and try to find meaning both in our living and in our dying.

I have noticed in Western culture a rising obsession with being youthful. We avoid telling people our age, we dye our hair, Botox away our wrinkles, whiten our teeth, drive sports cars, exercise to extreme, and chase after all of the exciting things youth do, particularly if we did not get our fill decades earlier. We seem to hold in high regard someone who continues to do the things of youth into old age. We resist aging, yearning for the energy, freedom, and exhilaration of being young again.

Perhaps not coincidentally, our culture does not value the more mature in our society. If you don't believe me, ask someone how tough it is to find work when your job has been terminated in your fifties! We do not see them as having anything to offer or contribute. It's as though nothing eventful or worthwhile occurs after your fortieth birthday. We are perceived to drift into a sad and pointless death spiral for which the only antidote is a return to the things of youth. We do not see old age as a distinct and important leg of the journey replete with its own unique and valuable challenges, goals, and contributions.

We do not appreciate the significance of slowing down to introspect and self-reflect. We do not value the cultivation of wisdom. Old age is when our bodies, including our brains, begin to deteriorate. But that does not mean that our minds do so as well. The pain of this deterioration, both physical and mental, is real and can produce suffering. But in the words of *The Torah: A Modern Commentary* by W. Gunther Plaut and David E. S. Stein:

Suffering does not heal, only suffering that has meaning and is accepted willingly has the power to heal and transform an individual.

I feel very blessed to have made it to sixty years of age given how many people I have known who have died far younger. None of them had had complete control of their fate, any more than I have had. I am overwhelmed when I think of the millions of things that had to happen, and not to happen, for me to be here today, and most were not under my influence. It is a privilege to get old, and we should be mindful of that. If we continue to cultivate mindfulness as we age—letting go of the things of youth and rethinking our heuristics, our values, and our priorities—then old age and death will not be things to fear. We have the power to not only transform ourselves but our society as well.

I would suggest that if we old folks care anything about the world we are going to leave to our children and grandchildren, it's time we changed. Racing around and only entertaining ourselves as we did in our youth is narcissistic and childish. Worse still is expecting to be entertained. We should be nurturing and mentoring our youth, not pretending to be like them. We need to do better than that. We need to conquer ourselves and role model the values we want our society to maintain after we are gone.

Perhaps if we did, we would be more highly valued.

But in order to do so, we must begin to understand the challenge facing us by delving directly into the concept of complexity.

Chapter 23

Complexity: Ethics

One cannot logically deduce "ought" from "is."

—David Hume

THE TOPIC OF complexity is so complex that I couldn't do it in one chapter. In this chapter, the first of three on complexity, we will look at the ethics undergirding the practice of medicine. In the next chapter, we will examine how difficult it is to discover truth by utilizing science in medicine. In the third and final chapter on complexity, we will explore the most complex part of the equation—the human organism, both body and mind.

Since the start of the Scientific Revolution almost five hundred years ago, we have been riding a wave of excitement about what science, particularly medical science, can do to improve our lives. The accomplishments are numerous and significant, so much so that many have come to view science as more than just a method of inquiry, its original purpose. For some, it has become a philosophical approach to life, almost to the point of becoming a sort of scientism. It's as though scientists have become the new masters of the universe, and they own the only lens through which we are capable of understanding our place in the cosmos.

The practice of medicine has to some degree followed this trend, which I find somewhat unfortunate. Medicine is much more than just a scientific inquiry into the functioning of the human body. It is a discipline that has evolved from a sincere, altruistic caring for one another. No other species does it to the extreme that we do. One could argue that no other behaviour we exhibit reflects our evolutionary progress to the degree that health care does: tending to the sickest and most vulnerable among us. It is an endeavour involving not just the chemical reactions of the physiosphere, nor just the organic processes of the biosphere, but one encompassing the noblest element of the noosphere—the mind.

This means that the heart of medicine is *relational, not physical or biological*. We value one another, we depend on one another, and we care for one another. And as I said earlier, ethical values are the foundation of mature relationships; they are what sustain and nurture them as well.

So as important as science is for the practice of medicine, we must never forget that the practice of medicine is ultimately an ethical, noospheric undertaking because it asks the question: how *ought* we take care of one another? Central to that discussion is the patient-physician relationship. Within it, and within all of the relationships between patients and all members of the health-care team, lay crucial values, some of which will inevitably conflict with each other from time to time.

Historically, as I alluded to earlier, medicine was a parentalistic endeavour: "doctor knows best" was the adage. In some parts of the world that may still be true, but in the Western world we tend to use the other three models, and in situations of greater importance, we tend to use the deliberative model as much as possible.

One of the biggest problems that can occur in physician-patient interactions is that the two parties use different models, perhaps without even realizing it. I refer to this as "ethical asymmetry."

Many years ago I had a patient, a young woman, come to see me because she wanted a tubal ligation to prevent pregnancy. She was twenty-three years old and had always felt some ambivalence about having children. Interestingly, she had been in a relationship with a young man for several years, and perhaps because he was interested in a family she began to consider the possibility as well. However, the day she came in to discuss sterilization with me was a couple of weeks after she had found out that he had been cheating on her. She was very hurt, yet thankful that no children were involved. To guarantee that that would never happen, and because she was fed up with men, by the time of our appointment she had already decided to have her "tubes tied."

The purpose of her visit was to clarify a few details about the procedure and have me make the appropriate referral to a specialist. In other words, she was using the informative model.

Not surprisingly, I was concerned, not because I had any problem with her getting her tubes tied, but because I wondered to what extent the pain she was feeling was unduly affecting her decision. Her previous mild ambivalence regarding having a family was likely influenced by her own childhood, family-of-origin issues. But now she was going to make a decision that might not be easily undone should she change her mind once this most recent heartache of her boyfriend's cheating had settled. I felt that I owed it to her to use the deliberative model for our interaction. I shuddered to think that she might meet a guy a few years hence, when she was still young enough to have children, and change her mind but not be able to change her body.

My duty is to the patient's best interests, but in such a dejected state could she or I be sure what her best interests, her deeply held values, really were? Further, might they remain unaltered permanently? We were on different wavelengths, so to speak. Consequently, the models we used for our interaction were not in sync. She wanted to use the informative model; I thought the deliberative model was more appropriate given what was at stake. There was an asymmetry in our ethical relationship.

I told her that I would be happy to make the referral, but I would like to discuss it with her a little more and perhaps have her see a therapist, as well, prior to proceeding with the surgery. She interpreted that as being inappropriate because her values and decisions were completely up to her. I explained to her that I was not questioning her right to her own values nor the content of them. Rather, I was concerned that her stated values at the moment might not stand the test of time if her disillusionment abated and that the two of us might both then come to regret her decision. I explained to her that what I do for a living is a little different than selling cars at a dealership. If I were selling a car to her, I didn't need to know anything about her values. As long as she had a license and the money, the car is hers. If buying the car would put her in the poorhouse, or for some other reason owning a car at this time was unwise, it was none of my business as a car salesman.

However, in my line of work as a doctor, I have taken a fiduciary (trust-based) oath, which entails a moral obligation to make sure that patients do not act against their own best interests. A salesperson does not have to assure herself or himself that you really can afford to buy their product or service. However, as a physician, I must be sure that a patient's stated values, and decisions arising from them, are not transient and situation-dependent.

She understood and agreed to think about it and return to discuss it once more before I made the referral. On the next visit, she stated unequivocally that she was sure that she wanted to proceed. After our pleasant dialogue, although still a little skeptical, I was sufficiently convinced to refer her to a gynecologist.

The specialist also had concerns and did the same thing I did, with the same results. About six months after her initial visit with me, she had the surgery.

Three years later she returned. She had met the most wonderful guy, and it was looking very serious. She wanted to know about getting her tubes untied. A little older and wiser, she now more fully understood what I was driving at three years earlier. I referred her back to the same surgeon, but we lost contact because she moved out of town. I hope that everything turned out okay for her.

A lot of patients don't realize the moral obligations involved when we take our oath as physicians. Many individuals who will offer you advice related to your health do not take such an oath. But we physicians are not allowed to function like a fast-food diner, providing your burger for you exactly as you ordered it. Because of the more serious ramifications of health-care decisions, we are expected to guide patients in decision making by insuring that they act in accordance with their values. Our first priority is for the patient's welfare, not for "the sale." That process takes time, but it also requires that patients know what their values are and that they have reflected upon them. It requires a certain degree of maturity and mindfulness. That's why, for the most part, parents make decisions involving the care of their children.

It is also why we have to will the good and growth of our patients as other. It is *their* values they must use in making their decisions around their lives, not ours. We must nurture their ability to not only reflect upon their values but also mentor them as they hone and evolve them.

How do we accomplish this, you may be wondering? We use a process referred to as "consent."

To consent to an action means that one is fully committed to it; we will it with our whole being without reservation. Because medical decisions involve our health and our lives, we want to feel very sure before we make up our minds. In medicine, there are three elements involved: disclosure, capacity, and voluntariness.

Disclosure means communicating to patients, in a fashion they can understand, all of the information they need and desire in order to make a decision. Centuries ago, doctors simply did what they thought was optimal, and everyone hoped for the best. With the recognition of rights, doctors were expected to explain the treatment to the patient but usually told the patient what the doctor thought they should know. Gradually we came to realize that perhaps we should share with every patient the information that most patients would want, not just what the doctor felt should be provided.

Only in the last few decades have we come to realize that because treatment is done to an individual, we should probably individualize the provision of information. In other words, we provide all information relevant to that particular patient's circumstances and further enquire if there is anything else the patient wants to know. It requires that we know the patient to some degree. For example, hand surgery for a concert pianist is going to cover a different, and more extensive, degree of information than it would for someone like me whose most sophisticated use of my hands involves eating chicken wings.

Capacity addresses a patient's ability to process the information provided in order to make a decision that is consistent with the patient's values. The default position is that all patients have capacity until proven otherwise. In the event that there is a question as to capacity, there are specific tools we can use to assess a patient's capacity. When the patient's capacity is in doubt, we may have to turn to the person the patient has designated to make decisions—a power of attorney (POA) for personal care. Patients can appeal to the courts if they disagree with the capacity assessment, and ultimately the courts will have the final say. Fortunately this is uncommon, but stressful when it occurs.

It is important for people who act as POAs to realize that their job is not for *them* to decide what should happen to the patient. Their job is to communicate to health-care professionals what *the patient* would say if the patient still had capacity, even if the POA disagrees with that. POAs are supposed to speak for the patient when the patient can't, not make decisions based on the POA's own personal values. It is always the patient's values that guide decision making, not those of the POA.

When there is no question regarding the patient's capacity, it is important to remember that although patients must demonstrate an ability to reason, they do not have to actually use reason alone to come to their decisions. In other words, as long as they convince us that they can reason, then they are at liberty to decide how they please. In theory, they could flip a coin if they want, provided they convince us that they understand the ramifications of what they are doing.

Finally, there is voluntariness. This means that we must be sure that the patient is not being coerced or unduly influenced in any way. The patient may seek or be offered advice from anyone he desires, and loved ones can try to persuade him through reason that a certain course of action is best. However, the patient must feel completely free to make the final decision himself, free of all types of threats, including emotional blackmail.

It is probably obvious that patients and physicians need to be educated about this complex process of consent. They both must learn more about the nature of their relationship and the unique fiduciary obligations involved. Those engaged in health care who must obtain licenses to do so are expected to follow a higher standard than people involved in other disciplines. The marketplace alone may guide unlicensed individuals who do not have to report to a governing body. For example, in the marketplace, guided in North America by capitalism, the motto is *caveat emptor*—buyer beware. Capitalism is neither good nor bad, moral or immoral. It, like all "things," is amoral—it has no morality of its own. It is a tool, like a knife, which can be used by creatures capable of moral behaviour, like humans, for actions that are either good or bad. A specialized knife referred to as a "scalpel" can save your life; a common dagger can take your life. The morality lies not in the instrument but in the user.

We can opt, for example, to apply capitalist principles within a moral framework if we choose, but we don't have to, and in fact we don't. But the same is not true for medicine. We embed within it a moral foundation that mandates, as we have seen earlier, a trust that physicians will care first and foremost for the health of their patients, not their own self-interests.

As I am sure you realize, this dynamic is a game changer. During years of training and countless clinical scenarios of all description, physicians are exposed to myriad medical problems. Some of these are uncommon, even to the point of being rare (canaries or black swans), and the public often has no inkling that they exist. This is why using the deliberative model for assisting patients in making decisions is so important, but it can be a tough tightrope to walk for physicians. In disclosing information, we don't want to be bullies or terrify patients, but we have to be sure that patients have really understood the potential consequences of their decisions, which is very difficult given how limited the medical experience of some patients can be. Not to mention, of course, the other understandable and universal factors related to naïveté and denial that complicate the process.

So it behooves us to explain medical information as accurately and comprehensibly as possible. This concept is referred to as "transparency," and it is an important ethical principle. But there is a problem inherent in this process. As we will explore in detail in the next chapter, medicine deals in probabilities and there is a difference between uncertainty and indeterminacy. If we are uncertain of something, we can attempt to gather more data and analyze it to decrease uncertainty and better delineate the exact likelihood of a certain outcome. However, in a complex universe, some things may not be able to be determined irrespective of how much data we accumulate. We see this in physics: we cannot simultaneously know precisely both the position and momentum of an electron; the more we know of one, the less we know of the other (the Heisenberg uncertainty principle). Some things are simply unknowable.

So this disclosure process is not always as straightforward as it seems. You might think that consent in medicine is like me deciding whether I want to order a dessert in a restaurant after my main meal is done. The waiter brings over the dessert trolley, and I peruse it to see if anything catches my eye. Ah yes, pecan pie, my personal favourite! Now I have to decide if I am too full to have it, does it look tasty enough to justify the calories, what is the cost, et cetera. There are a few variables involved in my decision but not that many. If I decide to go for it, the waiter will serve the piece of pie from the trolley, and I will joyfully ingest it, happy to have the cost tacked onto my bill.

But consent in medicine is quite different. If I consent to taking a cholesterol medication in order to prevent a heart attack, I don't know for certain whether I was ever going to have a heart attack, nor do I know for certain that this pill will prevent it. That's very different from getting the very piece of pecan pie on the trolley in front of me. It is more like buying a lottery ticket for a piece of pecan pie, lottery tickets the other restaurant patrons can buy, too, and none of us knows who is going to win the piece of pie.

Don't believe me? Well, then it's time to explore the ideas of risk and probability.

Chapter 24

Complexity: Decisions, Decisions!

When you know a thing, to recognize that you know it, and when you do not know a thing, to recognize that you do not know it—that is knowledge.

—Confucius

IT IS PROBABLY obvious that engaging in a medical investigation or treatment first requires making a decision. What may not be as obvious to both patients and physicians is the roles that risk and probability play in making decisions.

Our job as physicians is to predict the future, which means that all of our interactions with patients revolve around probability. There are two ways to interpret probabilities.

One is referred to as the "frequentist" approach, and the best example is the one we have used before—flipping a coin. If a coin is completely fair, then there should be an equal likelihood each time we flip it of obtaining a head or a tail. Although each flip is independent of all other flips, statistically speaking the pattern over time of a fair coin is to have the distribution of heads and tails approach a fifty-fifty ratio. If you flip a coin enough times, you will get a sense of how fair the coin is by the frequency of heads and tails. The same is true for a pair of fair dice. In artificial and simple environments like casinos, the frequentist approach works very well.

The other way to interpret probabilities is referred to as the "Bayesian" approach, after Thomas Bayes. It is more relevant to situations outside casinos because in real life there are usually many factors that affect the probability of something occurring, some of which are known and defined, and some of which are not. For example, we are aware of some of the many factors that affect your risk of having a heart attack, like smoking, diabetes and high blood pressure. This means we often have an a priori suspicion that some outcomes, like a heart attack, are more likely, or less likely, than others.

A good example is an exercise stress test. Before we do the test, we posit an a priori (beforehand) likelihood that you have heart disease based on risk-factor analysis—smoking, high blood pressure, diabetes, et cetera. It turns out that if your a priori likelihood of heart disease is either very low (which is common) or very high (less common), the results of the stress test don't help us much. If you are a low-risk candidate, a positive stress test is more likely to be a *false* positive than a true positive, meaning that, in fact, you do not have heart disease, and the test result is in error. Equally, if you are at very high risk, a negative test does not reassure us; it is more likely going to be a *false* negative, meaning you actually do have heart disease despite a negative test result. Only when your risk is in between does a stress test sway us one way or the other—either to reassure if negative or to suggest further definitive testing (like an angiogram) if positive.

This is not intuitively obvious to most patients and, frankly, to many doctors either. Statistics are tough to interpret, and it is easy to be mistaken or even fooled. I have seen many people who have felt very reassured by a negative stress test done during an "executive physical" at a private clinic, who were already low risk to begin with. The test was statistically speaking a waste of time because it told them something they already knew, though I doubt that was ever explained to them.

So why do we do these tests if they are often not very helpful?

Because our health is so important to us, it affects us at a deeply visceral level. Few aspects of our lives can incite the raw fear that the threat of ill health can. We know from quantum physics that even the best scientist cannot be completely objective—be outside of the experiment—and that is especially true if emotion is involved, as it is in health-care decisions.

No matter how much we try to con ourselves into believing that we can be objective, it is hard to maintain rationality when you are terrified for your own health or that of a loved one. That's why doctors are told not to treat themselves or their family. Fear can lead to a state of enhanced vulnerability for all of us and can result in some very unwise decisions. In fact, any time we are emotionally invested in something our objectivity takes a massive hit, although we hate to admit that. And there are people out there who capitalize on that, using vague statistics, anecdotal evidence, ambiguous terms, and frank hyperbole to mislead us. Often this is done quite innocently and with the best of intentions, but sometimes it is done in a consciously manipulative fashion.

We like to believe that because we live with our bodies all of the time that we understand how they work. We combine this gut feeling with a belief that we are reasonably intelligent and competent in many areas of life, like our workplace, and surmise that we can, therefore, assess our symptoms quite accurately with the help of Dr. Google.

By analogy, I drive a car, and I have flown in a plane many times.

I am reasonably intelligent and have some skill sets, like playing goal in hockey. *Ergo*, shouldn't I be able to fly a plane by consulting Captain Google?

If you see me in the cockpit, run for your life! The skill sets I have, like playing goal in hockey, and the understanding I have of the human body do not translate *at all* into understanding aviation. Neither does driving a car or having been a passenger in a plane. The reason why pilots have to study so long and fly many hours supervised before they can fly solo is because it is a unique skill set to learn and a difficult one at that.

When patients are afraid, they are more vulnerable and more easily swayed into believing anything, including what their vague recollection of grade ten health class is telling them. That's why it is important to obtain the guidance of someone knowledgeable who is not so viscerally influenced by your symptoms. They must still care but be able to allow rational thought to assist in making decisions. Most importantly, it must be someone you trust, who understands that it is your values that guide decision making and can mentor you in the process.

It behooves health-care providers to be cognizant of this at all times, individually and as a profession. We can unwittingly contribute to angst when we are careless or inexact in our attempts to educate. I am very concerned that as a profession we produce excess anxiety in the population with terms like "at risk" or "increased risk" or "high risk." What do those terms mean? How do they help? If your specific risk of an event is four times the general population's baseline likelihood of one in a hundred thousand, your risk is still pretty low (one in twenty-five thousand), even though you may technically be considered at risk or increased risk or even high risk. Data may be statistically significant but are they clinically relevant?

It's important to try to put these risks into perspective. Risk is everywhere; it is inherent in existence. Accordingly, medicine can only reduce risk so far. Cholesterol-lowering medications are a classic example. We are taught to follow guidelines that stratify patients as low, medium, and high risk. Please be aware that guidelines are often established by panels of "experts" who often have very close associations with companies that make drugs for conditions the guidelines are meant to address. Often these experts are also emotionally invested in being experts. If we are going to discuss with patients the possibility of taking a cholesterol pill every day for the rest of their lives, we should try to quantify precisely how much their risk will be reduced. We should do so in absolute, not relative, terms.

For example, if your risk presently is 15% and the cholesterol pill will lower that to 10%, then you have reduced your absolute risk by 5% (absolute risk reduction or ARR). But often the patient is not quoted this number but rather the relative risk reduction (RRR). The RRR in my example is 33% because 5% is one-third, or 33%, of 15%. This a ploy often used to convince someone to take the pill because RRR (33%) seems much more significant, and scarier, than ARR (5%) even though it is less meaningful to the patient. Why is this less meaningful?

Realize that two patients could have identical RRRs of 33% despite having very different ARRs: one having 1% (dropping from 3% to 2%), the other 20% (dropping from 60% to 40%). They might both opt for treatment if they only examined the RRR. But the ARR, if discovered, would likely convince one of them not to proceed. Tricky, eh? Maybe even sneaky?

Table 1. Comparison of ARR and RRR

	Current risk	Risk lowered by cholesterol pill	Absolute risk reduction	Relative risk reduction
Patient 1	3%	2%	1%	33%
Patient 2	60%	40%	20%	33%

Further, it is important to realize that there is an absolute lower limit to how much you can reduce your risk. Perhaps the lowest level you can bring your risk to, because of age and gender and other unalterable variables, is 8%. If so, is it worth it to take a pill to reduce your

ARR from 10% to 8% (2%), even though your RRR is 20%? Many times when you do the calculations for a patient with high cholesterol who also smokes, it turns out that discontinuation of smoking would reduce their risk far more than the cholesterol pill ever could. Wouldn't it just make a lot more sense on many levels—cost, prevention of other diseases, not having to take a pill—to only quit smoking instead? Problem is, if you only quit smoking, no one makes any money off of you—you no longer buy cigarettes, and you don't pay for cholesterol pills. Where's the fun (profit) in that?

No intervention we ever do in medicine works for every patient who receives it; zero per cent and one hundred per cent rarely exist in life, including the practice of medicine. This should come as no surprise; after all, there are seven billion of us on the planet, and although we share many similarities, we are not exactly the same. Even identical twins are not identical in every way. Our tendency to magical thinking wants us to believe that there is a magic exercise or pill or diet that will make everyone better; that's not very likely. So any intervention can be analyzed in terms of number needed to treat (NNT). In other words, if 50% of the people who receive treatment x improve, then the NNT is 2; you need to treat two people to make it worthwhile for one person. This means that for every two people taking the treatment, one person will take the treatment, pay for it, take the risks of it, suffer the side effects of it, but not benefit from it. Like golf, you want that number to be as low as possible, ideally one (but that never happens).

What do you think the NNT is for most cholesterol pills? The really good ones are 20. In other words, over the course of five years, one heart attack will be prevented among twenty people taking the drug. That means that nineteen people who take the drug do not benefit. They were either never going to have a heart attack anyway, or they had one despite taking the drug. Since none of us comes with an owner's manual, we don't know who will benefit and who won't. Very few patients are aware of the concept of NNT or its importance.

Equally, there is a number called number needed to harm (NNH).

It works the same way except it looks at how often someone is harmed by the treatment. You want this number to be high because you want lots of people to have undergone the treatment before anyone suffers significant harm. We don't tend to advertise this number much. I think we should. And it should be weighed in light of the NNT.

These concepts are used in discussing both treatment and prevention. However, many people do not understand that there is a significant difference between prevention and treatment. It's one thing to have a medical problem that is sufficiently annoying to prompt one to seek treatment. If you are already having a problem, it may be worth taking some risks for something that is very real in the present moment. However, it is quite another when you are feeling fine and you are simply worried that some risk factor you have *could* change that desired state of affairs.

It reminds me a little of the expression "Don't try to make a happy baby happier." When you do so, you risk making the baby unhappy; sometimes it's best to leave well enough alone. That's when NNH is more important—you should be more wary of taking significant risks right now for only *potential future benefit*.

This is a good time to explain the difference between primary and secondary prevention (remember that most prevention is really postponement anyway). Primary prevention is prevention done, for example lowering cholesterol, when one has *not yet* experienced any cholesterol-related diseases (and, in fact, may never).

Secondary prevention is done after one has, for example, suffered a heart attack, and we want to prevent another. Secondary prevention is a little easier to accept because you have already incurred harm: nothing predicts the likelihood of having a heart attack as much as already having had a heart attack. So it is easier to justify risks of taking medications to prevent another heart attack when you have already had one.

We would like to believe that the universe is very simple and that the future, therefore, is very predictable. But the universe is very complicated and complex, and despite our knowledge of risk factors, we are not nearly as good at predicting and preventing illness as patients would like to think.

For example, there was great hope at the beginning of this millennium that the cracking of the genetic code would result in unimaginable health benefits. We naively thought that simply knowing the genomic sequence of nucleotides would provide us with, akin to Willy Wonka, the golden ticket to understanding the human body, and disease would become a thing of the past.

Then we realized that there are innumerable epigenetic factors—factors of the environment in which genes reside—that influence the activation and manifestation of these genes. There are very few diseases we know whose sole and complete cause is a single gene abnormality. In fact, there are very few diseases that have a single cause of any origin, genetic or otherwise. The overwhelming majority are either known to have a multifactorial causation or we have no idea what causes them at all. (The fancy term for our ignorance is "idiopathic," which sounds impressive until you realize how much it sounds like "idiot.")

Beyond that, simply knowing the cause of a disease, including genetically influenced ones, seldom leads to an immediate and obvious cure. In medicine, the answer to the question why is often either elusive or unsatisfying if found. Most often it leads to the kind of annoying infinite regress that drove my father crazy when I was six and asked him why over and over again.

Our experience with the Human Genome Project should have humbled us into realizing how little we understand of the human body, but it appears we humans don't humble easily. In our medical training we learn about a lot of "canaries," uncommon or even rare conditions of which we know less than we would like, often because of their infrequency. They are often the ones that most terrify us; they seem to strike otherwise healthy people, often when they are young, in an unpredictable manner.

The problem is that although any individual canary is uncommon, there are an awful lot of different canaries out there. We hear about them constantly, and we trust that medical science has tests to detect them and treatments to cure them. But the truth is, for a lot of them we have neither. They are, in the words of Nassim Taleb, "black swan events," which are very uncommon or even rare events with an impact that is disproportionate to their frequency. Much like very infrequent but really massive (Richter scale 9.0) earthquakes, they are hard to predict but are devastating. No amount of preparation for the far more common smaller earthquakes (Richter scale 6.0–7.0) will help in either predicting or preventing the damage that a magnitude 9.0 earthquake will do. Medicine is much the same.

An example may help to explain this.

We do mammograms to screen for breast cancer in women over fifty, but the really aggressive breast cancers tend to occur in women far younger than fifty, women we don't screen. Obviously when a woman in her thirties succumbs to their disease, many more years of life are lost (in the prime of their life, I might add) than when a woman diagnosed at seventy (who usually has a far less aggressive cancer and far better prognosis). Only recently have we been able to detect a breast cancer gene that *may* be able to improve the situation, although the prevention is quite aggressive (prophylactic mastectomy). So we can continue to do mammograms for the overfifty crowd, but that will never help detect or prevent the black swans—the women much younger than fifty with the really aggressive cancers. The same is true for bowel cancer. (No studies have shown that screening all women younger than fifty helps, and there is legitimate concern that the radiation exposure itself could produce harm.)

Even when it comes to mammograms for women over fifty, the evidence is far from amazing, and the cost is significant. When we do not understand statistics well, we fail to appreciate how large a study has to be to confirm benefits of preventive strategies. You have to follow huge numbers of people for extended periods of time and monitor many variables (including potential for harm from these interventions, directly or indirectly) in order to prove effectiveness of a preventive intervention.

We are talking about tens of thousands of patients followed in incredible detail for many years, and that is both difficult and expensive to do. Often these studies reveal a reduction in mortality from the disease being screened, but overall mortality from all causes does not change nearly so much. In other words, often we can stop you from dying from that disease but not necessarily from dying of something else. We don't always understand why that is, and it is rather discomfiting.

Equally, although it would seem to make intuitive sense that there is an advantage in detecting something early, it turns out that that is not always true. We learned this with PAP smears designed to detect cervical cancer in women. We were performing far too many PAP smears, and in so doing found many abnormal ones that would have returned to normal spontaneously had we simply followed them. Instead we directed women to undergo countless invasive and unnecessary procedures with significant side effects. In the process, we spent a lot of money scaring and harming a lot of people needlessly.

Sadly, for many rare and aggressive diseases, and even for common ones, we have no easy way to detect their existence until they manifest clinically (unlike PAP smears). This is likely not going to change for a very long time. Why is that?

It is guesstimated that we have many trillions of cells in our body of which there are about 250 different cell types. All of them can become sickly, even cancerous. Our body does a great job of constantly eliminating most, but not all, foreign cells, like microbes, as well our own sickly cells, including cancerous cells. It's not until cancer cells become sufficiently numerous or out of control that we run into problems. So it is very hard to identify, and then find, the cells that are going to be a problem until, well, they become a problem.

Even if a dangerous group of cells could be detected with some blood test, that doesn't tell us where they are hiding. The resolution of our imaging machines is not down to the microscopic level. Even the best MRI has a resolution down to only about one millimetre, and that could represent thousands or millions of cells. By the time we have detected most cancers, for example, they are large enough to have potentially spread, and we have no way of knowing for certain if that is the case. A few exceptions are cervical cancers, where we can detect cells before they become frank cancers because of the ease of obtaining samples of cells through PAP smears. The same is true for skin cancers, where we can see the lesion with our eyes directly and remove them relatively easily.

However, when we say that a cancer patient has a recurrence, we are usually being a little dishonest. The cancer did not really come back again: often it simply never left after the first treatment. In truth, we simply could not detect it because we have no blood tests sensitive enough nor imaging tests refined enough to tell us that it was still around and where it was lurking.

If we look carefully at cancer treatment, we can see some evidence that the medical profession has been humbled over the last several decades, although we don't advertise that fact. When I was first in practice, there were regular reports of advances in improved *cure* rates for cancer; leukemias and lymphomas are good examples. But in the last twenty years, we don't seem to hear as much about new cures; we seem to have hit a ceiling.

The challenges of cancer detection mean that by the time we detect many cancers, they are often already a systemic disease, meaning that complete eradication is less likely. The treatments that are powerful enough to kill the widespread cancer cells are powerful enough to kill our healthy cells too. We may wishfully talk about finding a cure, but the reality is that the overwhelming majority of data provided from research treatment protocols today is about life extension, in other words palliation, not about cure or complete eradication.

In addition, research studies often use surrogate markers to illustrate that an intervention is helpful. We notice that a certain measurement is associated with complications from a disease and assume that any process that reduces that measurement will result in reduced complications. Diabetes mellitus (commonly referred to as simply "diabetes") is a good example.

Diabetes is a disease characterized by high blood sugars. High blood sugars can make you feel lousy, and very high blood sugars can be quite dangerous, so controlling blood sugars in the *short* term is very worthwhile. Further, we have known for some time that patients with diabetes have higher long-term risks of blindness, circulation issues, and heart disease (among others). We have assumed that the high blood sugars that cause short-term problems also cause these long-term complications. *Ergo*, if we want to reduce complications, we must reduce blood sugars through lifestyle changes or medications. In that vein, we follow a measurement, HbA1c (a blood test), which accurately reflects blood sugars over the previous two to three months. The reasoning goes that the lower that number, the less likely we are to see problems later in life. HbA1c is a surrogate marker, meaning that we don't care about a lower HbA1c per se; we care about what we hope it represents—fewer complications.

However, we have been disappointed that there is not always a precise, linear relationship between a lower HbA1c and fewer complications.

This should not be surprising. Linear relationships are not that common in a complex world. It also harkens back to the distinction I discussed earlier between correlation and causation. Just because two things happen together does not mean one causes the other. There may be a third thing that causes the two of them, for example. And often we don't know what that third thing is.

But there is more to it than that. One of the things we like to do in medicine is to isolate variables. For example, we do a study with a large number of patients who have myriad different characteristics (e.g., weight, age, gender, race). We divide them into two groups such that both groups have a similar distribution of all of these variables except for one, for example cholesterol: one group has high cholesterol, the other has low cholesterol. By doing so, we try to find out if high cholesterol is associated with an increased incidence of heart attacks, for example. (In fact, through complex statistical analysis that I have never been able to fully understand, people much smarter than me can tease out this information while looking at many variables.)

When we do these studies, we find this association to be true, that there is a *correlation*. We then proceed to develop a theory as to why that should be so, do some research, and discover, in fact, that high cholesterol may play a *causative* role in the development of heart disease. So far, so good.

However, factors do not exist in isolation—the biosphere is full of interdependencies. Flipping one coin does not influence the flipping of a second coin, but changing your blood pressure affects many things—your heart, your kidneys, your brain—all of which can affect your blood pressure in return.

We commonly infer that reducing this isolated variable—cholesterol—will guarantee a proportional reduction in heart disease and have no other undesirable effect. However, because the human body is complex, changing one variable may have other unrecognized effects that may mitigate the benefits. We see this in ecology all the time: we reduce one species (a pesky insect) in an ecosystem because we think it is a problem, but we fail to appreciate the profound ramifications that has on many other species, directly and indirectly, in a complex ecosystem. Small changes in the temperature of the earth affect all other aspects of weather, hence the concern about global warming.

In other words, isolating variables ignores the interdependency of multiple variables. I am sure you are as confused and frustrated as I am when the media reports unequivocally one week that a certain food is good for you, and the next week that it is bad for you, because it is good for one disease but bad for another. Mama Mia, what am I supposed to eat????

In addition, often a study will provide evidence that a particular drug is beneficial in preventing or treating a condition in a relatively healthy population. We then assume that it will provide equal benefit in very different and less healthy populations, as well. Or we assume that a drug that is taken in isolation will work just as well, with the same side effects, in patients who are taking multiple other medications. Starting to sound a little simplistic, you say?

We have no computer programs capable of measuring drug interactions involving more than three drugs nor can we be sure that each drug will continue to deliver the same benefit when many drugs are being taken simultaneously. Similarly, we occasionally see three separate interventions quoted as reducing the risk of a disease by 20%, 30%, and 40%, respectively. Does that mean that if you do all three, you reduce your risk by 90% (20%+30%+40%)? Not likely. Like linearity, simple addition is rare in complex systems.

Even in the situation of a drug that appears to be very effective, not all patients benefit nor benefit equally. We discussed NNT and NNH earlier. Some patients will be improved, but some will actually be made worse. Chemotherapy will prolong many patients' lives but will shorten some as well. We can quote percentages for different degrees of success (or lack thereof) of a therapeutic intervention for a population—some percentage will get great benefit, some medium, some minimal, and some only harm.

But like a lottery, no matter what the a priori odds may be, the only thing that really matters to any particular individual is how the person ends up. If a treatment helps 90% of patients it is of little consolation if you are part of the 10% it doesn't help. And we may not know that it doesn't help until after you have taken the drug for a while. Not only that, it may have harmed you in the process. As we saw earlier, most patients will not benefit from taking a cholesterol pill, so most will never be able to know whether they didn't have a heart attack because of the pill or because they simply were not going to have one anyway.

Sometimes patients want a better drug or a stronger drug. What do we mean by "better" or "stronger"?

A better drug is one that either has a better NNT or better NNH or preferably both. A stronger drug is one that has a similar NNT and

NNH at a lesser dose. A drug that is both better and stronger ideally has both a better NNT and NNH at a lower dose.

Suppose we have two drugs, *a* and *b*, with identical NNH. Drug *a* helps 33% (NNT=3) of people who take it, and drug *b* helps 50% (NNT=2). Drug *b* is a better drug. (If drug *b* also did this at half the dose, it would be stronger as well.) So if you are taking drug *a*, do you want to switch to drug *b* since it is better?

The answer is, it depends. If you are one of the 33% of patients who are helped by drug *a*, you do not want to switch. If you are one of the 67% for whom it is not helping, you do. The only exception would be if both drugs work for you, but you are being harmed by drug *a* and end up not being harmed by drug *b*. If that is the case, then switch.

Some would say that you should switch regardless because the better drug is the better drug even if drug *a* works for you. But think about it: there is absolutely no guarantee that because drug *a* worked for you that drug *b* will work for you. You could well be worse off because there is only a 50% chance that drug *b* will work for you.

Equally, even if drug *b* worked for you, you might suffer a side effect with it that you did not suffer with drug *a*. So beware of the temptation to simply opt for the "better" drug without thinking. If the drug you are taking is working with few side effects, you are likely better to stick with it.

As for a "stronger" drug, it is pretty irrelevant unless you are having side effects because the advantage of a stronger drug may only be a lower NNH. If you are not having side effects, it is often clinically irrelevant.

Finally, remember that a drug that is inferior but has been around a long time may be a safer choice than one that appears to be superior but has a less well-proven pedigree. I am loath to try new drugs with patients unless they are desperate because it takes time to know the full story behind a medication. Because of the nature of statistics, we often don't know the full story of an intervention until it has been studied in millions of patients (real life) not thousands (research studies). I am always leery of new drugs; I have heard too many miracle claims over the years only to see them fall well short of the hype or even be pulled off the market. Anybody remember thalidomide or Vioxx?

As you likely have perceived, it is easy to be confused by the science in medicine if you either don't understand statistics or the statistics are not presented well (or at all). A lot of this relates to how information is generally provided to patients: often by the lay media, whose understanding is not very good either. One of the biggest problems is that many studies are poorly done. They may not involve enough data (number of patients over a long enough period of time), or they are not properly randomized, for example. Without randomization, bias, which is inherent in any study, rises dramatically.

Often surrogate markers have been studied, and the results are conflated to apply to clinical conditions in a seamless, but potentially exaggerated, manner. Improving the surrogate marker does not guarantee that we improve the disease itself. A better cholesterol level does not guarantee that you will not have a heart attack ever.

Sometimes only favourable aspects of the study are released. Results are often overly hyped. It has only been in the last decade or so that *some* (but not all) of the major medical journals have required researchers to register their studies before they are done so that studies cannot be hidden if the results are not what people wanted. Often studies are done many times until one study finally shows the desired results, and then only *that* study is published, with no reference to the failed attempts. Registering studies before they are done is one way we can hope to cut down on this inaccurate reporting. Transparency is a crucial element of ethical behaviour no matter what the endeavour, so any time people are hiding something, beware. That is equally true for alternative and complementary medicine. It is tempting to be swayed by anecdotes, but ethical behaviour dictates that NNT and NNH be presented transparently no matter who is prescribing the health intervention.

Hopefully this chapter has served to educate not confuse you. The science behind the medicine we do is complicated and complex (as most areas of human knowledge are), but ideally we need to explain these concepts to every patient as part of the consent process. However, that is easier said than done; there are time constraints, educational limitations, et cetera.

In addition, there is one last level of complexity we need to explore, and we will do so in the next chapter. By way of introduction, let me give you a hint about what's involved.

Several years ago I attended a conference that included a session dealing with genetic testing. During that session, two siblings had been kind enough to speak to the audience about a fatal genetic disease that afflicted their family. They presented the case of their now deceased sibling who had died of this disease quite young and before testing was available. The two siblings expressed great appreciation for the thoroughness of the physicians who counselled and educated them about undergoing genetic testing to see if they carried the gene for the disease that took their sibling's life. The only option if the test was positive was an invasive medical intervention with potential for serious side effects.

Sibling 1 had clearly been very emotionally distraught by her sibling's death, so when she tested positive, she underwent intervention without hesitation. Fortunately, it was successful and without complication. Sibling 2 also tested positive, and although initially somewhat ambivalent, after much contemplation proceeded to have the same intervention but experienced significant complications. Interestingly, a third sibling of the deceased who was not present at the talk had opted not to be tested and, therefore, not to receive the intervention.

Sibling 1 was angry at the absent Sibling 3 for not being tested because that meant that Sibling 1 might lose yet another sibling to this disease if he had the gene.

At the end of the talk I spoke with Sibling 2, the one who did not do well after the intervention. I had assumed that a positive test for the genetic marker meant that there was close to a 100 percent chance of getting the disease. However, Sibling 2 informed me that if one tested positive, there was a 70 percent chance of getting the lethal disease between the ages of thirty and eighty. Now that is still pretty high, but it is not 100 percent as the audience, I believe, had assumed.

Even more importantly, I asked Sibling 2 what the distribution of the disease was during that span from thirty to eighty years old. Interestingly, despite the fact that both siblings had avowed having been thoroughly educated by the specialists, Sibling 2 did not know the distribution. I explained to her that the distribution might be incredibly important in decision making. For example, what if most cases occurred after age seventy? Or most occurred between thirty and forty-five, and because Sibling 2 was already forty-five, the risk of acquiring it now was much less than 70 percent? I was rather shocked when Sibling 2 had never thought about that!

I then asked Sibling 2 if the distribution had been calculated for different ages, how low would the likelihood of disease have to be with a positive test in order for them to have opted *not* to have the intervention. Again, they had never thought about that. They did eventually admit that if the probability of acquiring the disease had dropped down below 20 percent (in other words fifty of the seventy people in a hundred who would get the disease would have done so by age forty-five) they would probably not have had the intervention.

I refer to this mysterious method by which we make decisions as the "black box process" inside each of our heads. The three living siblings had all been provided with the same information, they all had capacity, and they were all free to make their own choices. And yet they all chose very differently; their respective black boxes processed the data but then came to very different conclusions about what to do next. Sibling 1 would have done the testing and if positive would have had the intervention no matter what. Sibling 2 was noticeably more reluctant. Sibling 3 chose to do nothing.

How do we humans weigh all of the risks, probabilities, and other data to come to a decision? Is there any way to assess what complex calculus we use? Or should use? Where does risk aversion or risk tolerance fit in when assessing consent? How can we know when people are making the right decision and processing the data properly? How much should fear or emotion affect our deliberation? How does someone really process, for example, a 5 percent chance of death or paralysis when contemplating surgery?

I don't think medicine can answer these questions at present and maybe not at all. I don't think we fully understand what motivates patients' behaviours. We offer a copious amount of information, hoping it will encourage a patient to choose what we think is the right course of action. However, we all know that data alone is insufficient much of the time. Not infrequently we resort to fear tactics, but as I said earlier, I don't think scaring university students about future risks of excessive alcohol is terribly effective.

That doesn't mean that the concept of consent is useless; it just means that it has limitations. We hope it represents the perfect way to make decisions, but it is an approximation at best. The black box mystery may be the unknowable factor that prevents us from ever being certain that we have done the right thing.

That complex organism called a human never makes it easy.

Chapter 25

Complexity: The Black Box

If you don't know where you're going, you'll end up somewhere else.

—Yogi Berra

IF YOU THINK things were complex in the last chapter, you ain't seen nothin' yet! Because now we are going to be talking about us, and us is complex: our physical aspects and particularly our mental aspects.

Every one of us is constantly engaging with our environment: we receive sensory input, process the data, utilize acquired or self-derived heuristics, make assumptions, engage episteme and techne, invoke deductive and inductive reasoning, and reflect in order make decisions upon which we act. There's a lot of information to digest, and there's a lot going on inside that black box inside our head.

I have to admit that in my experience, the black box inside of most patients' heads often has unrealistic expectations for what modern medicine can provide. In general, I think they overestimate the good we can do and underestimate the downsides. There are many reasons for this. Many relate to aspects of human thinking that we looked at earlier in the book. First and foremost, we are afraid. We all have a deep sense of naive realism; we like to believe in magic. Our left hemisphere likes to see patterns, even if they are not there. We see causation when there is only correlation. We see what we believe, and we believe what we want to believe.

One of the biggest traps that patients can fall into is their failure to appreciate how important their role is in getting better. It arises from a combination of magical thinking, naive realism, and fear. As I stated earlier, few diseases or conditions have a single cause, so not surprisingly few require only a single therapeutic intervention for improvement to occur.

In this vein, there are a number of things that make me chuckle in practice, and I am going to share them with you now. *Please don't be offended!* It's just that when I hear them, it is so obvious that either irrational fear or naive realism is talking (or both), but patients often can't see it as that (and they don't find it nearly as entertaining as I do).

For example, "Doctor, I want you to send me to the best specialist!" I am tempted to say, "Ah you're the one! Thank goodness because I am so tired of having all of my other patients request to be sent to a bumbling bozo!"

Or if I am having a grouchy day, I am tempted to ask, "What if this hotshot specialist doesn't want to see *you*?" or "What makes you so special?" (Patients often rate doctors; do you think doctors ever rate patients? How do you think you would be rated on a scale of one to ten? Are you the kind of patient doctors would recommend to each other? Bet you never thought of this stuff before, have you?)

I often wonder, too, what patients mean when they say best doctor? Highest IQ? Most knowledgeable? Most congenial? Most experienced? Most honest?

Occasionally, patients brag about being seen by the head of the Department X, implying that they are in the best of hands, as though because some poor sap had to take his turn at being department head that that automatically must mean he is better in his field of study. Being department head is seldom a recognition of clinical superiority. Even if the person is a great department head, that does not translate into clinical excellence any more than goaltending brilliance portends artistic prowess, or being a good CEO means you are a good mother, or a photographic memory implies great surgical skills. Being a great researcher doesn't mean you are a great clinician either. They are two completely different, and unrelated, skill sets.

Sometimes I will have sent a patient to see a specialist who said something the patient didn't agree with, so she asks for a second opinion. On two levels that request can amuse me. On the first level, they have already had a *second* opinion. They likely forgot that I probably offered an opinion, so technically *mine was the first opinion*, and the specialist I sent them to was the *second* opinion. Another specialist would actually offer a *third* opinion. Ha! Ha! The joke is on the patient—I went to medical school, too!

The second level that can occur occasionally is when a patient simply wants to keep seeing more specialists until they finally find someone who says what they want to hear. To be fair, there are many times when a third opinion can be very worthwhile, especially with conditions that are complex, rare, or require extraordinary intervention (or commonly when the relational aspect of the second opinion specialist just didn't feel right). But every once in a while, a patient just doesn't want to hear the truth (Mr. Smith, I think every lung specialist is going to suggest you stop smoking, sorry!). It is not uncommon in medicine to shoot the messenger.

But the one scenario that I find most telling is when patients say,

"I don't want to see Dr. Z. My friend had a terrible result with her." It never occurs to patients that the terrible result may have had nothing to do with the specialist.

I can think of very few times when I see patients that they don't own 90 percent of their treatment. A common mistake many of us make when we finish our medical training is to take too much responsibility for getting patients better. Any time a physician is doing more work than the patient, something is wrong. I may prescribe a blood pressure medication, but I also advise stress reduction, weight loss, a better diet, more exercise, and so forth. Even for a simple ankle sprain, the bulk of the recovery is in the patient's court, not mine. The patient needs to rest, ice and elevate the ankle, wear the brace, attend physio, and do home exercises. If the patient has already been following a healthy lifestyle, recovery will be quicker and more complete. It's mostly up to the individual.

Nowhere is this truer than with back pain. Back pain highlights a number of misperceptions that lay people have about medicine, so it is a great one to look into a little further as a way to explore the human body and how it works.

In order to treat a medical condition, for example back pain, it is best to first make a diagnosis. It may be a very preliminary diagnosis that will be fine-tuned as time goes on, but we usually have to have some idea of what we are dealing with. (In fact, we often begin with a differential diagnosis: a list of the most likely explanations for the patient's present symptoms and signs. The list helps us to focus our thinking so that we can come up with the final diagnosis.) So how do we make a diagnosis?

Remember I said that medicine is at its heart a relational discipline? When I was in medical school, I was taught that there are three things that contribute to making a diagnosis:

1. the history (in other words, talking to the patient, asking questions about their symptoms);

2. the physical examination (looking for signs); and
3. investigations.

In your opinion, what percentage does each contribute to making any diagnosis?

I'll give you a clue. The most important one contributes 80 percent, the next 15 percent, and the third 5 percent. (I was taught these in medical school, and after thirty-five years in the business I can attest to their accuracy.)

Well, any guesses?

Okay, I'll cut with the suspense. Eighty percent comes from *history*! Yes, as bizarre as it sounds, talking to patients is still the most important part of making a diagnosis (remember how much of our brain is devoted to communication?). That's why paediatrics can be so challenging—kids are not always good at expressing themselves. They may say their tummy hurts when they really mean they feel nauseated. It's particularly challenging when a parent brings a child to us from daycare because then we are receiving a history from the daycare people second-hand through the parents.

The next most important is the physical exam at 15 percent. The least useful is investigations. That's not to say that investigations, like blood tests and ultrasounds, have no purpose. It's just that they are seldom going to give you the answer if the history and physical haven't given you a pretty good idea what the diagnosis is and, therefore, the right test(s) to do to *confirm* that diagnosis.

Returning to back pain, if you do not do a proper history and physical exam when someone presents (that is, shows up) with back pain, back X-rays alone cannot give you the diagnosis except in rare circumstances. (For years, insurance companies ignored all sources of musculoskeletal pain if the X-rays were normal, meaning that the bones were normal. It is only starting to improve in the last decade or so by recognizing the many nonbony causes of musculoskeletal pain.)

Patients are infatuated with tests (and technology—the fancier the test the better), and they perpetually underestimate the importance of talking. Many times I have had a patient return after seeing a specialist, for example a gastroenterologist (a stomach and bowel specialist), complaining that "all she did was talk to me, she hardly touched me, and she isn't going to do a scope." Be thankful—it means she doesn't think there is anything seriously wrong like cancer or ulcerative colitis, you don't need to undergo a painful and risky procedure, and you don't need medications. You likely just need a better diet and stress reduction for your irritable bowel syndrome! Don't worry, be happy!

Making a diagnosis requires accumulating data and then processing it to produce a cohesive story that explains the patient's predicament. Logic is certainly part of it, but intuition, often gleaned from experience, is important too. And as much as it may surprise patients, the bulk of the data we use comes from talking to them. The better historians they are, the more quickly and accurately we can make the diagnosis. In other words, the more information they can give us from their observations of their symptoms (things they feel, like pain) and signs (things that are visible to them and us), and the patterns of those symptoms and signs, the easier our job. Wildly stabbing for the diagnosis in the dark by just ordering a pile of potentially expensive, painful, and risky tests is best avoided by taking a proper history. (Although sometimes we have to, for example, when a patient is brought in unconscious to the emerg. When patients can't talk to us, it is *much* more difficult to make a diagnosis.)

Although a lot of medical school is about cramming data into our brains, the most important part is getting to understand how the body works, patterns of disease and behaviour, et cetera. You cannot tell how a watch works by simply looking at the parts in isolation; you need to see how it is put together and how the parts interrelate to really "get it." This is no less true for the human body. In fact, although most areas of study in life involve specialized *information*, more importantly they require a specialized *understanding* of how things work. It's about learning how to think a certain way; otherwise, you are just going through the motions. (Ever listen to someone learning to play a violin?)

When doctors are first in training, we learn to "take a history," but in the beginning we do so in a very unsophisticated way, with a shotgun approach by just asking everything. As we gradually understand more about the human body and the nature of disease processes, we ask more focused questions, each with a very specific purpose, in order to tease out a diagnosis more reliably and intelligently. That's why, when we take a history from a patient, we ask pointed questions because we have to distinguish the signal from the noise.

There are many ways to look at the human body and how it works, but there is one perspective that is most often helpful as a starting point. In fact, it is so fundamental that the practice of medicine is essentially divided into two categories based on this perspective. We can look at the human body *structurally* or *functionally*. Historically, surgeons using scalpels handled the structure-oriented problems, and internal medicine specialists using medications, not scalpels, handled the function-oriented problems. That is still largely true today, but there has been a bit of blurring in this regard, like interventional radiology and cardiology.

Despite the limits of analogies, I will use one here to illustrate. Suppose you are buying a used car. The structure might look fine—there is no rust, the upholstery looks great, and everything the eye can see looks fine—but functionally, the engine could be a wreck, the fuel could be contaminated, and it could be a real clunker. Or the opposite could be true—it looks terrible but purrs like a kitten. You would want to both look at the car and take it out for a test drive before you would want to buy it. That's because both the functional and structural aspects usually matter when buying the car, and the two can be independent of each other to some degree.

So let's look at back pain. If you fall and break several of your vertebrae (bones of your spine), that is a structural problem, and as with most fractures of bone, you will need the advice, and perhaps services, of a structural doctor—a surgeon. The pain is constant because until the bone is stabilized, there will be pain. X-rays are good at diagnosing this because it is a problem of structure (the bone is broken) visible at a macroscopic (seen with the unaided eye) level, and bones show up well on X-rays. So we use screws and plates or casts to stabilize the bones, reduce pain, and protect the bones while they heal.

However, most back pain is not from broken bones but from non-bony structures. Ever since the discovery of X-rays, both doctors and patients have been mesmerized by bones. We often completely forget that there are lots of other structures (referred to as "soft tissues," as opposed to hard tissues or bones) in our bodies that cannot be seen with X-rays. Our *musculo*skeletal system does have bones, of course, but as the name clearly states, it also consists of *muscles* (and other soft tissues, like ligaments, tendons, and nerves).

Often patients are convinced that the only source of back pain is bones, or that only bones can cause really bad pain. I guess that's because we all know, or can imagine, how painful a broken bone can be. (Even when you break a bone, though, not all of the pain is just from the bone because, of course, all kinds of other tissues get damaged in the process too.)

If you do an X-ray, it will not reveal the source of most back pains because the source is usually from muscles or nerves that you cannot see on an X-ray. In fact, even if you did imaging that showed the muscles and nerves, like an MRI, you would still likely not see the cause of the pain because the pain is more functional than structural. The pain comes from spasm and inflammation of muscles or irritation of nerves, which are really at a microscopic (cannot see with the unaided eye) level. That is more a functional issue than a structural issue: how they work not how they look (remember the used car analogy?).

Muscles change—they contract and expand, on a microsecond-by-microsecond basis, at a microscopic, cellular, and biochemical level. Nerves get irritated by inflammation around them or sometimes malfunction on their own. Patients are often convinced that knowing exactly which muscle or other soft tissue is the problem will help, but imaging often adds little to a good history and physical. Imaging, even MRIs, are just *still pictures*, so they are very good at looking at static, that is, structural elements to see if they have structural integrity (like bones). Because they are still pictures, they cannot tell you how well a dynamic structure like a muscle works or a nerve works.

The analogy would be a golf pro looking at your golf club (MRI) as opposed to looking at video of your golf swing (physiotherapy) to explain your wicked slice. Physiotherapists look at dynamic structures like muscles in a dynamic way by listening to your story and asking pointed questions, and by examining how you move and where you are tender. Because most back pains are functional problems of soft tissues, surgery will not be helpful, and instead we use anti-inflammatories, heat or ice, muscle relaxants, and nerve-directed medications (all of which work at the cellular and biochemical level), and more importantly functional interventions like physiotherapy and back exercises to get better. However, if patients don't lose weight, watch their posture, do exercises, stretch regularly, et cetera, they cannot get better.

This dichotomy of structural (static) versus functional (dynamic) is a good example of the importance of *understanding* the human body. We humans tend to think primarily structurally because it is a level that we can see: it is macroscopic, more linear and concrete, and we like things that way. Functional problems, because they are more nebulous and microscopic, are less intuitive for us. For these reasons, patients are convinced that X-rays will help in the diagnosis; they seldom do.

In fact, the first thing you must do with any test result that is abnormal is ask yourself, Does this abnormal test explain the patient's problem, or is it, as in the case of Joe, a red herring? Back X-rays are a classic example of that. Yes, the bones may be tilted or twisted out of position, but they did not get there on their own. The soft tissues, especially the muscles, got them there because bones cannot move on their own. If you don't believe me, trying moving the bones of your back without using your muscles. So unless the bones themselves look abnormal, they are not the source of your pain. The things that got them into the unusual positions are the muscles, and they, or the nerves irritated in the process, are often the source of the pain.

Often it can be difficult to find the source of pain, or other unusual symptoms, because the problem is occurring on a microscopic level, where small nerves are being triggered. Sometimes nerves just do funny things. Tests can be disappointingly normal because the resolution of imaging and other investigations is not discrete enough to confirm the dysfunction. Sometimes we simply have to use trial and error in using therapies, assuming a nerve is being irritated by history but not able to prove it with tests.

Fortunately, we have often amassed considerable experience from seeing similar cases in the past so that we can clinically (that is, without tests) make the diagnosis and direct treatment even though no investigation can prove it for us. A good example is tic douloureux, a facial pain caused by dysfunction of the fifth cranial nerve (there are twelve cranial nerves—nerves that come directly from the cranium, not the spinal cord). The proof, as is often the case in medicine, is in seeing symptoms improve with time-honoured treatments, even if we do not completely understand them at a microscopic level.

Now there are three major exceptions regarding back pain. The first, although less common than muscular pain, is back pain from a disc bulge that puts pressure on nerves leaving the spine. Nerve pain has distinct characteristics, and if a nerve is being compromised, the history and physical exam will demonstrate this. Again, plain X-rays are relatively useless.

To confirm it, we can use specialized imaging that is capable of seeing soft tissues, like a CT scan or MRI, because disc related pain has a considerable structural component. (Patients often assume that any really bad back pain must be a "pinched nerve" from a disc bulge because that sounds really painful! Much like people with a tension headache will call it a migraine because everyone knows that migraines are always worse than tension headaches, right? Maybe not. Migraines can be quite nasty, but they are diagnosed not on the basis of the severity of headache but on multiple other clinical features. Tensions headaches, and other types of headaches, can be very painful, too.)

Nevertheless, a lot of the pain from a disc bulging is from inflammation that is produced when it bulges, and so only about 10 percent of disc problems require a surgical, or structural, solution. This means that the other 90 percent will improve with anti-inflammatories, ice, physio, et cetera. Disc disease is a great example for patients to understand that tests are almost always purely *diagnostic, not therapeutic*. In other words, they cannot directly make you better, so waiting for the test results before engaging in the therapy that is almost surely going to be necessary is not wise. The same is true while waiting to see the specialist. Do your exercises regularly and you might be able to avoid the scalpel!

The second exception is rheumatologic disorders like rheumatoid arthritis or ankylosing spondylitis, where X-rays are almost always normal or only subtly abnormal early on. That is because a lot of the pain is caused by inflammation in the soft tissues that occurs at a microscopic, functional level not a macroscopic, structural one. The treatment seldom involves surgery unless the disease has progressed over many years and produced structural changes.

The third exception is when back pain is a manifestation of some underlying sinister medical problem like cancer. People are often convinced that the more severe a pain, the more serious the underlying condition must be. We like to think in linear terms: more pain equals more serious disease. But as we know by now, linear is seldom true. Remember roseola? A higher fever does not automatically mean a more serious illness.

Sinister back pains are black swans; they are uncommon, but more importantly they have red flags (e.g., weight loss, pain unrelated to activity or position, other systemic signs and symptoms) associated with them. Physicians are trained to look for these; that's why you come to see us. The overwhelming majority of back pains are mechanical and have none of these features. That's not to deny the existence of these black swans, but we need to maintain a rational approach to back pain and not overinvestigate every back pain when we can, in fact, detect the worrisome ones clinically. That's where years of training and understanding the human body come into play.

In both structural and functional problems, the patient owns a lot of the responsibility for getting better. Even when major surgery is necessary, being fit, not smoking, having a good diet, and having a good attitude and social support are all critical for good results.

With back pain, a physician's job is to rule out serious but infrequent causes of back pain and then educate patients so they can fix themselves. Although back pain is one of the commonest reasons patients see family doctors, the average family doctor probably has at most one or two patients per year who require surgery (for a disc herniation) and perhaps only a couple who have an underlying rheumatologic disorder like ankylosing spondylitis or rheumatoid arthritis. Sinister back pains are even less common.

Our anti-inflammatories and mild analgesics will help, as will physical therapies, but the bulk of the work resides with the patient, and if they do not do their part, our part won't make much difference. They fix their backs by being very careful with their posture, being careful lifting, losing weight, keeping active, eating better, doing regular stretching and back strengthening exercises, seeing therapists to assist in all of this, using heat and ice, and reducing stress. Anyone trying to help you with your back pain is doing a disservice to you if they do not help you to find out why your back hurts so you can change your behaviours and prevent recurrent episodes. Equally, if they do not educate you about back care and prescribe home exercises in addition to their interventions, it will take you much longer to get better. There are one hundred and sixty-eight hours in the week; three hours of treatment per week can't make up for the remainder if you don't do your part.

You probably noticed above that I mentioned stress. What does that have to do with back pain? Or with any pain, you ask?

First of all, I am convinced that patients are far too busy and far too stressed these days. They don't find time to take care of themselves in order to prevent disease. They don't have time for a strep throat, so they want a quick fix. They want health care to be more convenient and less hassle, which I understand, but the hidden message then becomes "I don't have time for my health; I'll just have to squeeze it in when or if I can." Even workplaces can find it irritating when employees' health issues interfere with productivity through health-care visits and workplace accommodations. Sometimes I think a lot of people are more mindful when it comes to taking care of their lawn mower or laptop computer than they are of their own bodies.

Because we are so busy and have high expectations for everything, we dread the idea that a health issue might arise and complicate an already too-complicated life. This just adds to the existential angst, prompting us to scour the internet every time we have a new ache or pain. If websites presented information in a balanced fashion, it might be helpful, but in their attempt to cover themselves medico-legally and seem authoritative, they bombard the user with so much data that only the most discerning individual can differentiate the signal from the noise.

Secondly, stress management is an extremely important and often underappreciated aspect of healing. The strongest medicine we have for healing is our mind. Don't believe me?

Imagine the following scenario. Two patients are lying on stretchers in the emergency department. Both have identical fractures of their femurs, the largest bone in the leg. The emerg nurse, having already triaged the two patients, comes to you as the emerg physician with the X-rays, and the two of you comment that their fractures are identical and neither, apparently, has incurred any other injury. (Is this starting to sound like a thought experiment?)

The two of you step behind the curtain to see Patient 1, who, despite the pain of such a fracture, seems pretty calm about the whole affair. She understands that she will need surgery and that there will be a substantial recovery period, but she seems not only unfazed but almost giddy.

So you and the nurse proceed to the cubicle next door where Patient 2 is waiting. Patient 2 makes no eye contact, is weeping uncontrollably, and states that the pain medicine has not helped at all (even though it was the same as the one given to Patient 1).

Why the difference? The fractures and treatment thus far have been the same. What gives?

Some context might be helpful. Patient 1 has a supportive family, is in otherwise good health, and fractured her femur as she came running downstairs at home having found out that her lottery ticket had won her $10 million.

Patient 2 fractured his femur in a car accident caused by his drunk driving, and his best friend was killed in the seat beside him.

Do you think the pain they feel is different? Do you think the analgesics we use for Patient 1 might be more effective than for Patient 2? Their levels of *pain* may be similar, but their levels of *suffering* are vastly different. Do you think the prognosis for the two of them is different, too? Who do you think will heal more quickly and completely?

Patient 2 may blame the surgeon if his femur does not heal so well, but I am not sure that is fair. Equally, Patient 1 may praise her surgeon, but that likely isn't fair either. Doctors and patients alike often ascribe more blame and more credit to doctors than is likely justifiable. The universe is a complex place, and our minds play a big role in maintaining our health and facilitating our healing. So does luck.

We know that stress plays a huge role in our physical health. We also know that our physical health affects our mental health. Heart attack victims have a better prognosis the better their social networks. Equally, studies have shown that exercise can be as helpful for depression as most antidepressant medications.

Muscles, in particular, are commonly affected by stress; back pain is a good example. Why is that? When you think about it, the only way, apart from telepathy, that you can communicate what is going on inside your head is through muscles. You may smile, blink, nod, point, or talk. Your muscles are how we know what you are thinking and feeling. You can tell from a distance whether a person is relaxed or stressed just by the person's posture, for example. Asthma, irritable bowel syndrome, high blood pressure, migraines, tension headaches, back pain—the list is near endless—are all manifestations of muscle tension in our lungs, bowels, arteries, head, and back.

This means that our personal approach to our health, and our life, is critical for our well-being. Thousands of books and articles have been written about the mind-body connection; it is very real. Any time you have any kind of medical problem, it would be wise to ask yourself two questions: How is this medical problem affecting my mental health (because it always does)? And perhaps even more importantly, how is my mental health contributing to the development and manifestation of my medical problem (because it *always* does, too)?

In medicine, I think we often overlook the tremendous psychological affect that illness has on us. For example, the day you are told that you have diabetes you are a changed person. You now have an incurable and lifelong condition that affects every aspect of your life and does so every second of every day for the rest of your life. That's big. And I am not at all sure that classical medicine puts enough emphasis on the psychological aspects as it should.

Bigger still is how your mental health affects your physical health. We all manifest our stress through our body one way or another; there is simply no avoiding it. The mind-body connection is very real and very powerful. The more we understand our minds and the more we learn to be mindful, the better off we will be. I'll talk more about this in the chapter dealing with intimacy.

But for now it is important for each of us as patients to acknowledge and understand that reality. We always own part of our illness because we own our minds.

That is not to say that we have complete control. I have no doubt that I may have inherited some weakness in my electrical conduction system of my heart, and even if I had managed stress perfectly well, I might still have developed A-fib. But it might have occurred much later in life if I had managed my stress better.

There is always a lot of luck involved in life, too, often more than we want to acknowledge. I think the biggest struggle in being human is captured in the Alcoholics Anonymous prayer:

> *Give me the courage to change the things I can, to accept the things I cannot change, and the wisdom to know the difference.*

In every aspect of our lives, we struggle with the tension of bad luck and bad management. The mature person, the evolved person, knows and valiantly struggles with that reality daily, reflecting and introspecting constantly. It is a continuous struggle for me.

But we also exist in a complex universe, so part of our struggle as humans, and therefore as patients, is to recognize our role in the big picture.

It is often said that our world is becoming smaller because we are, through technology, becoming more interconnected. In other words, evolution is pushing us toward more interdependency. No one person controls or oversees everything anymore; it isn't possible. We are very impressed by those who are confident and who tell us what we want to hear; we love happy talk. We may want to believe that our political leaders know everything that is going on in our country and can control it, but that simply isn't so. Knowledge and responsibility in any organization must be distributed through many individuals because there is so much to know; we all own a piece of it. The minister of health is one person and cannot possibly understand and oversee all aspects of the health-care system. The few thousand bureaucrats that supervise the health-care system have some regulatory powers but can't micromanage everything. Health-care workers number a few hundred thousand, so although they have some control over health-care resource allocation and application, it will always be limited.

This means that the biggest and most influential group that is involved in health-care management is the users of the system. Individually, they may have less control than a minister of health, but by shear volume their impact as a group is huge. This means that how the public uses the system matters a lot in terms of how well it runs. And the person with the greatest control of the health of each user is usually the individual user himself. If patients take a passive role waiting to be rescued by "the system," they will never get the results they want, just like with back pain. Patients 1 and 2 with the fractured femurs have more control of their health than they may realize. Mindfulness goes a long way in determining our health.

Health care is a relational endeavour of the collective. When it reaches the complicatedness and complexity it has, it has to be that way. We can no longer manage with a mentality that "'father (physician) knows best." The parentalistic ways must be abandoned (except in uncommon scenarios of serious mental health issues or unconsciousness).

There is no one person or group that controls everything and on whom we can depend to rectify all deficiencies. We patients cannot simply act likely narcissistic consumers; we must understand that this is a joint venture and all resources are finite. We have to ramp up our level of sophistication. We have to become more critically analytical, reflecting intelligently on the information we ingest, not panicking and demanding more and more in a less than mindful fashion. We are going to have to make our health a priority, not something that we care about only *if* we can find time (and never do). And we are going to have to have those difficult discussions, including talking about things like death.

We must be prudent when we utilize health care. We need to acknowledge that many of us really don't understand the human body very well and admit that we cannot be objective about ourselves. It is for these reasons that we seek the help of well-trained practitioners (the same way doctors do) to assist us in making decisions that are wise not just for ourselves but for the sustainability of the entire healthcare system.

It is essential that we be prepared to grow, be open to change. That entails hearing and doing stuff we don't want to hear and do. Conquering ourselves is never easy. We need to let go of our naive realism and accept the fact that, despite our advances, we still understand very little of the human organism. In fact, there may be a limit to how much we can understand, and despite that unpleasant reality, we need to continue to work together to take care of one another in a morally justifiable fashion. In an increasingly complex world, where knowledge and responsibility are disseminated so widely, we can no longer absolve ourselves of our part in the grand venture of health care. We need to learn to take care of ourselves and each other as mature adults.

We would also be well advised to let go of the fear-based thinking that says our health is *totally* determined by how we behave so that bad things only happen to bad people who deserve them. There is a lot of luck involved in the genes you inherit, where and when and to whom you are born, as well as vagaries of a complex world with millions of variables we often know nothing about. Had I inherited an extra chromosome number 21 when my mother's egg and father's sperm met, I would not have gone to medical school. No one in my medical school class, or in any medical school class that I am aware of, has Down syndrome, Trisomy-21.

Further, every action we take in our lives is probabilistic; some predictions are accurate and some are not. So sometimes we get the elevator, and sometimes we get the shaft. Luck always plays a factor, and our denial of that is a reflection of immature fear.

This means, like it or not, that we all take risks. Often we are unaware that we are doing so or unaware of the exact amount of risk we are taking. There is no singular and unassailable risk comfort level we should all adopt, nor are there exact formulae for us to use in weighing risk with reward. Each of us must mindfully make probabilistic decisions every day about how we live our lives in the context of a world that is not only difficult to understand but likely impossible to fully understand.

We may want to believe that all of the good that has happened to us has been completely within our control and, therefore, deserved but luck plays a huge role in our lives. Equally, we may want to shun all responsibility when things go bad, but that, too, is inaccurate. Interestingly, many of us do the opposite with others—when things go well for others it was luck, but they deserve all of the bad stuff that comes their way. It's our insecurity and fear speaking; life is never that simple.

We must resist the binary thinking that we control either nothing or everything in our lives or the lives of others. It can be painful to admit to that truth, but we can't grow if we don't. We must be firm but gentle with ourselves and with each other, as we nurture one another's growth.

Physicians have to learn to step away from the role of omniscient and omnipotent healers, no matter how difficult that may be for us, and no matter how scary it may be for patients.

This is true not just with respect to the practice of medicine; it is true for all disciplines in our society. We have to stop waiting to be rescued by our politicians, our lawyers, our universities, and our institutions. We need to grow and mature and take ownership for our little corners of the world. But where do we start?

I think we begin with humility. There are many things we do not know and some we cannot know. We deal in spectra and probabilities, not in binary concepts that are assured. In this rather unnerving context, we contemplate as a collective what is the right thing to do, never being sure, always having to reevaluate, striving to love as evolution intends for us.

Searching for and sharing ethical truths is critical. We need to nurture and educate one another so that we all grow and benefit from being part of the collective.

The word "education" comes from the Latin *ex* meaning "out," and *ducare* meaning "to lead." So education is a leading out, from ignorance to wisdom, from immaturity to maturity. We need to lead our healthcare system away from decisions based on fear, overly simplistic biomechanical models, and greed, to a system that wrestles honestly with complexity in the context of relationships that promote the value of both the individual and the collective.

In order to grow, we must learn more and then teach better about consent, risk, and probability; the functioning of the human body; the complexity of our black-box decision making; and the challenges of doing all of this in the context of human interrelationships.

This lack of understanding the black box is not peculiar to medicine. We develop policies and pass laws without really understanding how people work. We think that documenting how we expect people to behave and outlining the punishments for misbehaviour will transform individuals. It may, and it may not.

Sadly, modern medicine not only doesn't understand the black box issue much better, but it doesn't seem very interested in it either. It tends to stay at the superficial levels of the physiosphere and biosphere to find the answers, utilizing biomechanical approaches to problems, not noetic ones. For example, most diabetes is lifestyle related, and yet our approach has been to produce new and "better" drugs rather than examining why it is we have so much more diabetes. Why, when we are so much better educated, do we still have so much diabetes? What is it about the way that our society functions that seems to produce such unhealthiness? Is there something about our attitudes, our perspectives, and our values that needs to be reexamined? Maybe mindfulness, not pills, is the answer? Maybe too much stress-induced adrenaline (an anti-insulin hormone) is part of the problem?

When the fentanyl crisis hit, we raced around providing antidotes to prevent overdose deaths but never asked what it is about our society that drives people, often young people, to such scary behaviours? It reminds me of the alcohol poster in the exam room, thinking we can stop the problem without understanding what's going on inside the black box first. We see this repeatedly in our approach to all addictions.

With the rising numbers of people afflicted by hepatitis C and HIV, we fail to ask why some people engage in some high-risk behaviours when there are safer ways to engage sexually that minimize the likelihood of acquiring these diseases.

It's time for us to look a little closer at teaching and learning.

Chapter 26

Teaching and Learning

A theory is like medicine or government: often useless, sometimes necessary, always self-serving and occasionally lethal.

—Nassim Taleb

I MAY NOT be quite as cynical about theory as Nassim Taleb, but I must admit that I have never understood the purpose of education, which is a rather embarrassing statement given that I have spent a lot of time in academic pursuits. Perhaps it is because the model that I have been most exposed to is rather old-fashioned. It is the pedagogical approach in which a learned person, the teacher, positions herself at the front of a classroom and regurgitates knowledge to an audience consisting of pupils who somewhat passively ingest said knowledge to become "educated."

Don't get me wrong, I think knowledge is important, but learning to think and to reflect are more important than merely accumulating raw data. In this day and age in particular, the ability to search for information is easy, which paradoxically makes learning more difficult. Why? Because the challenges in this age of information overload are to distinguish the signal from the noise and then to try to understand the signal in a meaningful way, not simply regurgitate it during an exam. The mere accumulation of more data is not intelligence (nor is it science).

I am of the firm conviction that the most important things any educator can teach you are to be skeptical, to question everything, and to be critically analytical. Only by doing so can we expect to develop the skills of introspection and reflection, including self-reflection. This is how we begin the process of becoming more mindful, rewiring our brains, and growing.

I find that a disproportionate amount of medical training is still rather pedantic. It is more an exercise in having the professor show off her prodigious ability to memorize than it is about teaching students to think and reflect. It is a worn-out model reminiscent of the parents at my daughter's grade school—just load up pupils with as many programs and files as possible and we have done our job.

All disciplines, not just medicine, suffer from this. At a deep level, we love theory and academia, the episteme of the Greeks, because it appeals to our sense of naive realism. We study something from this idealistic, objective perspective, where the problems are always easily defined and the solutions are straightforward. Kind of like the frequentist approach to statistics—a theoretical and perfectly fair coin flipped an infinite number of times. That may work for the disciplines of the physiosphere, like physics and mathematics, but for most human endeavours it fails because we are dealing with living things in the real world, not computers in a lab. Living things are far more complex and require delving into uncertainty at a far more profound level, a level that benefits from techne, where theory ends and craftsmanship begins.

I remember in medical school meeting a boy genius, several years my junior, who was helping in one of our labs. We thought he was interested in becoming a doctor, but to our surprise he had no interest at all. When I asked him why, he said that he could not possibly engage in a discipline that he did not fully understand. He could not imagine performing a procedure or prescribing a medication for a patient unless he completely understood every aspect of it first.

I found that rather perplexing. I certainly did not feel that I had to understand at every level why a cast helped in the healing of a broken leg if we found empirically, through techne, rather than theoretically, through episteme, that casts help broken bones heal better. Yes, it would be intellectually satisfying to understand all of the detailed physiology and more behind the success of a cast, but my goal as a doctor was primarily to help people, not to be intellectually gratified. If Grandma has found that ginger tea reduces nausea safely, we don't need her to draw the chemical structure in order to benefit from it.

Education is a wonderful and noble pursuit, but it has perennially struggled with its purpose. Is it simply a cerebrally rewarding theoretical pursuit divorced from reality or is it a practical instrument meant to improve the world we live in?

The answer, as it usually does, involves a tension of the two ends of this binary spectrum. My favourite high-school teacher said, "Knowledge is its own reward." However, I have come to realize that as we mature, we must ask ourselves whether this knowledge improves the planet and nurtures our evolutionary growth.

For example, I was always disappointed in how history was taught. The focus seemed to be on recounting battles, names, and dates. But I never walked away with much of an understanding as to why events occurred as they did. What aspects of human thinking and behaviour prompted the actions of historical figures? What did we learn about how humans think and act so as not to make the same mistakes and commit the same horrors? I found the study of history to be far too romanticized, using an idealized retrospectroscope that oversimplified the human condition and ignored the very real complexities of human behaviour. (Akin to the sentiment that the winners write history, not the losers.)

In the words of George E. P. Box: "All models are wrong, but some models are useful." All models are theoretical constructs that often use surrogates, not the real thing. We look at cholesterol in the hope that changing it will change what we really want to change, which is incidence of heart attacks. We are programmed to see patterns, and we are drawn to develop theories that explain those patterns. But theories can sometimes interfere with our ability to observe well. We can miss critical information because we dismiss it if it doesn't fit the present theory. We see only what we already believe. We often draw bull's eyes around the arrow after it has landed.

Medicine is trying to become more evidence-based, in other words more scientific rather than just doing what we have always done out of inertia or based on anecdotes. I applaud this, but we must recognize the significant limitations of searching for evidence:

1. It can be difficult and expensive to discover really good evidence (especially if there are hidden agendas).
2. No evidence will eliminate the fact that medicine is still a probabilistic pursuit (nothing is ever 0 percent or 100 percent).
3. Evidence is often easier to accumulate for issues that are quantitative rather than qualitative.

In addition, we must avoid thinking of evidence in a binary way: either having evidence or not having evidence. Just like justification in an argument, there exists varying strengths of evidence, and sometimes the evidence is weak.

This is why it is so important to be open-minded (which some people confuse with empty minded!). No process of deductive or inductive reasoning is ever foolproof. We never know the whole story, so we are forced to make assumptions and develop heuristics along the way. The challenge is to be open to reviewing them and then rewire our brains accordingly. In order to think outside the box, we must first admit that we created the box; it was self-imposed, often through the use of assumptions, and those assumptions often arose from binary thinking.

One of the best examples of using surrogate markers is in education itself. We use tests and exams to assess students' abilities. But are they an accurate representation of people's abilities to apply their discipline in the real world? In medicine we try to approximate real-life situations by using actors to portray patients or even involve real patients in exam scenarios. This helps to minimize the artificiality to a degree, but not completely. This might explain the old tongue-in-cheek dictum: "What do they call the person who graduates last in the class in medical school? Doctor." We may believe that he is not as competent as the person who graduates first, but his relative position is mostly based on his performance on surrogate markers called exams, not real life. (This is likely the origin of the cynical dictum: "Those who can, do; those who can't, teach.")

In my experience, what differentiates the more helpful physician from the less helpful one is not the amount of knowledge or episteme he has, but rather how much he enjoys his work. Does the techne still excite him? Has he maintained his passion for helping people? Does he still care?

So one of the most important things we need to do differently in education, including medical education, is to balance episteme and techne, theory and practice. This means that contrary to the thinking of my young friend in medical school, we cannot wait until we understand everything before we act. We may sound more convincing when we explain our treatments using a grandiose theory, but the proof is in the pudding. If it works, it works, theory or not.

I have found many times over the years that wise old family doctors have known of a treatment for years and implemented it in practice, without ever having understood why it worked. Many decades later, researchers trip upon this, develop a theory, and think they have discovered it. The best example I can think of is one I will discuss at length in the next chapter—breastfeeding. Many years after convincing us to formula-feed, "experts" then "discovered" that in fact breast milk was superior to formula. I am quite sure that every grandmother on the planet knew that fact long before the experts did because they were paying attention, not trying to develop self-aggrandizing theories.

Over my career, I have seen an explosion in the use of mnemonics, guidelines, and algorithms in teaching medicine. They can be helpful, but when applied mindlessly, we run the risk of adopting a reductionist approach that involves treating test results not patients. So often I have seen patients prescribed lipid-lowering agents purely on the basis of a test result, not in a context that appreciates the patient's values and uniqueness. Guidelines are designed for populations, but we treat individual patients, each of whom is unique, and it behooves us to individualize treatment accordingly.

We need to teach students to get a feel for how humans work, for the art they practise, and to get to know each patient as an individual. Many times during my career I have made a diagnosis based mostly on a deep and largely inexplicable intuition, in part because I had developed relationships with my patients over time. In these clinical situations, I just knew something was wrong, and I kept searching.

Years ago I had two patients with severe back pain that did not fall into any typical pattern. The first patient came to my office and could hardly move, his pain was so horrible; I could barely perform an examination. I knew something bad was brewing, although I did not know what. I arranged an urgent CT scan for three days later. The day before the CT scan, the patient called and asked me to cancel the scan because the pain was gone. In fact, he had just finished playing basketball with his children. I wasn't convinced, so I suggested he proceed with the CT scan anyway, and sadly it revealed a malignancy in his pelvis, one that was impinging on his nerves and giving him the pain.

The second patient also had excruciating, atypical pain. Her blood tests, plain X-rays, bone scan, and even CT scan were all normal. But I knew something was seriously wrong, and I had an inkling I knew what it was. I arranged the only test that would give me the answer, an MRI, which at the time was a very new investigation. It confirmed my suspicion—she had metastases directly in her spinal cord. It was rare, and only an MRI could confirm it. Often we know before we understand.

Nurturing this deeper understanding is important in producing well-rounded physicians, not just technicians. It takes time and mentoring to learn to distinguish paranoia or obsession from legitimate intuition. Discernment, good judgment, and wisdom are critical skills not often mentored during our training—we focus on accumulating lots of data and being thorough, leaving no stone unturned. However, often that can make it more difficult to find the signal among the noise. Information technology does not translate automatically into wisdom technology.

One of the most important things a teacher can pass on to her charges is not the confidence of thinking that we know, but the humility that we can always know more because we know so little to begin with. That requires that all teaching—be it in a classroom, a home, or a doctor's office—should be about willing the good and growth of the other as other, not about making the teacher the centre of attention. It is not so much about regurgitating data as it is about modifying our neural pathways, either adding new wiring or rewiring (or eliminating) old pathways. These processes are inherently scary for us because they involve the risk of losing something well known in exchange for something not so well known.

Naturally, some of us are more comfortable with risk while others are more risk-averse. Helping us to find our comfort zones and expand them in a safe manner is a large element of teaching well. Teachers should want us to conquer ourselves and grow, even to the point of surpassing the teacher. The best teachers are humble; they know that knowledge is a moving target. They admit to their deficiencies, realizing that a good teacher is also a good student who never stops learning.

I found one of the scariest situations in teaching residents was when they were so confident that *they failed to know that they didn't know*. Being ignorant is one thing, provided that you recognize it, because then you will work to correct it. But being ignorant of your own ignorance is dangerous because it leads to unjustifiable overconfidence. It would give me great pleasure if someone reading this book contacted me to offer insight or advice that would help me to grow. Teaching and learning should be joys, not burdens. By understanding our fear of change and our innate insecurity, we can cultivate the courage to rise above them, and that allows for the transformation of burden to joy.

If medicine as a discipline is going to care about maximizing its potential for good, then we must humbly learn to balance the episteme with the techne. This is true for all disciplines that impact our society—law, education, politics, business, et cetera. It means that our teachers have to have functioned in the real world in order for their offerings to be relevant to us and to make the world a better place. Both rational and nonrational modes of reflecting upon episteme and techne are critical.

I understand the safety and comfort of academia, but pure episteme can be dangerous. The same, of course, can be said of pure techne. Intuition can fool us because the complexity of the universe frequently produces counterintuitive results. Our various ways of observing and thinking can trick us if we are not careful. Irrational fear and other powerful emotions can cloud our judgment. For these reasons, the many well-established beliefs, traditions, and rituals that constitute culture, including medical culture, do not always stand up to intense scrutiny.

So over the years, I have come to believe that there are five areas that medical education (and all education) should focus on:

1. Understanding how humans think
2. Understanding relationships
3. Engaging in useful research
4. Applying business principles to the work we do
5. Understanding the bigger picture

How Humans Think

Given the importance of thinking in medicine, I thought I would explore some common logical fallacies that we fall prey to and why we make such errors. You may not know these fallacies by name, but you have certainly seen them and likely engaged in them. No doubt you will understand why we make them.

We fall victim to the ad hominem fallacy when we are scared that someone else has proven us wrong, and rather than just admit it, we attack the person ("ad hominem" meaning "to the person") instead of dealing with the facts. The opposite scenario is common when someone wants to bully his way through an argument with you, not by using reason but by bragging about his expertise. It's called "argument by authority," and you can usually recognize it when someone is not willing to be transparent. He is hiding something and wants to make you feel stupid or bad for questioning his genius.

The fallacy of the false dilemma is commonly used and is a great example of binary thinking. So often people want to make issues seem black and white; they are afraid of the grey zones, so they label a problem as having only two possible solutions—a dilemma (meaning two premises)—when in fact there are many possible choices. Beware arguing with binary thinkers because they are often unreasonable (literally). Seldom in life are there only two choices.

The naturalistic fallacy is a dangerous one in medicine. It confuses "ought" with "is." In other words, we think that because we *can* do something, that we *ought* to do something. Hopefully by now you have realized that that is not so; sometimes it is best not to do something even if we can (don't just do something, stand there!). Ethical reflection can help us in such situations.

It is common to see people use the cherry-picking fallacy, where they use only the data they want to use (Big Pharma is notorious for this, remember ARR and RRR?). People who use the false analogy fallacy can easily dupe the public. In these situations, an overly simplistic analogy is used to explain something far more complex in medicine in order to scare people into behaving a certain way. Very often we can fall into the trap of letting our emotions get the best of us by being swayed by arguments that appeal to a strong emotion, like fear or greed, but in fact have little substance.

Milgram highlighted how prone we are to fall for the *argumentum ad populum* fallacy—everyone else is doing it, so it must be right. Tribes count on this to keep people in line because no one wants to be a pariah.

I could go on for pages because there is almost no end to the ways our lower brains can be suckered into less mindful thinking. Fear, pain, and insecurity, as well desires for wealth, pleasure, power, and honour, underpin these fallacies. It's so tempting to see only what we want to see and believe only what we want to believe.

Any discipline would be wise to educate their students about these errors in thinking. This is particularly true in medicine because there is so much specialized information, and its interpretation is compounded by the intense, visceral emotion peculiar to health issues.

Beyond faulty reasoning, there are other human factors that complicate the practice of medicine. Patients and physicians have an incomplete or even erroneous understanding of our bodies and disease. All of us have imperfect memories making history taking a challenge. Commonly we fear that our symptoms portend something worrisome. Thanks to internet roaming, often we develop a theory and then self-diagnose long before we consult with a doctor. Alternatively, it can be tempting to minimize or deny symptoms when we are afraid, making diagnosis by the physician even more awkward. It is not rare for patients to have multiple motives (some of which can be obscure) in seeking a physician's counsel; the human psyche is a complicated place.

In addition, doctors are not machines; we have off-days. Thank goodness I was having a good day when I had to intubate that six-year-old boy. In some jobs we can fix our mistakes; sometimes medicine is not quite so forgiving.

Physicians suffer from the same medical problems and social

problems as any other person. None of us had perfect parents or a perfect upbringing; we bring our own shortcomings to the office, and we struggle with them. The terms "transference" and "countertransference" refer to the unconscious transfer of previous experiences, and their attendant emotions, from one person to another. In medicine, both patients and physicians bring, at unconscious levels, past experiences, feelings, and emotions to relationships, and they can be erroneously transferred from one to the other. I may remind a patient of their abusive father; they may remind me of someone who annoys me.

Except in psychiatry, I am not aware of any attempts in medical training for students or residents to understand and manage this ubiquitous reality. In fact, little attempt is made during our training to get to know ourselves better or to help us to "conquer" ourselves. It is simply assumed that if we learn enough data, that will be sufficient. It isn't.

Humans don't like getting bad news, but equally we don't like giving bad news either. Medicine was fascinating to study in medical school, but seeing real people with some of these fascinating diseases I found to be deeply troubling. Often we are not taught how to give bad news well, for the sake of the patient, and for our own sake as well. That is not likely going to improve until medical schools have courses specifically exploring the human, not technical, aspects of disability, death, and dying from both sides of the stethoscope.

All of these issues are intrinsic to the human condition, and their management falls within the realm of the art of medicine—the techne. Medical education (and all education) is doing itself a great disservice when it deals only in the episteme and ignores the reality of this techne, particularly when it ignores a deep understanding of how we work.

Relationships

Almost without exception, when I have had a patient express discontent with me or another physician, it is because we either did not communicate well or did not empathize well. I asked in the last chapter, What do patients mean by a good doctor? Because we have a difficult time assessing the competency of someone who is more expert in an area of life than we are, we invariably gauge their proficiency by how they treat us. Do they listen to our questions and answer them directly in a way we can comprehend? And do they seem to care?

The practice of medicine is primarily a noetic pursuit—one of the mind—because it is ultimately a relational endeavour not a purely technical one. Given that, one would think that social skills, an important element of techne, would be one of the most important things to teach in medical schools. In fact, I have often heard the expression "the doctor is the medicine." In other words, it is the way we behave as a person that ultimately results in successful therapy. You are likely going to consider more seriously the opinion of someone who cares about you and explains things well to you than someone who does not. It's very similar to why you remember your favourite high-school teacher and why you probably did well in that class. We are relational creatures.

But it may surprise you that socialization is not a high priority in medical school or residency; we are far too busy trying to impress each other, our profs, and our patients with the gargantuan volumes of trivia and minutiae that we have memorized. Why is that? When we enter medical school, even though we have all demonstrated considerable academic ability in order to gain admission, our deep-seated insecurity leaves us feeling overwhelmed in the face of becoming a doctor. Some compensate with false bravado, others adopt a laid-back image, and still others, like me, simply accept that we will spend four years with a deer-in-the-headlights look.

The truth is, none of us wants to fail, and at heart we are all pretty competitive or else we would not have made it that far. Furthermore, our professors teach us that being a good physician is about being intelligent, working hard, and being driven to learn more. Fostering that competitive edge, mixed with healthy doses of fear, is what fuels our passion to do a good job.

Given our competitiveness, physicians have been seen as the leaders of the health-care team. Historically, leaders have typically been portrayed as powerful, almost larger-than-life individuals who develop the vision for the followers and then lead this passive and somewhat hapless group to the Promised Land (the great man theory). I imagine by now you see the pathology in such a model.

Good leadership should be similar to good teaching: it is not about the aggrandizement of the leader but about the growth of everyone on the team. Each person and their contribution must be respected and nourished for the team to reach its fullest potential.

This means that doctors are only a part of the big puzzle. We are part of a team that includes janitorial staff in hospitals, health-care aides, various technicians, nurses—the list goes on. Our society values intelligence highly, but there are many kinds of intelligence. Some people have academic intelligence, others have mechanical, musical, or social skills, but academic intelligence seems to be revered the most for some reason.

Moreover, when we examine fair compensation for work done, we overvalue the academically intellectual occupations (episteme) and undervalue those with other unique challenges, such as the physicality of the job, the stress or danger involved, or the repetitiveness of the work (techne). Some responsibilities may be more glamorous, some are better paid, and some require more training, but we all have our role, and they all matter. If you don't believe me, imagine a hospital without cleaning staff? You wouldn't want to step foot in it! Given the plethora of infectious organisms, they are probably one of the most important people in a hospital setting, and we would be wise to appreciate that and respect them for the important work they do.

Interestingly, screening for medical school seldom involves assessing someone's ability to be a team player; instead, the search is often for Übermensch. But the complexity of the health-care system is such that being a good team player is critical. None of us can be leaders all of the time, and *being a good follower is just as important and just as difficult as being a good leader*. I wonder how many people reading this book who are nonphysicians working in health care feel that doctors are good team players? Conquering ourselves is never easy.

Research

There is less theoretical science in medicine than people think there is, and that is not a bad thing. It is simply an acknowledgement that a lot of what we do is based on techne. Although techne arises from intuition and creativity, it can also benefit from the scientific approach of careful observation and monitoring, even if a deep theoretical comprehension is lacking. In other words, if we can develop a theory or an explanation for why something works, that's great, but we don't necessarily need that to help people.

On a daily basis I receive Patient-Oriented Evidence that Matters articles, called POEMs (see appendix 3). Overwhelmingly, the articles discredit a lot of the beliefs and dogmas that have been guiding the practice of medicine during my career. They do so by exposing supposed truths to rigorous analysis to see if our intuitions and theories are valid. Sometimes theories hold water, and our intuitions are correct. But it is startling how often we are wrong; the universe is a complicated and complex place, after all.

In fact, the toughest thing I find these days with respect to keeping up with medical advances is trying to remember which of the many things I have learned over the last thirty-five years has been shown to be either inaccurate or completely wrong. How could that be?

You know the answer to that question by now: we see patterns that may not exist, we develop simple theories for complex things, our intuitions can occasionally mislead us, and we believe in magic. When so much is at stake—people's lives and health, vast sums of money, careers and reputations—unearthing the truth can be difficult. It's easy to fall prey to academic hubris, to deny that we can do harm, to forget how difficult it is to predict the future, and to be confused or disheartened by the placebo effect.

It's tough to tame the ego; we are all insecure and don't want to be the weakest deer in the herd. We are embarrassed when our intervention that appears to be so successful is no better than placebo. Shame prevents us from admitting when we unintentionally injure rather than cure. Iatrogenic disease, from the Greek *iatro* meaning "healer" and *genic* meaning "produced," is disease produced inadvertently by doctors. It is a far bigger problem than we want to concede and will likely continue to grow because of the issue of complexity we have been exploring together in this book.

As people age, more things go wrong that we try to fix. That means more investigations (some quite invasive), more therapies, more surgeries, more medications, and thus more opportunities for interactions that we do not, and perhaps cannot, predict or understand. As we were told in residency, using typical gallows humour, we know that patients are sometimes going to die from what we do, "just don't kill more than your quota."

This is why sometimes it is best to do nothing. Paradoxically, advances in anaesthesia and surgical techniques, like minimally invasive ones done through scopes, have made procedures so much safer and easier that we are driven to do more of them simply because we can. But as POEMs frequently point out, the benefits are not always better than doing nothing and letting nature do her thing.

Looking back at medical school, I don't think the healing powers of the human body were ever emphasized enough. Vague terms like "conservative therapy" or "expectant management" were, and still are, used. They are polite ways of saying that we have nothing to offer, but they minimize, or frankly ignore, the power of nature and the fact that patients to a large degree heal themselves even when we do have something to offer. There isn't a lot of fame or fortune to be made, however, in researching how nature works or how patients heal themselves. It's easy to get carried away with our own importance, but we can only hope to be part of the solution at best. My failed cardiac resuscitations are a good example.

If we are going to have students, and patients, trust what episteme we do have, then it is important to avoid pseudoscience. So often I see research that makes statements using terms such as "approximately 37.2%." Are you kidding me? You don't use the word "approximately" and "37.2%" in the same sentence; that's hubris. Saying "about one-third" is far more honest. In terms of usefulness *clinically*, statistics should be quoted as <1%, 5%, 33%, or 50% (or the complementary 50%, 67%, 95%, and 99%). Most other numbers are close enough to those four that the significance is immaterial *most* of the time. You are not likely going to change your mind because the likelihood was 3% versus 11%, 28% versus 38%, or 43% versus 59%.

The second biggest challenge I am facing these days in keeping up is a painful one for me to admit to: I am having a harder and harder time trusting what I read and hear.

For example, medical conferences and seminars can be fun to attend. You get a brief hiatus from your usual routine, catch up with some old friends, and maybe make a holiday of it with your family visiting someplace new. It's always nice to hear that what you are doing medically is what pretty much everyone else is doing, so there is a sense of safety in numbers. I am not sure it is always a good bang for your buck from a learning perspective in terms of time and cost, but I can live with that.

What I have a difficult time with is the lack of transparency. So often speakers are connected to commerce in such a way that I find it a challenge to see through their bias, similar to the issues I mentioned earlier with medical journals and publications. I am never sure if a presentation is generated by the speaker or the company sponsoring the event, nor what remuneration the speaker is receiving. Transparency, as I have said before, is a critical ethical principle. When you are hiding something, we all get nervous. And I just never get a sense that I am hearing the whole story.

The Business of Medicine

By business of medicine (BOM), I do not mean the impact of

capitalism, per se, on medicine. Rather, I refer to the fact that although we have theory (episteme) and knowledge in medicine, how we apply it is part of techne, and we can learn a lot about that from business. Why? Because medicine has a business element to it. A chef may love cooking and be very good at it, but no restaurant can ever succeed having just a good chef. It needs a team, and that team has to grow past just good food. A beautifully plated meal means nothing to the customer if it doesn't get to the right person's table at the right time in the right way.

This highlights one of the fundamental shortcomings in how medicine has been practised: it has been a very top-down system with what I refer to as a "flattened pyramid structure." Doctors have been reluctant to let go of their place on the hierarchical scale in health care and delegate until just the last decade or two. Few chefs welcome patrons at the door, seat them, take orders, make food, deliver food, and then wash up. For example, many jurisdictions have been slow to incorporate midwives onto the obstetrical team, and when they have, it is because family doctors no longer deliver babies. If a physician has more of a technical interest in her discipline and is not a good communicator, she should hire someone who is a good communicator (or business manager, et cetera).

Equally, in many disciplines within medicine, the challenge is not simply to accumulate knowledge but to manage knowledge and manage time. What information is useful, not just interesting, and how do we use it effectively to improve the lives of patients in a timely fashion? The medical profession has been slow to adopt the use of information technology to improve care, which is surprising given that our business is largely about data management.

We are two decades behind most businesses. Many doctors still use handwritten notes with physical charts that cannot allow for rapid searching techniques, monitoring of conditions, or reminders for improved care. Not only should we have been utilizing computers with programs that offer these abilities, we should have been dictating our notes for the last two decades and using computer programs to develop better scheduling systems, like Advanced Access. We are only now starting to use email and other electronic media for patient communication and education. It is a sad comment that we still often use a decades-old model for after-hours health care where oodles of patients show up and wait to be seen. There is no excuse for it as we have the technology to avoid such chaos and provide more timely and less frustrating care; we just have to use our imagination. Our refusal to acknowledge the importance of the BOM has compromised patient care for years.

This is particularly true in family medicine, where we must be the repositories for all of the information associated with patients' health. In addition, we family doctors generally see many patients per day for more concise problems and, therefore, shorter visits than specialists. Cutting to the chase quickly and making a treatment plan without missing anything is the biggest challenge. Family doctors do not have the luxury of leisurely academia; we are first and foremost pragmatic because patients, quite rightly, want answers to very specific problems, not professorial lectures. There is an art (techne) to that, which has not always been appreciated. There is a tendency within the profession, and within society itself, to worship the academic or the specialist. But seeing the bigger picture from a generalist perspective is important, too.

Specialists have dominated medical teaching, and it has sometimes skewed people away from entering family medicine. However, with the burgeoning of information that is available to nearly every patient, visits with family doctors are becoming busier and more complicated. This fact, combined with increasing anxiety in the patient population, has resulted in more challenges for the life of a generalist. In my first few years of practice, patients presented with one problem; that is seldom the case now. It takes a lot more time to manage four concerns than one or two, especially when trying to use the deliberative model for decision making.

Given this reality, and the encouragement toward specialization, what then draws people to family medicine?

First, we are relational people. In other words, we are less concerned with the mechanics of diagnosis and treatment (like doing procedures and prescribing medications) and more concerned with the interactive process involved in coming to a resolution.

Second, we like the variety; I have always relished the challenge that no matter what your concern is, I have an approach to dealing with it. I may not have an immediate solution necessarily, but I do have a process whereby we will find the best solution possible. It may well require a referral to someone who will come up with the final diagnosis and treatment, but the process of getting you to the right person at the right time is a talent.

There is a tendency both outside of medical circles, and particularly within medical circles, to think that the students in the lower half of the class go into family medicine. In other words, only the really smart ones in the class can become specialists. But being a nonexpert holds unique challenges and, not surprisingly, its own skill sets, too. Much of it is practical wisdom, and it is just as difficult to master as any specialty.

Being able to switch gears quickly and efficiently is paramount as a generalist because on any given day one sees patients with a limitless breadth of complaints running the full gamut of life expectancy. (You would be surprised how many times family medicine residents are told that they are wasting their skill sets by becoming family doctors when they are doing specialty rotations during their training.)

Third, given the scope of our discipline, family doctors must learn humility early on and be far more comfortable with uncertainty than any other discipline. We are experts at nothing, and because we see patients who have not been screened by someone else first, we more often see problems that are undifferentiated and will remain mysterious. All physicians see patients for whom they cannot either make a diagnosis or for which they have no cure. This is especially true in family medicine, and teasing out the definable from the indefinable is difficult; humans are not comfortable with uncertainty, so we always want answers.

However, in a complicated and complex world, answers are harder to come by than we often want to admit, and not just in medicine. Often all we can tell patients is what something is not, and that can be reassuring. Equally, we can advise about what to look for: if a symptom or sign does not change, that is usually a good thing because bad things tend to progress and cause more disability.

Being efficient with our resources, knowing what problems are worth spending a lot of energy on and what are not, is going to become a bigger challenge in the future in a health-care system that is getting more expensive every day.

Let me share one of my fantasies with you (a medical fantasy—what were you thinking?). I have often wondered how much better our health-care system would be if we took all of the time, energy, money, resources, and personnel that we spend on research and present methods of education and spent all of it on improving the *delivery* of health care? In other words, rather than trying to advance our knowledge, what if we just learned to apply the knowledge we already have in a more efficient, scientific, and sustainable way?

What if we researched better teaching methods for both students and practising physicians, educated the public more about medicine and how the human body works, worked on more efficient scheduling, took fuller advantage of information technology, developed better protocols for investigations and treatments, eliminated the backlog wait times, monitored more closely the effectiveness of our interventions, and understood the nature of the patient-physician relationship better and applied it more diligently?

I have this sneaking suspicion that a lot of the research we do is not all that useful in practical terms (although it keeps researchers employed and us ever hopeful), and the resources would be much better applied in improving how we provide medical care and monitoring our failures and successes. I have no proof for this; it's just a gut feeling. But having run a business, I think there is at least a small bit of truth to it.

No business would ever function the way we do in medicine because it would go bankrupt. Successful businesses are always analyzing what they do to see if it works. We don't do that in health care. For example, no one is keeping track to see how much of a difference MRIs, as we presently do them, actually make in terms of improving patients' lives. In other words, there is no doubt that some MRIs help a lot, but many do not, other than alleviate anxiety. But given that they are expensive tests, is there a cheaper way of allaying anxiety? Are we getting a big enough bang for our buck?

When I was first in practice, CT scans were just becoming available, and I worked in a remote location. It was a five-hour adventure to get to the nearest CT scan, so we ordered them judiciously. The pickup rate for finding clinically significant abnormalities that would change patients' lives was about 50 percent. I suspect that the rate for present-day MRIs in terms of picking up abnormalities of clinical significance is much, much lower. Unfortunately, I can't give you a number because no one is keeping track, as far as I can tell. We do a lot of tests today; what percentage is abnormal? Of those, what percentage is meaningful and changes patient care? Maybe we should be keeping track and use that information to guide us in the utilization of all kinds of expensive or invasive procedures.

As I mentioned above, because anaesthesia and surgery are so much simpler and safer, we are doing more of some types of surgeries, but is it making enough of a difference? Are we using precious operating room time and personnel for procedures that offer little benefit, leaving less time and resources for ones that provide great benefit?

In other words, we are not using scientific or business principles to monitor what we do. Because we can do something, we simply do it.

In addition, many patients and physicians don't realize that most doctors are not just running a practice; they are also running a business. Very little attention is given to this during our training, and it shows. I personally think doctors worry too much about money. No business does well if its primary goal is to make money. A business does well when its goal is to provide the best product or service possible. Do that and the money will flow accordingly.

I have witnessed far too many physicians try to keep overhead costs down by cutting corners, and it makes no business sense. You spend many hours a day in your office, so make it comfortable and inviting. It doesn't have to be palatial, but a miserable physical space depresses everyone—staff, physicians, and patients. Computerization is critical for effective data management. Money invested in a welcoming and well-run office is money well spent. A happy office begets better care.

I think we could learn a lot about how to hire and treat staff because they are always the biggest assets in any business. Good staff members are critical to good patient care, and their jobs are not easy. Not only do they have to have a wide range of skill sets but they need to be patient and compassionate because they deal with patients every day, who by definition are scared and not feeling their best.

Having a team mentality is critical; as employers, doctors must listen to their staff and involve them in decision making in matters that effect their performance and job satisfaction. Doctors need to support their staff, particularly emotionally, and remunerate accordingly. You get what you pay for, and keeping good staff is the best investment any physician can make in his practice. Doctors should take pride in being good employers. I have always tried to do that, and it would give me great satisfaction to know that my staff feel that I succeeded.

There is no other business quite like medicine, so business principles should not be applied willy-nilly. Too often business principles have been applied by people who do not understand, for example, the patient-physician relationship or the intense emotion of the work we do. However, I think a strong case can be made that a better balance of episteme and techne, partly in the form of BOM, would likely result in a better system overall. I think business can teach us better ways of servicing patients than the present walk-in clinics that are so common, for example.

We spend a lot of money on health care, and at the present rate, given the reality of an aging population in the context of increasing technology, the cost is not likely going to go down. We are going to face some difficult questions about priorities because the present system is not sustainable. I don't think people appreciate that sustainability is a critical ethical principle. Imagine a family that spent all of its money in the first half of the year, only to have nothing left for the second half? Our thought experiment in chapter 19 should give us pause to examine the present way we manage the BOM.

The Bigger Picture

The specialist perspective is an important one, but it relies heavily on a biomechanical approach, and so it is often reductionist in its application: it analyses the parts of the watch without seeing the watch as a whole and integrated system. The generalist tries to understand the patient more holistically. Given the intimate connection of the brain and the body, we can benefit from both the specialist and generalist perspectives.

So often we see patients being "cured" of one problem only to have another problem crop up; their ulcer heals but their migraines get worse. We brag about our successes, but often they are shallow and short-lived. Why? Because we fail to see the person behind the ulcer or the migraine or the atrial fibrillation. We help a patient kick one addiction, only to find that they then engage in a different one. When we focus too much on one pixel we can fail to see the complete image.

This means that there is a bigger picture, and in fact there are two levels of this bigger picture.

The first is that we are integrated beings with a mind that functions beyond the physical limitations of the brain and the body. Classical medicine is only starting to understand this, but alternative medicine is often ahead of us in this regard. All illnesses have some level of non-physical element to them. The truth is that our minds are intimately involved in our health and our sickness. The better we understand the black box inside of our head, the way that our mind manifests in the world, the more likely modern medicine will be a deeply transformative discipline.

The second is that we are an integrated species; we affect one another, directly and indirectly. The health-care systems we develop to care for us are an endeavour of the collective, and it behooves us to remember that it is not always just about us individually. That can be tough to do when you are scared or feeling lousy.

We can do a better job of educating both providers and users of the health-care system about both of these truths. Evolution has taught us to conserve our energy and take the low hanging fruit first. So it is not surprising that both health care professionals and patients alike are drawn to the quick fix of medications or surgery rather than the more challenging route of lifestyle changes and personal transformation. But we can lead ourselves out from a tendency to react based on fear, denial, ignorance, and naïveté to a more critically analytical and ultimately a more ethically justifiable and sustainable approach to caring for one another (see appendix 1 for a primer I developed for medical students, and appendix 2 for a primer for patients).

It will require us to become more mindful. One of the greatest challenges is our reluctance to first understand ourselves, our own black boxes. We need to get to know ourselves, and each other, better.

In other words, we need intimacy with ourselves and with one another.

PART III: WHERE WE ARE GOING

Never Say Never

Chapter 27

Intimacy

I do not know the man so bold
He dare in lonely place,
That awful stranger, consciousness,
Deliberately face.

—Emily Dickinson

SOME PEOPLE THINK intimacy has to do with our bodies, especially some of our more private biological functions. It is true that many people feel awkward talking about their bowel habit, their urine flow, or their sexual performance, even with a physician in the confidentiality of a medical office setting. But that kind of intimacy is a rather shallow one.

Others feel that intimacy is about sharing our innermost thoughts and feelings with others, and to be sure that is a deeper intimacy. For that reason we struggle a little more, often needing to use alcohol or other mind-altering drugs in order to feel comfortable enough to do so. The classic example is when men can only tell each other that they love them when they are significantly intoxicated, slurring "I love you, man!"

But the intimacy that this chapter focuses on is deeper still. It involves intimacy with oneself. Before we feel safe to share, we must first be able to introspect and self-reflect in our own minds, and that we find difficult. We would much rather simply ignore some of the confusing parts of ourselves: our irrational aspects, our labile moods, our insecurities, our conflicting values, and our endless pursuit of pleasure that never fully satisfies, to name a few. It leaves us feeling unsettled. So we resort to using the denial that we have been using for millions of years since the acquisition of full consciousness and self-awareness. Although denial may have facilitated our survival in the early days, when applied routinely today it contributes to our suffering.

How so, you wonder? Well, it's complicated.

The Great Buddha said that desire is the source of all suffering. The problem is, evolution has programmed all living things to avoid pain and seek pleasure, and we are no exception. So are we destined to suffer? Is there any way out of this conundrum?

Life always involves both the presence and absence of pain and the presence and absence of pleasure. And Buddha knew that pleasure is more enjoyable than pain, so it is not surprising that we want the former but not the latter. However, as soon as we depend on that scenario, we are setting ourselves up for suffering. If we could let go of these desires and accept pain and pleasure with equanimity, we would be blissful. If we could enjoy every moment for what it is, a moment of life, without worrying about its content, we would be much better off.

I don't know about you, but I find that really hard to do (remember I told you I was a wimp). If we could ever reach complete enlightenment—nirvana—we would be content with whatever life threw at us and yet be perfectly at peace with having it all end at any moment. Few of us will ever reach such a state I suspect.

Aquinas said something similar: the more we chase after wealth, pleasure, power, and honour, the unhappier we will be. He didn't mean that we shouldn't enjoy them; it's just that they come and go and the more we rely on them to make us happy, the more we are destined for disappointment. Enjoy them, yes, but don't become attached to them. Instead, make your focus sharing your good fortune with others rather than accumulating more attachments. Buddha would not have disagreed.

That's because with full consciousness there is not just self-awareness but awareness of others, too, and when we share, it gives us a deeper, less selfish satisfaction. We can, of course, allow ourselves to be dominated by our lower brains that mindlessly avoid pain and chase after pleasure for ourselves alone, but we don't have to. That's part of what Buddha and Aquinas were driving at.

They acknowledged the centrality of our interconnectedness, wherein we can practise compassion and loving-kindness. When we share our pain and our pleasure with others, it eases the suffering for us all.

But it must start with personal intimacy. We must stop denying the existence of our reptilian survival instincts to avoid pain and lower mammalian desires for pleasure and realize that those beasts cannot be slayed. Obsessing on wealth, pleasure, power, and honour for ourselves alone can drive us to be narcissistic and selfish, and we will suffer. They can interfere with our ability to grow and interconnect with others, but we can rise above them even though we cannot eliminate them.

So how can we improve intimacy with ourselves in order to suffer less? There are lots of ways.

Let's start with health. There is an intense interdependence of mind and body. I have atrial fibrillation, and I can produce EKGs to prove that it is in my heart, but it is also partly in my head. Do we acknowledge the inescapable reality that all symptoms and medical conditions have both a physical and psychological component? Often bodily symptoms are a manifestation of psychological distress. When extreme, we refer to this as "somatization," from the Greek *soma* meaning "body."

One of the most extreme cases I have ever seen was during internship. An older woman presented with what appeared to be a stroke as she had complete paralysis and sensory loss in one of her arms. She could not move her arm, and pinpricks with a sterile needle that caused small bleeding did not affect her. Investigations revealed nothing objective to explain her symptoms. It turned out that just days before, her husband of nearly fifty years had died suddenly and unexpectedly from a massive stroke that had started with weakness in his arm.

It is wise to see a doctor if you have symptoms that are distressing you. You may in advance want to reflect upon the role of your mind in your symptoms. When you speak with your physician, it is perfectly reasonable as part of your deliberation to discuss the role of investigations and referrals to specialists. However, before doing so, it might be worthwhile to reflect upon your requests. Do you always want tests and referrals? Have the tests and referrals in the past generally been helpful in diagnosis and treatment, or have they mostly been useful to allay your anxiety? If the latter is true, maybe it is time to discuss that self-observation with your doctor, as my friend Joe usually did, in order to avoid painful, risky, and expensive tests and referrals that may not help and could harm. And it may help you to suffer less with the uncomfortable symptoms that have a psychic more than physical origin.

I feel as though I have seen an explosion in anxiety and anxiety disorders during my career. Paradoxically, it may be so because in many ways our lives are so much safer. We still have the same brainstem neurons and neurochemicals that our ancestors had, but not nearly the amount of real, external threats. Just look back to the first settlers in North America: little in the way of formal government or police oversight; no health-care system; no workplace, disability, or life insurance; no pension plans; no businesses open 24/7 to cater to every need; and the list goes on.

We had every reason to spend our days in terror worrying about all of the many things that could go wrong in our lives at any minute. (In the same way, perhaps, we hear more about random acts of violence in our society because we don't have as many wars for people to vent their anger as we used to.)

Now we look for things to worry about. Never have human beings lived longer, healthier, safer lives with access to so much pleasure, and yet we worry now more than ever that we are not going to live long enough or have enough. It saddens me to think of how many people will live long lives only to realize in retrospect that they spent far too much of their lives worrying about living to be old. We worry that our food isn't high enough quality; we used to worry that we would not have any food at all. We complain when we wait in the emergency department too long to receive top-notch professional help any time of the day or night; we used to have to fend for ourselves. We grumble because we don't have a perfect workplace; we used to beg for any work at all to feed our families.

There is nothing mysterious or unnatural about any of this; it is part of our evolutionary journey. However, with introspection and self-reflection—intimacy with ourselves—we can grow beyond our angst by rewiring our brains.

This is not easy, of course. The path to maturity involves immature steps, and often painful ones. That is not to deny the very important physical and biological aspects of anxiety or any mental illness. We inherit through our genes and our environment our neurochemistry and neuronal structures; none of us has a clean slate to start with. We have little control of much of this, and it varies greatly from person to person and during different times in each of our lives.

But contrary to popular opinion, I do not think the primary difficulty we have with disclosing and dealing with mental illness, for example anxiety disorders, relates to the stigma associated with it. Rather, I think that we avoid discussing mental illness for the same reason we avoid discussing death—it is too intimate.

Our mental health is primal because it speaks to what makes us who we are, and for that reason we find it intimidating to address. It's one thing to have a problem with your kidney or your leg, but it is a wholly different matter when the problem involves the neurochemistry of your brain that can affect your mind so directly. For this reason, I often find that patients are less likely to follow up with me about mental health issues than physical health issues.

We may not be happy when we need knee surgery, but because we want to get better we take time off of work to be operated upon and accept the necessity of crutches and weeks of arduous physiotherapy in order to heal. We are not nearly so enthusiastic when our problem is psychological, not physical. We are much more likely to spend thousands of dollars on alcohol or other nonprescription drugs to deal with our anxiety rather than spend it on psychotherapy.

Equally, couples will pay big bucks for an exotic holiday to get away from it all, hoping it will solve their marital problems (or worse still, spend even more on divorce lawyers), yet they recoil at the thought of spending far less for marital counselling.

Years ago I did a little experiment in the office. I made a point one day of asking every patient I saw if they thought their problem might benefit from some psychological counselling, irrespective of the nature of the problem. The less likely their problem had a psychological component, for example a sprained ankle, the more agreeable they were to considering counselling (although I am pretty sure that many of them worried that I was losing it).

However, from my perspective, the more likely their problem was a reflection of underlying psychic stress, often the less likely they were interested. Usually the response would be, often in a less than appreciative tone, "So you think this is all in my head, Doctor?" We avoid intimacy, sometimes to our peril. On many death certificates I suspect that the cause of death could read 'denial', although we will never see that written.

So why do we avoid intimacy? Why do we prefer to deny that there is a problem?

None of us is perfect; we all make mistakes. Provided that no serious or permanent harm is done, we should be able to accept errors more graciously provided that we are prepared to learn from them. However, we have been programmed to avoid errors because for our ancestors they could be lethal. Sure, when things go well, it's easy. We simply assume things turn out well because things are supposed to go that way or we did something brilliant to cause it to occur. So we don't bother to question it; we just roll with it. But when things don't go as planned, we often judge our errors harshly; we are too hard on ourselves.

To cope with such intense pain and shame, we often use denial—problem, what problem?—or attribute unfavourable results to bad luck, fate, or other people—why poor me? But the mature mind, the one that can be intimate with itself, will avoid denial and ask if there is anything that it contributed to the undesirable outcome that is changeable. The mature mind will do the same when good things happen, too. Lots of our good fortune is simply luck, and the mature mind knows that.

Shame and self-flagellation explain why we hate being judged when in fact we only hate to be judged negatively (especially by ourselves). If someone pointed out some aspect of ourselves that we were proud of (or at least neutral about), we would not react to being judged the same way as when we secretly feel shame. We might still be upset that the other believes she is better than us, but that, too, arises from a primal fear that we are not good enough, that we are the weakest deer in the herd.

Once we have come to peace with our own shortcomings, we are no longer ashamed of them, and being judged bothers us much less. We learn to forgive ourselves for our humanity, and part of our growth includes not forgetting. Not forgetting keeps us humble; it helps us not to make the same mistakes again. But being humbled is painful, and we often avoid pain, no matter how helpful it may be.

We worry that mental illness, because it speaks so deeply to who we are, reflects some serious, maybe even lethal, defect in us, so we feel scared, shamed, and stigmatized.

I think in general we have come to accept the illness of depression better in the last decade or two, but I am not sure that we are quite as enlightened about anxiety. Paradoxically, I suspect it is because we are not wired for depression as strongly as we are wired for anxiety.

Worry about potential risks and threats was protective in the unforgiving world our ancestors inhabited, so anxiety was a primal tool for survival. Some argue that depression may have had some survival advantage in that it allowed us to see the world more realistically, not through rose-coloured glasses. However, anxiety likely conferred a more immediate and continuous benefit in the big picture. This is why I think we seem capable of having more empathy for someone afflicted by depression; it feels more like an alien invading us than an internal defect whose existence we should deny.

Witness how our society worships being cool: heroes in movies face no end of extreme danger and laugh in the face of death. We wish we could be like them; we wish we could control that deep, anxious inner reptile and we are ashamed when we can't rein it in. That's why I think we have a harder time having empathy for those with anxiety disorders; they remind us too much of that part of us we can perhaps tame but never eliminate. To some degree, the words of Winston Churchill ring true: "We have nothing to fear but fear itself."

Mental health illnesses, such as depression, anxiety, bipolar disease, and schizophrenia, are very real and can be very disabling. We know from studies that there are neurochemical changes that occur with various mental illnesses. However, all of us have minds, not just brains, and those minds are capable to some degree of rewiring by observing and then controlling the various parts of our brains. These processes are not going to eliminate or cure mental health problems, any more than they alone can do so for afflictions of the rest of our bodies. But the intense interplay of brain and body and the control that the mind has over them ought not be ignored.

Becoming more mindful starts with slowing down, introspecting, and reflecting about how we work; it leads to self-intimacy that can reduce our suffering. It is not easy and is best done when our emotions are not running at full tilt. It is particularly hard to rewire our brains when intense pleasure or fear are raging inside of us. With time, however, our rewiring will serve us well when our emotions are at a peak; we will make better choices, ones that are less narcissistic or selfish that we may regret.

How intimate can you be with yourself? Want to try?

Do you crave drama in your life? Do you have a need to feel special? Do you feel compelled to please everyone? Do you hate to rock the boat or be unpopular? Are you always the peacemaker, no matter what? Do you avoid confrontation at all costs?

Or do you like to be different and not fit in? Do you like having a reputation as a bad boy or bad girl?

Maybe you engage in self-defeating behaviours to prove that you are not worthy? Do you find yourself entertaining self-fulfilling prophecies of doom and gloom? Are you too harsh with yourself?

Or maybe you always need to be centre of attention? The always-confident leader? Maybe you never want to own any responsibility when things don't go well? Always looking for a scapegoat?

Well, if any of these sound familiar, then welcome to humanity. Our insecurity is at the root. I know that this is going to sound blasphemous, but it's okay to be ordinary. If you do want to reach nirvana, you can't do it by grasping at illusions. Our unrealistic striving to be constantly special can produce severe anxiety, and our failure to achieve or maintain the summit of specialness can leave us depressed. Self-intimacy requires balancing the tensions of the good and bad, the ups and downs of everyday life, of being ordinary.

The pseudointimacy of social media contributes to the stress to be Übermensch. There is so much pressure to be happy that it has become a burden. The desire to be unique and special, to stand out above the crowd, promotes anxiety.

Do you ever worry that you are too sensitive? Do you have a tendency to hyperbolize: everything is a catastrophe or awesome?

Do you feel that you are resilient, that you can cope with adversity well? Or do you need everything to be insured and guaranteed or you can't cope?

If any of this sounds familiar, don't be surprised. Evolution programmed us to fear. When we have fewer natural disasters to worry about, we can become overly sensitive to any misdemeanor no matter how minor (we are referred to as "snowflakes"). All injustices can feel like a holocaust.

Do you confuse being wronged with being harmed? Does every wrong need to be righted and every harm compensated? Or can you let go and perhaps even forgive?

When we are afraid, we can devolve into binary thinking: the evil perpetrator who must be punished and the innocent victim who must be rescued. Life is seldom that simple. You are not bad just because you sometimes do bad things.

Do you ever get angry that the world is not fair? Do you rage against all types of hierarchies? Must everyone get a gold star? Are you ever accused of feeling entitled?

You are not alone; all of us are programmed to seek pleasure, and most of us want to see others experience pleasure, too. But at any given moment, life may not seem fair. Accept that although we are all ontologically equal, there are hierarchies of talents, gifts, and experience. Our binary thinking sees only disability and ability, not the true spectrum from disability to impairment to lack of ability to ability to expertise along the journey of life. We always want to be at the summit; but we must realize that life is mostly about the constant climb.

Ultimately, our gifts are not about ourselves anyway; they are not about our self-aggrandizement, but about helping others. On a hierarchical scale, I may have more knowledge and skill with respect to medical treatment than my mechanic, Claude, but he has more know-how with respect to automotives, thank goodness. Hierarchies are amoral things that can be used for good or for evil. If utilized for the good and growth of others, they are loving.

Of course, we have seen a lot of abuse of hierarchies during our history, so it is no wonder that the very idea of hierarchy can leave us with a bad taste. Some of the worst abuses have involved people who are supposed to love and protect us—our families. The appeal of being part of the small tribe called family allows some members higher up on the hierarchical scale to get away with behaviours that are completely unacceptable elsewhere in society. The scars that such abuse leaves are deep and difficult to heal because they usually occur at a time when we are most vulnerable and impressionable. They can leave us with faulty heuristics about healthy relationships and degrading self-images. It can take years of therapy to rewire those foundational neuronal networks.

Even as adults, we are bombarded with abuse of hierarchies. Movies and shows on television role model bombastic behaviour, and the more dysfunctional, the more we tune in. Perhaps they appeal to us because of some primal urge for power. Maybe they add that drama we feel is missing from our lives. Or possibly they make our lives seem better by comparison.

Whatever the reasons, I find it uncommon to see people behaving well in most of the popular entertainment. There is a preponderance of violence in word and action, and abuse of all kinds of hierarchies. I heard Denzel Washington, who I think is a wonderful actor, state that it is easy to play a villain but tough to play a true hero with authenticity—that takes talent (which he has). These forms of entertainment, replete with a plethora of sociopathic role models, affect us more than we think. If they didn't, corporations wouldn't spend so much money making them.

I seem to be seeing more abuse of hierarchies in the workplace as well. I think a lot of this is based on an immature understanding of leadership. Being a good manager is very difficult. Too often people get promoted to the managerial level because they are very skilled or clever, or confident or extroverted. But none of these have much to do with knowing how to help people grow in their work. Narcissistic managers or CEOs, no matter how talented, are scary because they do not know how to be transformative in their leadership. Sometimes they have a lot of episteme, but not much techne. For that reason, they often undervalue techne, even to the point of feeling threatened by underlings who want to grow. In order to manage people, you have to be further along in your personal evolution than they are, secure enough to support the evolution of others and open to evolution yourself. We need to learn to both give and receive, because both are equally important. In other words, you need to have made more headway in conquering yourself, especially in the power and honour departments. That's intimacy.

Studies show that employees are happiest and function best when they feel appropriately challenged in their work, have a sense of satisfaction that they are doing something useful, are appreciated, and are growing. The paycheque is often much less important.

Unfortunately, many companies manage employees very poorly, bordering on bullying, and think that paying them well can make up for it. Employees can get suckered into believing it for a while, but not for long if they want to be happy. Teaching managers and employees about engaging in assertive behaviour, as opposed to the more typical passive-aggressive type, is a good start. Few people understand what consensus is, but it generally provides much better results in any team endeavour even though it takes longer to do. Dialogue produces a happier work environment than debate or edicts from on high.

The workplace is a good example of the dwindling value of deep and meaningful relationships. Organizations strive to be bigger and more efficient and therefore "better," but in the process they tend to minimize direct human interaction in favour of electronic forms of communication that lack intimacy. So it is not surprising that there is much less dedication between employers and employees than there used to be.

We are a much more independent people because we can get away with it. We don't need others like we used to. We can shop online with credit cards, engage in our work, superficially socialize, and in fact live our entire lives all without leaving our homes. We can care less about other people because we don't need them, and this ease of access to all of the stuff we want fosters more narcissism. The problem is, when things go south, we are also on our own.

Part of the trouble arises because Western culture is largely built on the self-made man model, the Übermensch who wins at all costs. We very much tend to worship extroverts in our society for this reason. The book *Quiet*, by Susan Cain, does a wonderful job of exploring this phenomenon and is well worth reading. It's reassuring to know that Einstein was an introvert. He probably didn't need to be managed.

Susan explores Western culture's love affair with extroversion and shares the struggles she had as an introvert. Introversion is almost seen as a disorder, even though it describes a substantial percentage of the population. Facades and false bravado easily fool us because we are very influenced by first impressions. We envy those who seem confident, no matter how little justification there is for their self-assuredness. Our attitude toward it highlights how much human beings have a tendency to compare themselves to one another.

We may not realize it or want to admit to it, but we gauge ourselves by comparing ourselves to those around us. Our values are largely determined by our social milieu. Do we have enough stuff? Enough money? Have we done enough travel? Are we successful enough? Do we have enough friends? Are we popular enough?

If we come up short in our self-appraisals, we can feel miserable, no matter how good our lives may be. Don't believe me? Think of someone in your town or city who is not very well off and feels dejected because of it (maybe even you?). Now imagine that person transported to a very poor part of the world, or to a time a few hundred years ago when many had much less than we do now. In that place or time, the person would likely be considered wealthy and most fortunate. And no doubt he would have a very different, and better, view of his life situation as a result.

Our attitudes can be so crucial in determining our priorities, behaviours, and happiness. How self-absorbed and narcissistic are you?

To a large degree, we gauge our happiness based on others and what they have. We want to fit in, and we want to know where we are in the pecking order; we don't feel comfortable just being ourselves. In order to grow, we must first accept as our starting point who we are at this moment. That's intimacy.

Do we take ourselves too seriously? Can we laugh, especially at ourselves? Because our work involves some very serious matters, I think physicians often fall into the trap of taking themselves too seriously.

Most people love drama and like feeling important, and so we can fall into the trap of taking ourselves too seriously. We convince ourselves that anything we are good at is important and any aesthetic preferences we have are special, which means that we are important and special too. We like being in on secrets because we like being on the inside, not outside, of an elite tribe. The problem is, secrecy and transparency are at odds with one another.

Do we have obsessions or compulsions that get in the way of our growth? Medicine tends to nurture obsessive thinking and compulsive behaviour in its practitioners. Because a doctor's job is to worry about the future of their patients, she is always on the lookout for the black swan or canary. Fair enough. But when taken to an extreme, when episteme is not balanced with techne, we can do more harm than good with overinvestigation and treatment. *Primum non nocere*—above all do no harm.

Obsessive-compulsive disorder is common and involves deep primal emotions, fear being among them. Perfectionism can be crippling: as long as we do everything to the very best, we feel as though we can keep the beast at bay. But the moment we fall short, we can be overwhelmed and experience catastrophic thinking. If I don't get top marks in a course at school, then I won't get into graduate school, and then I won't get a job and…then…disaster! Panic attacks start this way, and they are like a five-alarm firing of brainstem neurochemicals that can overwhelm the best of us.

It is true that we often admire intense dedication, the grit to never quit. But it can be pathologic if we lose balance in our lives, when we see ourselves as just that small sliver of achievement, when it is all about us. Addictions belong in this category; they have been described as "licking honey off a razor." The list of addictions is near endless. Any one of Aquinas's big four—wealth, pleasure, power, honour—can be taken to an extreme. More and more our society worships people who turn a talent or interest into an obsession. We revere experts because we want to believe that someone has the answers for us; it is a bit of magical thinking. Or we are convinced that the fame and fortune obtained in nurturing a gift to the max will guarantee a blissful life.

However, even a shallow survey of the lives of the rich and famous tells us that happiness is not that simple. Numerous psychological studies have revealed that because most things lose their lustre after a few months, once our basic needs of living have been met, having more seldom equates to greater happiness. In fact, sometimes it is the opposite. The more we have, the more we have to worry about, and the more we have to lose. How many people who win huge lotteries don't end up any happier? It can be hard to know when enough is enough.

In a world where you have to battle for safety, sustenance, and sexual partners, you need powerful neurochemical signals just to survive. So we are all wired for addictions, to take as much as we can get when it is available and to hoard it for ourselves: more is better, bigger is better, better is better. No wonder we can confuse needs and wants. Are you really twice as happy with a thirty-dollar bottle of wine as a fifteen-dollar bottle of wine? Do you really need an expensive car, or do you just want it or need to think that you deserve it?

Science has provided us with unprecedented opportunities for wealth, pleasure, power, and honour through technological advances. This means it is easier to lose our balance and become addicted if we are not constantly mindful of our brainstem neuronal impulses. I think addictions are on the increase for that reason: when we have not conquered ourselves the attraction of such opulence can be hard to pass up. We need intimacy to feel fulfilled, to feel loved, but you cannot have intimacy with things. Things are poor surrogates for the loving relationships with others that give our lives meaning.

I think two of the most challenging addictions involve eating and sex: the two behaviours we are wired for in order to sustain ourselves individually and as a species.

Eons ago we were programmed to never pass up a free lunch because food was not always plentiful. Now, for most of us in Western society, the opposite is true: it is too available, and the nutritive value is questionable. So the epidemic of obesity should not surprise us. Unfortunately, we have tended to focus on losing weight as opposed to not gaining weight. In other words, we have not been mindfully watching ourselves eat, so we end up overweight. Then we search for magical diets or exercises that will bypass the need to be mindful so that we can lose the excess weight far more quickly than we gained it. Mindlessness got us into the problem, and mindfulness can help to get us out of it.

What has been driving us to eat excessively? What has been distracting us from monitoring our diet and eating habits? What's been eating *at us*? The answers are not easy to find, and the solutions may require digging deeper into our psyche to deal with unresolved stress or faulty heuristics. That requires time, introspection, and the courage of intimacy. The same is true for all addictions, when we lose our balance, when we don't know when enough is enough.

We have to be patient; change takes time and seldom moves in a straight line. That is not to deny important physiologic and neurochemical aspects of weight gain and loss that may require medication. But overwhelmingly, my experience in practice is that patients are not prepared to make the small but significant fundamental changes that will pay off eventually because it could take several years, the time frame over which they gained the weight.

Yes, that can be disheartening; I am not by nature a patient person, so I fully understand. But never adopt any change in eating or activity that you cannot maintain for the rest of your life. Patiently and consistently follow that mantra, and you will succeed. Be always mindful of the food you buy, of every bite you put in your mouth—both the nutritional quality and the quantity. And be more active doing things you like to do, and do them with people you like to be with; that makes a huge difference. Exercise, when done mindfully and not to an extreme, can be powerful for our bodies and brains.

Now, what can I say about sex? Like anything else that is pleasurable, sex can devolve into an addiction if not engaged in mindfully and perhaps even more so because it is so primal to all forms of life. So again, it should not be surprising that many people obsess about it. Pornography is big business.

In my line of work, I have seen a lot of people naked (literally and figuratively), and I have made two startling observations:

1. With rare exceptions, we arrive in this world with one of two types of standard equipment. And there is less variation in genital structure than in the structure of almost any other parts of our body, and for good reason. Evolution demands uniformity for procreation to be successful. (I'm still upset that my Betamax lost out to VHS—I wish we could be as smart as nature.)

2. Trust me that almost all of us look better with our clothes on (myself included).

So, because we are all structured and wired to engage in sex, it means that sex is mostly a mind game. I would like to see us mature and engage in sex in ways that are loving, not narcissistic and selfish. I am not sure that we have much control over what turns us on sexually. Like most aesthetic preferences, it can be difficult to explain. However, although sexual thoughts may pop into our heads in the same way as any other thoughts do, we do not have to focus or obsess about them, and we certainly do not have to act on them. If we simply observe them as a thought—a neurochemical process in our heads like any other—then we don't have to let them define us or run our lives. That's being mindful.

I am personally unconcerned with what genitalia you have or what genitalia you want to have. Equally, I really don't care what thoughts enter your stream of consciousness that turn you on sexually, but *please* realize that you can be hurt and hurt other people with sex—physically and psychologically—so *at the very least* be ethical and loving with your sexuality. Otherwise, sex becomes an addiction that harms yourself and other people.

Child pornography is particularly harmful. Even if people do not act on their thoughts, involvement with child pornography still hurts innocent and helpless children. These people should get medical help if they have urges that they cannot control. To avoid harming, no one should engage in sex with someone who does not consent to what they want to do. That includes children and anyone incapable of giving consent because they lack capacity (i.e., mental illness, disease, head injury, intoxicants).

All addictions arise from desires for pleasure or from avoidance of pain. So often we focus on the harmful effects of the addictive behaviour, not on the underlying causation, like the alcohol posters I spoke of earlier. Drug and alcohol addictions, as we noted in an earlier chapter, often have their origin in social anxiety: we want to fit in, to feel like we are good enough, and these substances help us to do so. That doesn't make us bad; it reflects, rather, that we are sad. Often we find a certain kind of shallow acceptance in tribes who use substances as a means to deal with their existential angst. But such relationships are not truly loving; they encourage stagnation not growth.

Life is difficult; no amount of technology or other advances is going to eliminate that reality. We all find life challenging on a regular basis, and we all find ways to escape: hobbies, work, reading, movies, et cetera. In moderation, they can be healthy, but in excess they can become obsessions that make us lose our balance.

Sometimes we simply find the world too much to bear, and we turn to something that will ease the pain; licit or illicit intoxicants or other forms of escapism. I have often sincerely said that if I had to be stranded on a deserted island, I would choose to be stranded with an alcoholic because in my experience they are often very sensitive individuals. I just wouldn't want there to be any alcohol available!

So often I see individuals with addictions be too hard on themselves; their embarrassment is often the biggest impediment to getting better. This is particularly true with health-care workers because we often expect too much of ourselves, to be Übermensch. We deny our emotions and pretend that we can see misery and suffering and not be affected by it. We don't dare reflect on why bad things happen to good people, why life isn't always fair, or why there is suffering in the world. We just keep really busy and kid ourselves into thinking that we are doing okay, often as we sink into deeper cycles of addiction.

So many people need our help that we can be overwhelmed and lose our balance. We forget that you can't give from a dry well, no matter how much you want to help. No amount of denial can eliminate our humanity, and our insecurity is often at the heart of the problem. Health professionals often push, or are pushed, to the breaking point before they finally relent or are offered the same help we would provide to patients.

This highlights the importance of our attitudes to people with addictions. It is easy to get into "us and them" thinking when we see people suffering form addictions. Smoking is a great example. So often I hear people who do not smoke railing against those who do: we shouldn't take care of them, or we should punish them. But it would be prudent to realize that most people start smoking in their early teens, at a time when we are all very insecure and scared, and we want desperately to fit in. Smoking helps people be part of a tribe and relaxes them. They have often learned it at a vulnerable age from people close to them, like their parents (who in turn learned it from their parents).

Tobacco companies are powerful—they have managed to convince us not to make smoking illegal for minors in the same way as alcohol. True, minors cannot buy cigarettes, but they can walk down the street and smoke them, even though none of us can walk down the street drinking alcohol. Why do we allow that?

The craving for addictive substances and the withdrawal effects from them are powerful and both may well need pharmacological intervention in order to cope with the pain. For these reasons, we have tended in the past to focus more on the biomedical aspects of addictions and not enough on the underlying reasons for turning to these substances. We have often failed to appreciate the social circumstances of people with addictions, particularly the social circumstances they return to once completing a rehab program. We all tend to hang around with likeminded individuals, so it is hard to resist the superficial intimacy of tribal inertia that comforts us to wallow in immature, even self-destructive behaviours. For that reason, there is now more focus on aftercare and social support. We have finally come to realize how tough it is to change tribes.

But more than anything else, people with addictions of any type need to learn mindfulness so that they control the addiction and not vice versa. So often you can see that a patient will be successful because he has finally come to believe that he deserves to be happy, he is as good as anyone else, and with help he can control his lower brain cravings and become continent, in control, again. Blame and shame are of little help to people with addiction; we need to love them.

How we respond to adversity is so critical for our lives. Malcolm Gladwell's book *David and Goliath* explores the reality that many of the world's most accomplished people have faced huge adversity and by overcoming it have made massive contributions to society. They persevere in situations when many of us would falter.

Nassim Taleb, in his wonderful book *Antifragile*, goes even further. He explores the fact that some systems and individuals actually need adversity to flourish. It's more than resiliency, because they don't just survive or rebound, they excel. In other words, so much of our lives relates to our attitudes and approach to the inevitable mix of good and bad we encounter. We are all likely familiar with post-traumatic stress disorder. But there is also something called post-traumatic growth.

Sometimes our greatest transformations have their origins in adversity. I think we often forget that antifragility is a key feature of evolution.

This brings me to the topic of stubbornness. So often in our lives we can feel stuck, seemingly unable to extricate ourselves from unfulfilling life circumstances. There are usually extenuating factors beyond our control, but almost always there are factors we can control, but don't. Why is that?

For years I have struggled to understand stubbornness, and I still have no definitive answer. However, I am becoming more convinced that stubbornness is really fear amplified to such an extreme that we feel paralyzed to overcome it.

So we stay the course, refusing to change and to grow. The problem is, if we always do what we've always done, then we'll always get what we've always gotten.

Einstein said that insanity was doing the same thing over and over and expecting a different result.

It is only through intimacy that we can challenge our stubbornness, rewire and do things differently.

The remainder of this book looks at how we can do that in the health-care system, in our individual lives, and beyond. But not by using blame and shame. We can do better than that.

Chapter 28

Blame and Shame

Everything should be made as simple as possible, but not simpler.

—Albert Einstein

DO YOU EVER notice that whenever something unfortunate happens in the world, often our first reaction is to find someone to pounce on and attribute blame? That is quickly followed by experts claiming that the system responsible for said problem is broken and, of course, they alone have the solution to prevent all further unfortunate events from occurring. They can fix it.

This pattern is universal, but I probably notice it more in medicine because it is an area I understand a little better. Sometimes problems we have ignored finally rear their heads, and everyone recoils in horror. How could the people responsible possibly have ignored the warning signs for so long? It is called denial, and we all do it, sometimes even after we are caught.

Other times a black swan event occurs, and we are convinced that someone, somewhere, should have seen it coming and acted sooner. And, yet again, the experts or politicians or lawyers assure us that they will find solutions—through commissions, laws, punishments, more money and, of course, shame—such that no black swan will ever catch us off guard again. Ah, if only life were that simple!

When these events occur in medicine, I have often observed that someone remote from the problem, and frequently outside of the health-care system, gravely announces that the system is broken. Honestly, how can a system comprised of imperfect human beings expect not to be broken? We are all broken, aren't we? We don't start our lives completely mature, do we? None of us has conquered ourselves, have we? How can a chain be expected to be stronger than all of its weak links?

Of course, there are times when people have legitimately and innocently erred and correction is possible. Equally, there are times when narcissism or selfishness indicate that the error was not so innocent and must be dealt with accordingly. But until we humans become perfect, we are going to make mistakes, innocent or not, and it is self-aggrandizing hubris to claim otherwise, particularly about rare and thus difficult to predict events. (Even more so when we know that we are not responsible, and we can blame and shame someone else!)

Too often we oversimplify and find one scapegoat to take the blame for the inevitable failure of complex systems. Pain and fear are at the root of such attitudes and behaviours, and anxious individuals who find it difficult to keep their emotions in check often run the agendas. Often we fail to realize that it's much easier to make a drug error when you have to know details of thousands of drugs, not a hundred, and when patients are taking ten drugs not two.

As the world becomes more complicated and complex, not only is error more likely, but the ramifications for mistakes escalate, so stress increases for us all. Misfiring a rifle harms far fewer people than misfiring a nuclear weapon, so narcissistic and selfish individuals become more dangerous and powerful.

Yes, we do need to be held accountable for our actions in order to grow. However, when very anxious people demand nothing short of perfection in an increasingly complicated and complex world, and experts promise that they alone can assure such perfection, they are both living in a binary world of naive realism. The former want to be perfectly safe, and the latter want to be the centres of attention, our saviours, and we might be wise to take them both with a grain of salt.

I hate to say it, but the medical profession is as guilty of this as any. We often feel the pressure, sometimes self-imposed, to fix everything even though we know that we can't.

We medical types like to simplify things sometimes to the point of being simplistic. We take complex concepts and reduce them to atomistic levels and think that we lose nothing in the process. Like taking apart a watch and thinking that it still tells time. When using the kitchen drain analogy to describe the heart, we forget that our blood and our arteries are complex living things that interact with each other in ways we do not fully understand. (Of course, we are not alone. Many of us assume all things natural must be benign, forgetting that arsenic is a naturally occurring element, that you can drown in water and that oxygen is actually highly toxic to the lungs in excessive amounts, which is a constant struggle in ICU's.)

When I was first in practice, we started to get a glimpse of the complex interplay of blood and arteries. At first we suggested that everyone over age forty, particularly men, take two regular strength (2 x 325 mg) Aspirins per day. As we began to look more closely, however, we realized that there were risks to that, so we then suggested taking only one aspirin. Then we realized that perhaps not everyone should do so. Then we discovered that 81 mg was just as good. Now we tend to suggest it mostly for secondary prevention, not primary. With each iteration, we were sure that we had finally found the definitive answer. I am waiting for the next definitive answer.

I suspect this oversimplification is a manifestation of our deep tendency for binary thinking—this is food or it isn't; that is safe or it isn't. Einstein's quote opening this chapter reminds us of this: when we oversimplify something, we often lose its essence.

I can think of no better example of this than medicine's embarrassing promotion of infant formula over breastfeeding, particularly in the fifties and sixties.

On four levels it is very telling of the profession, but more importantly, it is telling of the way humans think and behave. I am sure I could find similar examples in any field of study, not just in medical practice.

On the first level, we thought that we could come up with a mode of nutrition that would rival, if not exceed, breastfeeding. Now just try for a moment to think like a scientist. Nature has been experimenting with breastfeeding for hundreds of millions of years using literally trillions of test subjects, not the least of whom are we humans. This business of breastfeeding appears to have been rather successful thus far.

Now in order to prove that you have a process better than breastfeeding, you would have to perform an experiment that would produce a volume of data of similar orders of magnitude. For example, if you want to prove that a two-sided coin is fair, you have to flip it more than once. Statistically speaking, even with a perfect coin, there is a very good chance that you would not get fifty heads and fifty tails after one hundred flips. The more flips you do, the more likely you are to reach a fifty-fifty split *if* the coin is fair. Naturally, you would have far more trust in a coin that flipped fifty-fifty after one trillion flips than a coin that did so after only one hundred.

So to prove that formula is just as good as breast milk, you would have to compare millions of infants over thousands of years to have the same level of confidence as we have in breast milk. Before we duped mothers into opting for formula, did we have that kind of data? I think not.

Nevertheless, we pushed formula to young mothers so much so that entire generations (including mine) were not breastfed. We were far too sure of ourselves, and the public trusted us far too much.

That's not to say that there isn't a role for formula as either a supplement or for women who choose, for a wide variety of often very good reasons, not to breastfeed. But from a purely statistical perspective, we should have made it clear that formula feeding should not be the default position on the basis of it being just as good because we simply could not prove that. Medicine (and commerce) believed what it wanted to believe, made the data fit, and then convinced us with minimal evidence. I am reminded of essayist Anaïs Nin's observation: "We don't see things as they are but as we are."

On the second level, medicine fell prey to its own need to be Übermensch. I appreciate the importance of health care and the noble foundation upon which it has been built: to help others. It is part of what attracted me to the profession. However, our Hippocratic oath also reads: *primum non nocere*—above all do no harm. It speaks to the issue that sometimes the best thing to do is either nothing or act simply as an assistant to nature. We don't have to be Übermensch. When we overplay our hand and exaggerate what we can do, we risk losing our credibility and thus the trust of patients.

Breastfeeding is completely natural, but that does not mean it is easy and without pain. Lots of very worthwhile endeavours in life that are natural come with a price; just look at an infant learning to walk! However, medicine often wants to play the role of hero, but when we do so, we deprive patients of the opportunity to grow—we give them a fish rather than teaching them to fish. We see people having pain or fear, and we just want to get rid of it for them, rather than helping them to conquer their fears and pain.

We could have invested the same amount of time, research, and money into assisting women with breastfeeding through more promotion, more education, more mentoring, funding more lactation consultants, and better breast pumps. Instead, we chose to come to the rescue of the poor damsels in distress who were struggling with breastfeeding and just bypass the entire process. In other words, we got so wrapped up in our own ego needs to be the great fixers that we forgot to love our patients.

Thank goodness we have come to our collective senses and now encourage and assist women in this challenging, yet supremely rewarding, process by focusing on them (and their infants), not on us.

The third level highlights the shallow degree of science that we do. We have no appreciation for how complicated and complex the universe is—we oversimplify. How could we possibly have missed the fact that the formulae we produce contain *no bioactive* organic ingredients, and breast milk is loaded with them (like immunoglobulins)? The benefit of these factors is enormous as evidenced in studies confirming myriad advantages, including fewer infectious diseases in infants, for example.

The fourth and perhaps most important level is one that illustrates the limited depth of the scope of medical practice. Modern medicine adopts a very biomechanical perspective of the human species. The major reason for that is that it is easier. In the physiosphere, things are more distinct and defined and therefore more quantifiable. That's why we use analogies from the physiosphere like kitchen drains for biospheric entities like arteries without realizing the severe limitations of them. To make matters worse, we persist in doing so even when it comes to the noosphere.

When we compared breastfeeding and bottle-feeding, we simply examined the effects of delivering nutritive contents into a baby's stomach (and as noted, we didn't even do that very well). It never occurred to us that *how* it was delivered mattered. We may as well have advocated having a robot tube-feed the formula into the infant's innards because we did not recognize the phenomenal difference between that process and the tender, intimate, and loving engagement of mother and child.

While trying to come up with a miracle breast milk replacement, we missed the intangible benefits of the real miracle called breastfeeding that were right before our eyes. We could not see it because it was too close. And because we could not measure such factors quantitatively, we simply chose to ignore them. They didn't seem to matter. I am reminded of Einstein's comment: "Not everything that counts can be counted; not everything that can be counted, counts."

Of course, we are starting to realize that these matters do count. I wonder if that's because more physicians themselves happen to breastfeed since more physicians are now women? Is it possible that the male-dominated medical profession of the fifties and sixties didn't value the contribution that women made to society by breastfeeding (not to mention their other contributions)?

Equally, we have finally realized that the human touch of parents in neonatal intensive care units improves prognosis. You mean we're not just robots? Recall my relationship with Jane—touch matters. Ever been hugged?

To be fair, Western societies, and I suspect lots of other societies, have not valued child-rearing nearly enough, so anything associated with it was not valued much either (particularly motherhood, and to a lesser degree, fatherhood). We have explored this concept earlier with respect to the great wisdom writers; they rarely write of parenthood in their exploration of the meaning of life or the search for eternal truths. It has only been relatively recently that women were granted maternity leaves of up to one year, and even more recently that men have qualified for paternity leave as well.

Similarly, as with our bottle-feeding versus breastfeeding experience, we have chosen to ignore the possibility that there may be a significant and important difference between a child being raised by strangers with college degrees compared with the child's parents or other family members raising the child. We make it difficult for parents to work part time if they choose to balance work with parenthood. We don't find creative ways for parents to bring their infants to work to allow for some substantial and intimate contact throughout the day rather than just the mad rush at the end of an exhausting one.

The medical profession has done little to open up this dialogue. In part, that is because we have not valued it within our own profession. I have been as guilty of this as most of my peers; it is the culture we were raised in. (I remember doing a rotation in neurosurgery during clerkship and one of the staff men saying, "If you recognize your kids, you're not working hard enough." No exaggeration.)

I think it is time for us to rethink things. Yes, what we do in our professional lives is important, but it is not so important that it should always trump raising our children. I become more convinced every day that a very large amount of illness in our society relates to unhealthy lifestyles, particularly ones that affect our mental health.

The mental health of our families, however we define a family, matters greatly and has tremendous impacts not only on the family's physical health but the physical and mental health of our entire society. For example, seldom do I hear the profession speak out about the negative effects that shiftwork has on our health, both physical and mental, and how that adversely affects our relationships, especially with spouses and children.

Now I don't want to be too hard on the medical tribe; we fair no worse than most tribes, and better than many I suspect. Despite our imperfect humanness, I can think of few tribes nobler, and none I would be more proud to serve in. Every tribe falls prey to the same errors we do, in one fashion or another; we can all get carried away with our own importance. So how do we avoid making mistakes like we did with bottle-feeding? (And how do other tribes avoid their mistakes, too?)

I think we are beginning to realize the extreme limitations of the biomechanical model of medicine. Medicine is recognizing qualitative as well as quantitative analysis. We are starting to appreciate the importance of our feelings, intuition, autobiographical self-narratives, and nonrational selves. It's very tempting to limit ourselves to the binary thinking of our brainstem or the concrete thinking associated with the left cerebral cortex because they feel so definable, so safe.

I suggest that we become more humble. Despite its limitations, we did not even use the scientific method in medicine until a little over a century ago. And the application of ethical principles to the practice of medicine dates back barely over a half century. Despite good intentions, the history of medicine at times reads more like a horror story than a tale of altruism. And that goes not just for medicine, but for all human undertakings: law, education, politics, business, and others.

I suspect that you are getting tired of me saying that the universe is a complicated and complex place. But it is, and we constantly get overexcited when we discover something new and blow it out of proportion; we lack humility. How often have you read that a new discovery is going to revolutionize something really important, never to hear of it again? How often do you get confused when one study says that x is good for you, and two weeks later we are told that x is really bad for you?

There are several reasons why this happens, and you likely know them. We always have more than one motive for doing something, and although the one obvious motive in medicine is for improved health of the population, the more opaque one may be the more important one. Just look to Aquinas's four temptations—wealth, pleasure, power, or honour. As we have explored earlier, we are attracted to these four things because they make us feel good or special or put us centre of attention. This is true for all professions, not just medicine.

Money, in particular, is a great motivator in our society; when we say that someone is successful, we invariably mean that he has a lot of money. It saddens me to think that money is often the final common currency for all of our life values. Most new drugs, for example, incur costs in excess of a quarter of a billion dollars on their way to the marketplace. That's a lot of money, and those involved, including shareholders, expect a healthy profit for that kind of risk, sometimes to the exclusion of other more noble values.

Several decades ago, 80 percent of medical research occurred in academic environments, and 20 percent took place in business settings. The ratios are now reversed, which means that the motivation underlying most medical research is not a noble quest for understanding but for profit. The influence of money on the medical profession has grown enormously, and we should be on high alert for its corrupting influence.

Whenever you examine any research, find out what was going on behind the scenes. Are the physicians (sometimes referred to as "experts") who are advocating for a certain treatment also board members of companies that manufacture that treatment?

I often get the sense that we have unbridled enthusiasm for all research. I suspect that both fear and our childlike sense of awe account for this. But a significant amount of research in any field yields very little value beyond padding the resumes (and potentially wallets) of the multiple authors involved.

In order to stay humble and maintain our integrity, it behooves us to avoid magical thinking and do proper science when we do research. That requires using the null hypothesis as our starting point, not the financial bottom line.

We would like to find a treatment for a certain disease, cancer z for example, and we are wondering if drug a might be helpful. Perhaps we choose drug a because it has worked on cancers similar to cancer z, or it was successful in treating cancer z in animals, or perhaps from a theoretical biochemical perspective we think it may work. Our starting point is one of hopeful ignorance, in other words, the null position—we have an inkling, but we just don't know *for sure,* at least not enough to risk people's lives.

Further, no matter what the result, provided that we are satisfied that we do the experiment properly, we will be happy because then we will know one way or the other what the truth is: to what degree a drug is helpful. Science should not be invested in any particular outcome; it should be interested in the truth. (Not surprisingly, journals of all types are more likely to publish positive results than negative ones. Equally, the Nobel Prize is far more often awarded for positive discoveries than negative ones, even though both may be of equal value.)

It's easy to fall prey to naive realism, but we do ourselves a great disservice when we don't question or examine information more closely. Yes, we should be excited when new discoveries are made (even ones with negative results), but that should not preclude developing a healthy skepticism that encourages us to examine data very closely. In the process of being critically analytical, we do not have to fall into nihilistic thinking or cynicism in the process.

One of the best examples I can think of in terms of understanding this point is the discovery several years ago by one group of physicists that neutrinos were found to travel faster than the speed of light. It caused quite a stir in the physics community because for almost one hundred years we had believed that nothing could travel faster than the speed of light. The implications would have been enormous; it challenged the very foundation of modern physics, Einstein's time-honoured theories of relativity.

Despite this, people kept an open mind. They wanted to know the truth, not protect the status quo, so they performed more experiments and in the end found out that the original results were faulty. But the open-mindedness to whatever outcome is what defines true science. We must constantly guard against the truisms that we often see what we want to see, we can only see that which we already believe, and when we tell ourselves something often enough we start to believe it is true.

Science depends on the principle of falsifiability. In other words, real science has doubt and uncertainty at its very core: something is not considered scientific if there exists no experiment by which it can be proven false. (Some would argue that evolution is not science because there is no way to test it!) This means that engaging in the scientific process requires humility, open-mindedness, and courage. One can be confident, but there is no room for arrogance.

We must also remember that absence of evidence does not constitute evidence of absence. In other words, just because we haven't proven that something is so, does not mean it is not so. As Nassim Taleb would say, "Just because you haven't come upon a black swan does not mean that they do not exist." That's what falsifiability means, and why the neutrino discovery, even though it was in error, was so illustrative of what science is all about.

In the nonbinary world that we inhabit, everything lies along a spectrum, and there is a tension in all of this. At one end of the spectrum, as I explored in medical education, is theory (episteme) and at the other end practice (techne). We need to balance living in the here and now, where we don't know for sure, with the desire to understand the world better and improve upon it. It's what the child prodigy I met in medical school didn't quite get. We may not fully understand breastfeeding and want to do better, but empirically we know that it has worked for millions of years for countless species.

This means that in order to advance our knowledge, we have to take risks, live with uncertainty, and come to peace with the fact that we are going to make mistakes. When the stakes are high, such as disability and death, that's a tough pill to swallow. The experts, as well as politicians and lawyers, don't always get that. They, too, want to pretend that they can rescue us from all of this, but like doctors, they can't either. We all live in the same probabilistic universe, as scary as that may be.

Many people fault the health-care system for being focused too much on disease and not enough on health. In fairness, using highly trained personnel and very pricey facilities like hospitals to encourage someone to stop smoking, for example, is very inefficient. By all means educate and encourage healthy lifestyles, but save the specialized and costly resources to do what they are good at when prevention is either nonexistent or fails (which will always occur in an imperfect world).

I fully understand why patients turn to alternative or complementary medicine. These disciplines may not always use science the way standard medicine does, but they know that practice provides answers, too. They understand the big picture better sometimes. I don't know if alternative medicine can withstand the scrutiny of hard science, but a lot of classical medicine can't either. Regardless, all of these disciplines, classical and alternative, share a few things in common.

First, they all deal with probabilities, none of which are ever 0 percent or 100 percent. Acknowledging this is fundamental to truth telling in any field or endeavour. Second, patients are frequently motivated by fear, and that can interfere with critical analysis. This is particularly true when patients or clients are relatively ignorant of how the body works and have a tendency, in their gullibility, to oversimplify. Third, the human organism often heals itself, and sometimes believing that you can heal yourself is the greatest medicine there is, even if the "real medicine," classic or alternative, is not that effective. Just look at the success of placebos. They are not a manifestation of simply duping oneself into feeling one is better; our mind can actually help us to heal, and so can the minds of others.

Because we are an interactive species, our relationships matter a lot. This is perhaps the greatest attraction that alternative medicine offers to patients, something that I think it provides better than classical medicine does. I do not want to imply that alternative medicine treatments are not potentially valuable in and of themselves, but when patients are listened to, feel understood, given hope and insight, and offered practical wisdom, in other words they feel cared for, I think that makes a world of difference.

Every second our bodies fight off all kinds of infective organisms and destroy myriad abnormal or malfunctioning cells, and we can influence these processes. Nature heals in part by destroying. Patients can be the healers when they rid themselves of unhealthy thinking and behaviours. As Malcolm Gladwell's book *David and Goliath* illustrates, attitude matters.

As I said earlier, I have paroxysmal atrial fibrillation, and I am convinced (though I have no episteme to prove it!) that my handling of stress has contributed to its development. I do take medications, and they help, but they cannot cure. A cure may not be possible, but I can make it better when I take care of myself, physically and mentally.

Part of this is acceptance. You may think it absurd, but I would say that developing my condition has been a gift. It has forced me to face my own mortality. It provided an opportunity for me to reexamine my life and lifestyle. I have slowed down, I eat better, I avoid all caffeine and alcohol, and all of these have been good things, things I might not have done had I not developed A-fib. The realist does not look at the glass as half-empty or half-full, but rather as a glass half-full of life-giving water and half-filled with life-giving air.

And that's the challenge: how to manage the good with the bad. Everything in the universe lies along a spectrum, where everything includes within itself its own opposite. We live in a world where we must learn to balance the opposing tensions. Yes, the health-care system, like all human systems, is broken and always will be; we can't fix it any more than we can fix people. We are all broken; I am and so are you.

However, we must not allow ourselves to fall into a nihilism that prevents us from reflecting and introspecting about how we can grow. It is true that we have a tendency to say that someone "deserves" her misfortune when we find something she did that likely contributed to her woe. But that is fear talking because life is never that simple. Every decision we make, whether it is followed by action or inaction, is probabilistic. Some actions are riskier than others, but none are without risks, and often it is luck what differentiates those who get good results from those who don't. People may be foolish and take risks we deem unreasonable, but that does not mean that they deserve their misfortune.

Accountability is necessary for maturation, but self-serving or arrogant blame and shame are seldom helpful. Therein lies the tension: there are no *easy or simple* solutions, but there are solutions when we learn to love well.

In that vein, in the following chapter, I will explore the challenges for the medical profession from outside the tribe and from within the tribe. Many of these challenges are not peculiar to the practice of medicine because all human endeavours involve humans. The details may be different, but that's about all. While reading the next chapter, ask yourself if there are any applications in what you do in your life because no doubt there are. When you fall short of the best that you can do, you might want to ask yourself, What is the best path for you to do better: the one of blame and shame or the one of compassion and love?

Whatever path you choose, it might be good to reflect upon Kant's first categorical imperative:

> *Act only in accordance with that maxim through which you can at the same time will that it become a universal law.*

Otherwise known as the golden rule.

Chapter 29

Asymptotes

Losing our illusions is painful because illusions are the stuff we live by. Beyond the illusions is a fuller truth.

—Parker Palmer, *The Promise of Paradox*

IF WE ARE going to evolve as a species, we need to understand ourselves better and grow past our illusions. Compassionate mentoring is more likely to nurture us than simplistic blame and shame.

In that vein, this chapter explores areas where our health-care system can mature by looking at factors that are both outside and inside the profession. Much of it follows from our exploration of intimacy. Often the two perspectives, outside and inside of the profession, are like two sides of the same imperfect coin, so let's avoid blame and shame. We are all human.

Challenges from Outside the Tribe

Today the plethora of information for patients to access from so many sources feeds anxiety. Patients are presenting with more concerns during every visit, and they are well aware of all of the black swans out there and want to be assured without a shadow of a doubt that they are not afflicted by one of these rare birds. That can be tough to do.

For example, these days a very large percentage of babies born with abnormalities have developed them in utero, not during the birthing process. In other words, to some degree we are maxing out how much better we can make obstetrics (and part of that involves an increased rate of Caesarean sections) in terms of providing a "perfect outcome." The next step involves more prenatal screening, so the next level of lawsuits is going to be related to failed detection of these uncommon or even rare abnormalities, not in suing for "bad deliveries."

(To be fair, we have probably always attributed too much blame to the delivery process. Studies have clearly shown, for example, that the majority of children born with cerebral palsy had nothing in their labours and deliveries to clearly prove that the damage occurred during delivery. Given that the brain is the most complex and least well understood part of our body, it should not be surprising that a multitude of factors we do not yet understand, from conception to labour, have affected its growth and development, not just labour and delivery. Our self-important arrogance backfired when so many parents sued us for "damaging" their newborns and giving them cerebral palsy.)

We often turn to technology to lessen our anxiety and reassure ourselves that there isn't a black swan lurking. Our love of technology is growing, but it is not new; we have always been suckers for it.

Years ago two interesting experiments were done. In the first, patients who were bedbound and afflicted by bedsores were treated with a new apparatus that was designed to speed the healing of their bedsores. Every two hours the patient was turned in order to have this machine deliver its healing rays on the skin ulcers. The results were amazingly good, and there was tremendous excitement that this new technology was a medical breakthrough.

But the machine was a complete sham. The healing occurred because the patients were turned every two hours, relieving pressure on their skin and thus minimizing the development of bedsores and facilitating their healing.

In the second, a new medication was tested to see if it reversed dementia. The medication had to be taken several times per day, and patients were monitored for side effects as well as improvement. In the course of a mere few weeks, patients' mental statuses improved remarkably.

The drug was a placebo. Why the improvement? In the processes of delivering and monitoring the drug the patients received considerably more social interaction than those who did not. That's what got them better; people were the drug.

Medicine will always remain primarily a noetic pursuit, not a technological one, because human interaction is always going to be the most important part of medicine, no matter how much technology we develop. (I suspect that is true for all human pursuits.) It is important for patients and doctors to remember that. New technology is always expensive, so we have to budget carefully. On the other hand, talk is cheap (in a good sense).

The cases mentioned above illustrate that it's hard to avoid tunnel vision, and not just with respect to technology. Patients don't always appreciate that most illnesses have many symptoms that can overlap with symptoms of other diseases. That's why it's best to seek the perspective of a physician prior to doing all kinds of tests and before you figuratively have yourself dead and buried.

Of course, it's always easier to see things clearly with the retrospectroscope than it is to see them in advance; black swans are always much easier to see in hindsight. Experts and lawyers may deny this, and their binary thinking can lead us into naive denial as well. For this reason, it is not surprising that the fear of lawsuits and disciplinary action often drives decisions by physicians. We want to please, and we don't want to miss anything. In a society where we are so often guaranteed 100 percent satisfaction in all aspects of life, mistakes and errors of judgment are poorly tolerated, especially medical ones.

One of the great challenges facing the profession is that it is no fun giving bad news, and patients don't want to hear bad news either. Many years ago I had a patient who was being followed by an out-of-town oncologist, so I had not seen her for over a year. I noticed that she had an appointment with me, and I reviewed the latest note from her specialist. In it he stated that there was no further treatment they could offer, but if she were still alive in two months, he would see her back for a CT scan. Not surprisingly, I wasn't looking forward to her visit.

She came in with a couple of family members, and to be safe I asked her about her most recent visit with the cancer doctor. Enthusiastically, and supported by her family, she stated that she was pleased with her most recent medical visit and was looking forward to the CT scan in two months when she would see her oncologist again.

I was flabbergasted! I didn't know what to say. I have since come to realize that many patients are not ready for the whole truth (and sometimes neither is their family), and although we must not lie, we must dole out the truth in a way that patients can manage. Disclosure is not meant to be punitive. We often take cues from the patient in this regard. (Here is my advice to all patients, particularly cancer patients: if you are someone who wants to know the *whole* truth, even if it is not pleasant, then make that clear to your treating physician. Otherwise, it is often assumed that your silence indicates that you are not quite ready, and information is parsed out accordingly.)

At the other end of the spectrum, I had a patient with a smoking-related cancer with a poor prognosis, which she knew, who was offered an expensive experimental treatment that she could not afford as she had no supplementary medical coverage. Her family was angry. In a genuine spirit of trying to find solutions, I commented that if everyone in the family gave up smoking and contributed the savings, they could collectively pay for most of her treatment. I thought the idea of both reducing their own risks of developing cancer as well as helping their mother beat hers was a win-win. However, they didn't see it that way. *Not at all.* I was *persona non grata.*

Now a lot older and a little wiser, I understand the human elements of both of these scenarios better than I did then. People don't always think or behave rationally, especially when stressed. And they don't always welcome the opportunity to do so either.

Often I hear patients complain, and rightfully so, that physicians don't educate them well enough. There are many reasons for that but the one reason that is sometimes the most honest is that we simply can't explain things. It can be difficult for doctors to admit when we don't know or understand, and even more unsettling for patients to hear that. When we ask deeper questions, we run the risk of the pain of shattered illusions, our Ubermensch letting us down.

Human behaviour is complex and hard to predict. I am not sure that we always appreciate that; in particular, the legal system sometimes expects more than is realistic. I often feel sorry for psychiatrists in this regard.

Other challenges for the profession? We can all deceive ourselves. Tell yourself something often enough, and you'll start to believe it is true. How often have I seen someone with an alcohol addiction convince herself that everyone—her spouse, the police, her boss—is conspiring against her? She can quit drinking any time, and would, if everyone just got off her back.

There can be many hidden agendas lurking beneath the surface of any story. Some people are just unhappy and are never satisfied. Desperate people can lie. Some people get so into the role of being sick that it can become their identity. I think that some patients become addicted to their disease. Physicians take fiduciary oaths and are regulated by professional bodies of oversight. Patients do not take oaths; there is no organization to report unreasonable patients.

Although all of us have had unpleasant or even scary encounters with patients, they are fortunately very uncommon. For the first twenty or so years of my career, there were no repercussions for misbehaving patients, and I found that quite unsettling. Yes, we want to be compassionate, knowing that illness, physical or mental, underlies such behaviour. But our compassion must have limits, otherwise innocent people, including fellow patients, can be harmed. In the last several years I have finally noticed signage in medical settings indicating that unruly behaviour and language will not be tolerated.

However, there is, at least in Western society, a growing sense of entitlement that can be just as unnerving. I understand where it is coming from. The many advances in our society—scientific, political, social—have made our lives much better. Everything seems guaranteed these days. I refer to it as the "thirty-minutes-or-less-pizza syndrome" (if you don't get your pizza delivered in thirty minutes, it is free). Business, law, politics, and even medicine all promise not only to make every dream come true but to compensate you—and punish someone else—if they don't come true. But it's not realistic.

A colleague of mine, after a particularly trying day, said he was going to get a T-shirt made and wear it to the office. It would read

> Life is difficult.
>
> You're not special.
>
> You don't always get what you want.
>
> Get over it.

We all have days like that, no matter where we work. The practice of medicine, however, is a little unique for three reasons.

First, society often expects us to solve a lot of problems that cannot be solved or that are not primarily medical. For example, businesses expect doctors to police the sick policies they have developed. That is not our job. Businesses must come to realize that when you hire human beings, they are going to get sick occasionally and miss work. Most of these illnesses do not require a visit to the doctor; a cold is a cold. If you can't accept that, then don't hire humans, hire machines.

Of course, machines can't replace a lot of the things humans can do, so businesses will just have to accept that humans get sick and accommodate for that. If an employee is missing too much work, then there may be a more serious medical problem lurking, and then we are happy to see the patient and get to the bottom of it. But I don't need to see you for a cold just because your boss wants a note as a way for me to police his company's sick policy for him. I have a fiduciary relationship with the patient, not with the person's employer. If there is no underlying serious medical problem, physical or psychological, then employers are going to have to deal with excessive work absence as a performance issue, not a medical one.

Second, physicians must take care of the sickest people before we deal with the less sick people. Sometimes you will have to wait because a doctor is occupied with someone with a more serious, and often unexpected, problem. We all know what a hassle that is, but we do not prioritize people based on how much we like them, how long we have known them, or how much they yell at us. Medical need is always paramount, as frustrating as that can be.

Third, medicine is an enterprise of the collective. Although I have a fiduciary relationship with the patient in front of me, I also have the same relationship with every other patient with whom I interact (and so do all of the other physicians with their patients). So I have to weigh and balance everything I do with all patients in that context, including utilizing collective resources.

We may kid ourselves into believing that privatizing medicine is the answer, but almost every aspect of a patient's care, even when privately paid for, is based on the resources of the collective. The doctor who sees you was trained at a university supported by funds from many sources, as are the roads that lead to health-care facilities, the utilities those facilities use, the talents of all of the support workers, an so forth. We all benefit from the contributions of many other people over many decades.

Further, private facilities often claim that their motivations are purely for greater efficiency and thus improved patient care. In other words, the assumption is that publicly funded medical facilities are inefficient, and without the bureaucratic constraints endemic to these large institutions, more patients can be cared for at less cost. That may be true to some degree, and if it is, then the physicians running them should not have to charge more than what the public-pay system provides. After all, by their own admission, more efficiency means more profit, too. So why is it that they all charge so much extra for care? In other words, we need to be careful with privatization, despite the public pressure.

Challenges within the profession

I remember the first time I ever wrote a real prescription, one that did not need the cosignature of a "real doctor." I was an intern working in emerg, and it was for an antibiotic for a child with an ear infection. I experienced an innocent excitement, as the many years of study had finally allowed me to do something tangibly useful in the world, not just pass exams.

All of us need to feel that we are useful, that we matter. But it would be wise for us to monitor what we do, and as I said earlier, I am not completely sure that we do that enough in medicine. In particular, I don't think that we monitor the harm that we do.

When we disseminate medical information and statistics inaccurately, or exaggerated with excess drama, we can generate a lot of anxiety. Paradoxically, giving people the impression that we know more than we do and that we can control more than we are able, can produce more angst because we provide a standard for quality and quantity of life that is unattainable. Black swans exist and by definition are unpredictable, often unpreventable, and frequently difficult to treat. In general, the harder it is to diagnose something, the harder it is to treat; rare conditions imply that we have less information upon which to make decisions and test treatments.

We have a duty, I think, to help the public come to peace with uncertainty and guide the use of finite resources wisely. We need to admit when we don't know, explain NNT and NNH, and educate about the limitations of testing.

We have become enamoured with experts, but expertise is transient because our understanding is changing all of the time. Sometimes it's the big picture that matters more. As I stated earlier, often I see studies where one discipline has cured a symptom but not the problem. For example, a treatment may ameliorate one set of symptoms (headaches) only to result in the patient developing a new set of symptoms of another body system (irritable bowel syndrome). Why? Because the real cause of both sets of symptoms was unresolved stress, and until it is addressed, the body will continue to manifest it one way or another. Generalists see the forest; specialists see the trees. Both add value.

This is why it is so important for physicians to understand what it is they do for a living, and for patients to understand it too. My job as a doctor is not to tell you how to live your life; only you can and should do that. Each one of us constantly does so on the basis of our internal value system whether we realize it or not. We may be very explicit in our understanding and vocalization of those values, or we may do so at a very tacit or subconscious level. We each choose our level of mindfulness.

This may shock you, but I don't tell people to stop smoking. Now before you light my book on fire for saying something so heretical, give me a moment to explain.

I don't know when I am going to die. So if I don't know that about me, I certainly don't know that about you or anyone else, including any of my patients. It is true that smokers tend to die younger than nonsmokers and also true that smoking cessation is perhaps one of the most beneficial lifestyle changes one can make to improve quality and quantity of life. However, I don't know if a specific patient who smokes is going to die of a smoking-related illness. Perhaps a car accident will kill the patient long before he gets lung cancer. Maybe he will develop a non-smoking-related terminal illness before he has a heart attack.

I have known patients who have defied the odds and never had a smoking-related illness; it just isn't very common if you live long enough. The point is that for any given patient, I just don't know his particular fate, nor does anyone else, including the patient. All I can give any patient are the probabilities; the rest is pure speculation.

That is my job, essentially: to assist and support patients in dealing with the odds, offering my compassion, knowledge, and skills to help them in decision making with the hope of improving their lives. The rest is up to the patients. I can help them clarify or even modify the values they use for making decisions. But I cannot predict the future, and I cannot fix patients on my own. I do not *tell* patients what to do (except in the unusual circumstances of unconsciousness or incapacity and only so as to secure their safety).

This brings me to an important point about being a doctor: there is a world of difference between taking what you do seriously and taking yourself seriously. How often have you seen a celebrity develop a medical condition that she never knew existed or cared about—until she got it! All of a sudden, it is the most important disease on the planet. Lots of people take themselves far too seriously and feel the need for a lot of drama in their lives. I suspect it stems from that need to feel special.

I think doctors should take what they do seriously because it involves the health and lives of other people. I also think that car mechanics should, too, for the same reason. Ditto for crane operators, police officers, parents, teachers, and utility workers. In fact, I think everyone should take their jobs seriously if it has a potential to impact the lives of fellow humans (which means almost any job that is legal).

I always chuckle when someone applying to medical school or recently entering medical school is asked why they are doing so. Invariably, the answer is something along the lines of "I want to help humanity" or "I want to make the world a better place."

Now I don't want to be mean to these individuals because I know they are speaking sincerely. But in truth, everyone who does anything that is contributing positively to the collective should feel the same way. The only people who don't we regard as sociopaths or psychopaths because they suffer from intense narcissism, but they are a very small percentage of the population.

In other words, unless you are part of that small group of sad and lonely individuals, whatever you do should be at least in part about making the world a better place. We should generally choose a path that we also enjoy if at all possible. Is that selfish? Of course it is! But that's okay because we tend to be better at things we enjoy (and are proficient at) as well as being happier and better people, from which we all benefit.

So to answer that you chose medical school because you want to make the world a better place can border on undue self-importance, as though no individuals other than physicians think that way, or physicians help the most, or we alone have no other motives. If we are mature and honest, we should answer that, like all people, we want to make the world a better place, we just think our interests and talents are inclined to medicine as opposed to other activities (like running a daycare or fixing unsafe cars). As I said earlier, I am not sure what else I would have done if I had not been accepted to medical school. Lucky I wasn't born five hundred years before they existed!

Each of us has gifts that we can, and should, bring to the collective. It's what evolution planned for us when it gave us the profound and varied abilities we have, not the least of which are our abilities to interact with and care for one another. Sharing has always been part of the plan. Humbly sharing our gifts and revelling in the good fortune of being able to contribute is the sign of a mature mind.

Doctors often feel, or are led to believe, that we are natural leaders. But so often we are taught that leadership is about being an Übermensch, that unique kind of individual who can lead and rescue the mere mortals. Mature leadership, however, involves humility, knowing that none of us is smarter than all of us put together. Kierkegaard put it succinctly when he said, "We must safeguard each person's power to become fully themselves; when we do we are acting morally."

We are part of a collective, and we are meant to contribute to it, not dominate it. Being mentored to reach your full potential, be that in university or the school of life, is not so much about finding a job as it is about finding your place in the world. We grow out of the necessary narcissism of childhood into a self-giving adulthood, where we pay back the care we were given as vulnerable children by in turn contributing to the care of the vulnerable in the collective—the young, the old, the disabled, the disadvantaged. All of us, not just doctors, must lead to our fullest ability.

Leadership is a moral act because it is about how we treat others. In order to be mature and moral leaders, we must start with humility. Yes, physicians are generally academically bright and have other talents as well. We often have a strong work ethic. But we also bring our own pathologies with us. Like everyone else, none of us came from perfect families or had perfect childhoods. And none of us have yet conquered ourselves. We can be swayed by the lure of Aquinas's four temptations.

In Western society, when we say that someone is successful, we usually mean that t he person has acquired a lot money, power, honour (fame), or pleasure. Physicians are considered successful, and so they often feel that they should be at the top of the income scale and are often bitter that people doing jobs of "lesser importance" make more money than they do. But they are not unique in this regard; anyone with a special talent tends to feel the same way since we are all built the same way. Any of us can fall prey to the big four.

None of this, of course, should be surprising. Our lower brain tells us that if we have enough stuff or high enough social status, then we must be doing the right things (we are successful), and then we feel safe. But what is perhaps a little disappointing is how little time we spend reflecting on whether we are happy.

I have always been a little surprised how seldom doctors ever speak among themselves about happiness. I think this is rather universal in today's society. We talk about how busy we are, how stressed we are, or how hard it is to make ends meet. The busier we are, the more useful or important or better our lives must be, right? For example, there are a lot of legitimate reasons why physicians run behind every day: patients are late, problems take longer than we could have predicted, and surprises lurk around every corner. But when we are running really late every day, then that signals something else rather different: it's either poor organization (which can be solved with a little humility and business of medicine training) or insecurity.

Insecurity? Yes. If we could accept the limitations of what we can provide for patients, let go of the need to be Übermensch, then we would balance our practice and our lives better and focus more on happiness than on success. We try too hard to pretend we are superhuman. Medicine is not alone in this regard. So often I hear the term "burnout" in the workplace, and it tends to have a wistfully romantic element to it: we burn out because we give too much; we are too devoted and demand nothing short of perfection. But love is willing the good and growth of the other as other; it is not meant to be self-destructive. The other must love, too; we must be both givers *and* receivers. Not just give fish but teach to fish *and* allow fish to be received reciprocally.

We must be honest: a lot of investigations and treatments that medicine has advocated in the past have been shown to be of little help or sometimes even harmful. Antibiotics can't help viruses no matter how lousy you feel. We have relaxed some guidelines for high blood pressure and diabetes, for example, because our previous aggressive strategies haven't proven as helpful as we thought. Annual physicals have very limited value in terms of picking up diseases early or preventing disease (refer to appendix 3).

Without sincere introspection and self-reflection, it is easy to simply keep ourselves really busy and so convince ourselves that what we do is important and by extension so are we: we are successful. However, when we set expectations for ourselves that are not just unrealistic but unreachable, we burn out. If doctors, or anyone driven to be successful, could learn to focus on humbly sharing their fortuitous talents and gifts in a sustainable and *balanced* way instead, I think they would be happier and ultimately more helpful.

Asymptotes

This idea of trying to find a balance led me to explore a mathematical concept referred to as an "asymptote."

An asymptote is a line or curve that continues to approach another line or curve without ever touching it.

Figure 1. An example of an asymptote curve

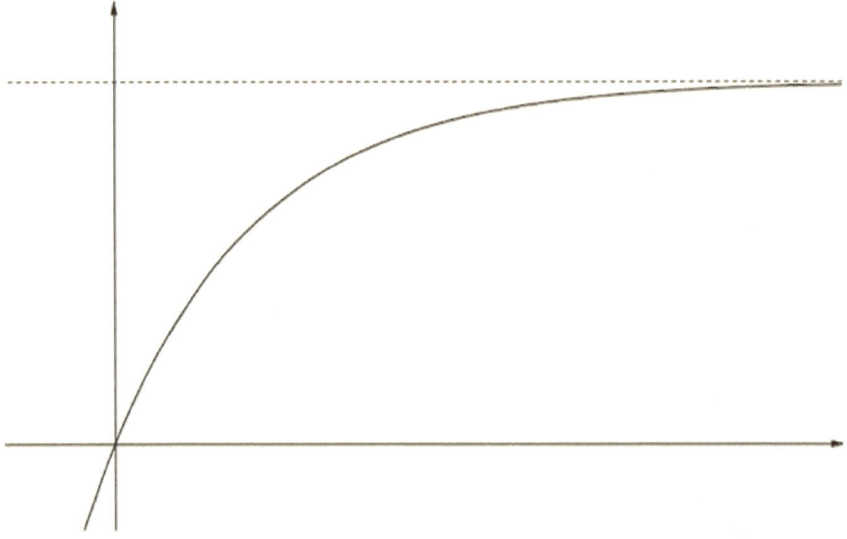

No matter how far you keep going, you never reach or surpass a certain ceiling. More importantly, the gains made as you proceed become smaller and smaller. For example, how much faster can a human run the one-hundred-metre sprint? When the previous world or Olympic record is shattered, it is measured usually in *hundredths* of a second, not in seconds. Even a tenth of a second in a roughly ten-second race is only a 1 percent improvement. In many human endeavours, the same is true: we are seeing incrementally smaller improvements, smaller tweaks. It's a lot more work for very little gain.

I am wondering if I am seeing evidence of asymptotes in medicine?

I have noticed fewer big breakthroughs in the last couple of decades of my career. As I mentioned earlier, cures for cancer have been replaced by treatments that turn cancers into chronic conditions. There are fewer and fewer radically new drugs or drug groups; the biologicals used in many autoimmune and other disorders are the rare exceptions. We do develop newer medications for high cholesterol, diabetes, and depression, for example, but they are not cures, and they are only incrementally better.

We have not developed any radically new imaging techniques since the MRI about twenty years ago. I seldom see blood tests ordered that weren't around twenty years ago, either. Surgical techniques improved a lot with the advent of fibre optics a couple of decades ago, and we are using them more liberally. We are doing more surgeries using vascular catheters, but again, these are two decades old as well. We are getting better at them, but they are no longer new.

The same is true in other areas of science.

We have not had a person on the moon, or any other celestial body, for over forty years, and it will be several decades more before we put a human on Mars. Leaving our solar system seems like a pipe dream.

We are reaching the limit of what a conventional computer can obtain in terms of power and speed; the next level, if we get there, is a quantum computer.

We have seen advances in physics in the last several decades, but nothing that rivals relativity or quantum mechanics, both about a hundred years old. And that is surprising given that we now have more people spending more money on research than ever before. Physics is still searching for the grand unified theory; string theory has not panned out as expected. Progress is measured in far smaller amounts as we delve deeper into the profound complexities of the universe. Paradigm shifts are rare.

I often feel that family medicine is reaching an asymptote. We now have excellent computer programs that help us manage the vast amount of information that we accumulate for our practices. The rate-limiting step in my practice is no longer the software of my computer; it is the internal software of my own brain. The pressures are mounting: patients live longer and acquire more medical problems and need more visits, there is more to remember, more rules to follow, more documentation to do, more issues to discuss each visit, more balls to constantly juggle, more black swans to be on the lookout for, and more diseases to prevent and recognize earlier. As anxiety rises, expectations do as well.

As I near retirement, I wonder whether younger physicians will have as long and satisfying careers as I have had. As we push closer to the ceiling, incrementally improving patients' health, is our own happiness compromised? Are we edging closer to burnout? I think doctors are much better at living balanced lives these days, but that also means that they don't work the crazy hours we used to. However, with patients living longer, being more anxious and demanding more, something has to give. I see a worrisome asymptote heading our way.

I see the same in most areas of work. Technology has allowed us to escalate efficiency and productivity, but that often equates to less margin, with no room for error, unpredictable and uncontrollable factors, or balance in our lives. Workers are often expected to function like the machines and computers that dominate our lives, and that stress is reaching an asymptote for many of us. On the other hand, nature is prolific and always allows for margin. It is not focused on ruthless efficiency. We have two kidneys, two lungs and can function on far less than half of our liver. Maybe we need to step back and re-examine our priorities, pull back from the asymptote.

On reflecting back on my career, what I have treasured most is that the issues people have shared with me have mattered to them in a deeper way than many other issues in their lives because health is so foundational. I liken the exam room to a confessional—patients frequently reveal their innermost thoughts and fears.

Often all I have been able to offer patients is support or reassurance, but it has been a privilege to do so. Although I envy people who work with their hands and can see something real and concrete that they have contributed to the world, I nevertheless hope that I have used whatever talents I have to compassionately improve the lives of the people I have touched. I wish that all of us, no matter how we contribute to the collective, can feel that way too.

We have certainly made progress in the human condition since I graduated from medical school in 1982. It is true that more of us are living to old age and are healthier in our old age than we used to be. It would be easy to attribute this to medical advances, but apart from immunizations, most of the improvements in quantity and quality of life relate to social factors, not medical ones. You may look at the statistics and disagree, but as the adage goes, "There are lies, damn lies, and statistics." You have to interpret the data to make sense of it.

People have always lived to old age, and it is true that more people are surviving to a healthier old age. But a lot of that is because we don't die in infancy and childhood from diseases prevented by immunizations (as well as better nutrition, safer housing, et cetera). Ditto for influenza epidemics. Equally, young people don't die in wars as much as they used to, and workplaces are considerably safer. All of those add up to huge numbers of individuals adding many decades to their lives and, overall, making life expectancy seem much longer. By contrast, further medical advances will only add small increments to life expectancy.

If you live long enough, you will eventually fall prey to some disease. When you don't die of a heart attack in your sixties, you are likely to die of cancer in your eighties, and that gives the somewhat artificial appearance that cancer is on the rise. After all, you can't avoid death completely. More and more, the things that take us from this world prior to reaching old age are black swans and canaries that are difficult to predict, prevent, and treat: a severe genetic disease in infancy, a car accident in your twenties, cancer in your thirties, a heart attack in your early forties. Yes, we can sometimes in hindsight identify risk factors, but any event outside of a couple of standard deviations of the norm is tough to see any other way than in hindsight.

Are we approaching a ceiling for all human endeavours? How much faster can we compute? Will faster computing really result in a true artificial intelligence? Is that a good thing?

How much higher can we jump? I have seen the question asked: no matter how much more we train, will we ever be stronger than an ox or faster than a cheetah? Why would we want to be?

Is it possible that we are hitting an asymptote for prolongation of human life once we exclude the black swans? How much happier will you be if you know that you will likely live to be ninety-five instead of eighty-five? Is that particular ten-year stretch of life that important to you?

Those are tough questions to answer. So ask yourself: How much has your life improved because computers are one hundred times faster than they were a few years ago? How much did your life improve when you reduced your marathon time by five minutes? How much less sad did you feel when your grandfather died at eighty-five instead of eighty-three?

Even more importantly, how much will faster computing, higher jumping, or living longer make in terms of creating a better, happier, or safer world? Are the major problems facing the world today going to be solved by more advances in the physiosphere or biosphere?

In truth, social issues, not medical ones, have always been key determinants of health, safety, and happiness. History has shown us repeatedly that the greater the divergence between the haves and the have-nots, the more problems there are for society. If that is true, and I think it is, then how much more can medicine now contribute to our health and happiness? We are an interconnected species by design, and simply approaching the asymptotic limit of what medicine can do is not going to make much of a difference in the big picture if we do not learn to care for one another and share those advances in an ethical fashion.

Remember Thought Experiment 1? A large part of what gives our life meaning lies in the fact that we share it. I suspect that the greatest threats to my children's and grandchildren's health are global warming and global political instability. If that is so, then maybe the greatest contribution that medicine can make to any society's health is ultimately to limit its importance and focus not on itself but on more pressing social issues—sharing the world sustainably and peacefully—endeavours of the noetic realm.

This leads to two more important and uncomfortable questions that must be asked. First, how much does our focus on medicine distract us from other far more pressing social issues? Second, how much is medicine contributing to the discrepancy between the haves and the have-nots in our society now? Whenever one individual or group is revered, automatically other individuals or groups are denigrated.

Just as too much emphasis on the profession puts too little emphasis on patients to mindfully heal themselves, too much aggrandizement of any group, no matter how talented or unique, results in the debasement of those outside of that group and their contributions to the collective. Harry S. Truman once said, "You can accomplish anything provided it doesn't matter who gets the credit." This means that mature leadership, *transformative* leadership, is about nurturing the good and growth of everyone as they bring their individual gifts and talents forward for the good of the collective without losing individuality in the process. We all matter, no matter how few or many letters after our name. Leadership is ultimately about love.

Medicine can exhibit leadership. It is founded on caring for the sick and vulnerable. We should not forget that it also includes the disadvantaged. Not only should we be advocating for the disadvantaged, we should be careful that we are not, through our own self-aggrandizement, helping to create the disadvantaged. With the pressing opioid crisis, have we the courage to ask why our fellow humans are turning to drugs to ease their pain? It is good of us, like white knights, to come to the rescue of those afflicted, but are we getting to the root of the problem? Is there something about our present social milieu that is contributing to this crisis and are we part of the problem? Harm reduction strategies may only be cloaking, not curing, deeper issues. We should be advocating not for more money and privilege for ourselves but for more equitable sharing of resources for all of society and for better treatment of each other and of the planet. No medical advances will improve the health of our societies more than caring for one another as equal members of the one tribe: fortunate *custodians* of planet earth.

Social issues are issues of the noosphere. We may be approaching a ceiling for what we can do for humans in the physiospheric and biospheric realms, at least in terms of what it can do for our happiness. But we have a long way to go in the noetic one, and it is far more important; it speaks to what it means to be human. Making more advances but not sharing them well is ultimately not going to help us. We see firsthand every day what allowing sociopaths to control our assets has done for our planet and our species. Any new development can be manipulated and monopolized, often by those who behave either narcissistically or selfishly. We try to improve our safety with better security or more weapons, but malcontents don't take long to find novel ways to destabilize us.

This necessitates that our next level of evolution involves the noosphere.

By all means we should enjoy our abilities, nurture them and benefit from them. But to stay connected, we must rise above our reptilian reflex to hoard for ourselves only and see our talents and fortunes as gifts that we need to share with one another, not as advantages to be lorded over those less fortunate.

This entails that individuals and tribes strive to make sure that they do not have far more than enough until everyone and every tribe has enough.

So although I enjoy practising medicine, it is not, in the words of philosopher and theologian Paul Tillich, my "ultimate concern." I enjoy helping people to live longer and healthier lives, and I hope that I have done so throughout my career. But as I turn sixty, I question whether the world will be a *much* better or happier place if we eliminate obesity or develop great cardio or guarantee fourscore and ten years for all. It's not that any of these goals are bad; it's just that they are not enough.

Even though most of the laws of physics work in either direction, evolution, like time, seems to go only forward not backward, from less complex and interconnected, to more. In other words, as a scientist studying the human species for most of my adult life, I have been impressed that there is a *telos*—a direction or purpose—to the universe and therefore to each of our lives. Helping people to live longer and be healthier is a good start; but ultimately, I want them to live meaningful lives during which they grow and conquer themselves, irrespective of their health or life expectancy.

There are hidden levels of paradox in all of this. Can you see them?

If you are having a tough time, I fully understand. It's because paradox is not outside of humanity; it is embedded within us. It's almost too close for us to see.

Chapter 30

Paradox Revisited

Perseverance is different from stubbornness: stubbornness is a refusal to re-examine the facts or to reappraise one's position with regard to them. Perseverance means not to allow oneself to be dissuaded or diverted from any worthwhile goal, but to meet every difficulty creatively, with new solutions, until one's ends have been achieved.

—The Essence of the Bhagavad Gita

WE HUMANS ARE a funny species, aren't we? I think that we are living paradoxes. But in our defence, I think we have to be in order to survive.

As I said near the end of the last chapter, I don't believe the universe is a place of purely random accidents; there is a telos to everything that exists.

Disagree? Well, there are twenty amino acids that constitute all proteins in humans (nine of which are essential; we can't make them ourselves). For a protein that is fifty amino acids long (which is not unusual), there are twenty to the fiftieth power possible combinations (20 x 20 x 20…fifty times). For evolution to work *randomly* (like flipping a coin) through all of these possibilities to find the right structure for a particular fifty-amino-acid protein for an organism, it would require a very long time. How long? The universe is ten to the eighteenth power seconds old. So trying a billion (ten to the ninth power) combinations every second would require many times the age of the universe.

How could that be so? It is simply unimaginable. In fact, so much of our world is unfathomable that we have to have a nonrational part of ourselves to be able to appreciate and cope with it. Logic—pure rational thought—is simply overwhelmed and thus insufficient for the task of living. That's where the nonrational—the creative and imaginative part of us—comes in. It's where we experience awe. We need it to survive and flourish.

In a complex world, we also need fear in order to survive; there simply isn't time to leisurely contemplate when danger presents itself. This means that at times we are ultimately going to behave irrationally, doing things that would not stand up to reason if we had time to reason. As we explored earlier in the book, denial, although frequently irrational, may well have been necessary for us to get this far, and it still has its place.

So I think it is no accident that we have irrational, nonrational, and rational parts of ourselves; we need them all. I think evolution has had this as part of its plan since the beginning.

Paradox is the embodiment of this reality. Paradox reflects the reality that everything manifests along a spectrum composed of the tension of opposites: proton and electron in the physiosphere; birth and death in the biosphere.

The tensions of opposites in the noosphere exist because we balance the rational and nonrational on a powerful and ancient foundation of fear and insecurity. As a goalie, rationally I want to make the save, and nonrationally I want to make a great save on a great shot. Both are undergirded by the irrational part of me that is embarrassed by letting in an easy goal and fear of getting hurt by a great shot.

It's easy to succumb to social pressures that lead us to shallow narcissism, searching for experiences in life—travel, career, accomplishments, accumulation of pleasure and wealth—in order to feel fulfilled. But we fail to realize that we cannot achieve self-actualization alone; we need relationships to make us feel truly complete.

We are communal creatures, and yet we struggle with intimacy: we share in sexual closeness but stay emotionally distant.

We want things to be better, but we don't want them to change. We want our lives to be better by having everyone *but* us change. We claim to want a better world, but we avoid the truth and disallow freedom of speech through political correctness. We ignore the elephants in the room that can hurt us, and we frequently persecute those who force us to acknowledge them in order for us to grow.

We fear being judged, yet we ruthlessly judge those judging us. We claim to detest judging, but we love being judged positively.

We become more affluent, and yet take on more debt. Life has never offered us so much safety and pleasure, and yet we find more drugs to help us to escape. The most commonly prescribed medications in our society are antidepressants. Wealth hasn't seemed to improve our happiness even though we are programmed for pleasure.

We spend more money on health care, and yet we have more angst about our health. The birthing experience is without parallel, and it has never been safer to give birth, yet fewer and fewer physicians practise obstetrics for fear of lawsuits because expectations are so high. We are living longer than we ever have before, and yet we worry more than ever that we are not going to live long enough. We all know that we are going to die some day, yet we can't talk about death (or sometimes even say the D-word).

The world is becoming more interconnected, and yet there is a trend for isolationist and protectionist public policies. We think we can succeed and flourish if we look solely after ourselves, but in an interconnected world that is not possible. We value the aesthetics of our own culture so much that we are willing to ignore or defy the ethics of our culture and war with those who differ from us. Our cultures value confidence to such a degree that we avoid humility to the point of "the killing certainties."

We advocate for rights and ignore the reality that rights entail obligations. Leaders think they can help the world by elevating themselves rather than helping others grow. We struggle with assertiveness, engaging in passive-aggressive behaviour instead. We tend to want to appease rather than to challenge to grow. We give a fish rather than teach to fish.

We keep so busy that we confuse human doing with human being. We think rituals are ends in themselves, so we end up in ruts.

We simplify in order to understand but do so to such an extreme that we become arrogant and lose our sense of awe.

We say we believe in evolution but fail to appreciate that evolution advances by both creating and destroying.

We seek more unique experiences, more extreme adventures but miss the simple miracles that surround us. We miss so much because we are too close to see it.

We fear bullies, yet they operate from their own fear, and they succeed only when we cannot face our own fears of them. We rail against the minor wrongs and ignore the major harms. We conflate being wronged with being harmed. We avoid hearing truths if they are painful, even if we need them to grow. We much prefer happy talk.

We protest against mothers choosing to abort their fetuses but defend gun laws that allow a stranger to kill her children, support capital punishment for the state to murder her youth and engage in wars that facilitate the death of her teenagers by a foreign power.

We want to make a grand impact on the world but fail to realize that the most good we do every day is with people we can touch. We allow guilt from our past and worry about our future to obscure the present moment, the place where love resides.

We mistake affection for love. In so doing, we often hurt the people we claim to care for the most, sometimes because we are more interested in being right than being loving.

Why all the paradox in us? Einstein developed the cosmological constant in order to make his theory of relativity work. It defines the energy that is stitched into the very fabric of space-time. I think paradox is the same: it is intrinsic to the entire universe. It is the tension of opposites that is stitched into the very fabric of existence, including our existence.

In quantum mechanics, one cannot completely define the location and motion of matter in any instant. The more we know of one, the less we know of the other—always the tension. The same is true for life: nature marches forward by utilizing an evolutionary process that both creates *and* destroys. In the noosphere we live in tension, balancing the rational, the nonrational, and the irrational along a spectrum to manage the grey zones. We cannot escape being living paradoxes.

One of the biggest paradoxes is that despite having to deal with this inescapable and harsh reality, as a species we continue to flourish.

Yes, our minds give us the ability to oversee the functioning of the brain. But something deep inside of us, something deeper than the mind, supports it, suffuses it, and guides it. That something is responsible for driving us in the face of incomprehensible adversity. What is it?

When my son was two years old, he did something curious that told me a lot about the human species. We had just returned from shopping, and we were unpacking the minivan. I realized that I had not seen, nor more importantly heard from him, for a while. Those of you with children know that when you have not seen or heard from a two-year-old for more than a few minutes, it means he is getting into trouble.

I shouted out to him to no avail. However, I saw the bathroom door mysteriously close and decided to check it out. I tried to open the door but felt some resistance. Now remember, he is two years old, and I am a brontosaurus, and yet he was trying to stop me from getting into the bathroom to see what he was up to. I gently opened the door, pushing him backward in the process, to find that he had poured most of the contents of a large bottle of soap onto the floor and was playing with it.

At two years of age, I doubt that he was capable of a deep level of mindfulness. We had never told him specifically not to do what he did, yet he knew that what he was doing was wrong. How did he know that?

Why does a three-year-old get upset when another three-year-old steals his toy? How do five-year-olds know that it isn't fair when they get a smaller piece of cake than everyone else? And do so with such intense passion and righteous indignation? How do we know when to feel scared and when to feel safe, even as infants?

We appear to be born with an internal moral compass. It may not know exactly what is right and what is wrong, but it knows that right and wrong exist.

Although I have seen people exhibiting immature and narcissistic behaviour, overwhelmingly I have borne witness to mature behaviour that has inspired me, including acts of true heroism: individuals donating organs to loved ones and to strangers, people finding joy in a life marred by disability, and families surviving the loss of one of their members.

I continue to be amazed, and reassured, by the courage and mindfulness of patients in facing misfortune, and often with profound equanimity. I have learned much from patients over the years. They have taught me to fish.

Nothing helps us more in dealing with hardship than connecting with one another. We are a social species; we have been designed that way over millions of years. The black boxes inside of our heads are as powerful as they are mysterious, particularly when shared. I may not always comprehend what goes on inside of them, but often they will mesmerize me. Imagine if Thought Experiment 1 had instead stipulated that you could engage in any activity you wanted, but you could not do so with anyone you were fond of or loved?

All of this attests to the presence of an unseen will or force that transcends, but includes, the mind.

My friend, Joe, despite his eventual suicide, inspired me because he fought the good fight for so many years at a time when society had much less to offer those with serious mental health issues. His partner, and other loved ones in his life, were a large part of that. Jane and her grandmother Mae overcame tremendous adversity and supported one another against the odds. I could write several books chronicling the many patients I have known who exemplified the best of what it means to be human and without exception the stories involve relationships.

When we are mindful, we utilize our observer self to understand the way we think in order to better control how we act. So mindfulness is important, but there is more to it than just slowing down, living in the moment, and juggling our various brain functions. Mindfulness without a moral compass would be incomplete. You've likely read or heard about Robert Fulghum's *All I Really Need to Know I Learned in Kindergarten*. We understand these simple but profound truths when we are five years old. How?

Recall that when the physiosphere became sufficiently complex, it gave rise to the biosphere that transcended but still included it. Life utilizes the physiosphere to grow.

The same is true of the noosphere. As life evolved, consciousness evolved. As consciousness evolved, it became more interconnected; mammals are more social and interconnected than reptiles.

As consciousness evolved further, the interconnectedness became more altruistic. Mammals travel in herds and raise their young; dogs will protect their human caregivers.

When consciousness reached its pinnacle, the potential for altruism did too. Only humans build hospitals, establish social institutions to care for the less fortunate, and create laws to guide our behaviours based on mutually derived ethical principles.

In other words, when consciousness becomes sufficiently complex, it allows for the development of a robust *conscience*, the source of morality, and the source of love. Love, a morally based interconnectedness, is what evolution has been striving for.

This helps to explain the penultimate paradox: humans.

Since the rise of the biosphere, all living things have had to struggle simply to survive. The challenges and threats posed to them by the physiosphere have been huge: floods, droughts, extremes of heat and cold, to name a few. But that is just the beginning. Even more challenging has been the biosphere itself: survival of the fittest is the guiding principle behind evolution. The biosphere feeds off of itself in a savage but amoral fashion. The greatest threat to any form of life has always been other life.

When the noosphere arose with the appearance of humans, the threats from the physiosphere and biosphere could be managed to a large degree. However, survival of the fittest has remained deeply engrained in us; we transcend but still include the biosphere, so we retain all of those primitive instincts within us, despite the development of our intelligence and our minds.

So it should come as no surprise that we can be a violent species; evolution advances by both creating and destroying.

However, once consciousness developed, behaviour was no longer only instinctual; it could also be mindful. In other words, morality came to exist because we could now choose how to act; sentience, self-reflection, and introspection gave rise to free will. Once that occurred, we left the innocence of an amoral world and entered into a realm where we know that right and wrong exist. As adult humans, we can no longer claim that we don't know the difference; the narcissism of a reptile or infant can be replaced by selfishness if we let it.

With mindfulness, we can become aware of the difference between right and wrong in order to make more mature and loving choices, the goal evolution has in store for us. We know that fear, insecurity, and the quest for pleasure can drive us to engage in morally wrong acts. But what drives us to do the right thing—morally desirable acts?

The answer to that question involves the ultimate paradox and its attendant bucket list.

Chapter 31

Bucket List

A human being is part of the whole called by us universe, a part limited in time and space. He experiences himself, his thoughts and his feelings as something separate from the rest, a kind of optical delusion of his consciousness. This delusion is a kind of prison for us, restricting us to our personal desires and to affection for a few persons nearest to us. Our task must be to free ourselves from this prison by widening our circle of compassion to embrace all living creatures and the whole of nature in its beauty.

—Albert Einstein

THANKS FOR HANGING in to the end of my book. I hope it has been worth it for you.

I have tried to be honest with you throughout the book, so now I want to know, can you be honest with me? Do parts of my book irritate you? Maybe the whole book does? Perhaps it even makes you angry?

If so, that's great!

It means that I have reached a profound part of you, a part of you that really matters. I have touched a deep nerve, a place of fear or confusion, perhaps. Or challenged a lifelong heuristic that you haven't thought about for a while (or ever).

Strong emotion is like rocket fuel used in spaceships: you need it to reach the heavens, but you must control it to get there. Let it motivate you to explore yourself, to be the observer where your mind—your true and integrated self—can mature.

Realize that any time you are exposed to information that doesn't challenge you, that doesn't make you feel at least a little uncomfortable, you may be missing an opportunity to grow. Why? You know the answer by now: growth implies change, change involves loss, and loss contains pain. You cannot create without destroying in the process; you can't have an adult daughter or son without losing the baby they were.

Growth, like baby to adult, is a critical and defining feature of all living things: they self-organize and they become more integrated within their milieu. Even the smallest seed germinates by sending out small shoots and roots in order to connect with the universe around it. The entire life of a plant is about becoming more entwined with other living creatures: other plants with which it hopes to reproduce and animals that may aid in that process or feast off of its bounty. But such venturing into the unknown entails risk.

Now before we go any further, I want to warn you: those of you who have found parts of my book (or all of my book) uncomfortable, this chapter may be the toughest. It's about growth, and so it is risky. Hang onto your hats!

As I said in the last chapter, from our inception, we humans have faced incredible obstacles—the rigours of the physiosphere and the threats from fellow creatures of the biosphere. Our burgeoning intelligence, however, has diminished much of that. We can protect ourselves from the harsh elements, from plants that are poisonous, and from animals that would like to have us for lunch.

However, a greater threat we have come to face is each other. That same intelligence that has protected us from the rest of the world has become our potentially greatest foe.

So given all of this adversity on so many levels, how is it that humans have been able to not only survive, but flourish?

I have read that 99 percent of all species that have ever existed on the planet are now extinct. Further, at present it is estimated that there are about ten million species alive on the planet (and likely more). If these numbers are accurate, it means that there have existed on the planet about a billion species!

Humans have been around in some form or another for at most a few million years. This means that for the overwhelming majority of the life of planet earth, humans have not existed. In other words, earth and nature got along just fine for hundreds of millions of years without us. Presumably that state of affairs could have continued indefinitely, and all would have been well.

However, evolution seemed to have other plans. It continued unabated, producing one species, and only one species in one billion, with full consciousness: *Homo sapiens*. As far as I can tell, it didn't have to, but it did. Why?

Given the horrors of human history, that's a legitimate question. On the basis of the last century alone, some argue that humans are evil and wicked and are a plague upon the planet, and at times it would be hard to offer a legitimate retort.

Looking at the damage to our environment, others avow that it is only what we do that is the problem; if we could just behave more like all of the other animals and stop being so different, all would be right again. There are occasions when it is tempting to pine for a return to the days of the caveman.

Various individuals lament the rise of technology, or even science itself, and yearn for the simpler bygone days of our forefathers.

So I ask you: did evolution make a huge cosmic mistake when it created us? Did it not see what it was getting itself into?

Is it possible that full consciousness is an overrated goal? Did evolution succumb to its own narcissistic ambition? Did it arrogantly flaunt itself and take things one step too far?

For me, the answer to all of these questions is an emphatic no!

Why do I feel so strongly? Because there is an ultimate paradox that we have not yet fully explored, and it explains a lot.

Our narcissistic behaviours arise from the parts of our brains that are literally billions of years old, so when we behave badly, we should not be so shocked. As annoying as that may be, we are never going to be rid of the potential for their manifestation. Our ancient yet immature lower brains are here to stay.

Equally, our selfish behaviours, ones where we know better but do worse, are a natural culmination of our fear, insecurity, and desire for pleasure winning out over altruism. Again, the path to maturity involves immature steps, and along the way we will falter, giving in to impulses below our higher brain functions. Our powerful brains, both logical and creative, offer a rich smorgasbord of options to pursue, and often we simply explore and act on what we *can* do, rather than mindfully contemplating first what we *should* do. Sometimes we selfishly choose actions that make us feel good but hurt others.

Yes, when we are young and don't know better, we can be very narcissistic, and when we are older and do know better, we can be selfish. But most of the time most of us are neither. We are caring and actually strive to become better people. So I don't buy the argument that humans are fundamentally evil or fatally flawed. We are products of our evolution, and much of what we do that is not desirable stems from immaturity, from lack of control. In some respects, we have been granted tremendous abilities and a license to do with them as we please without first proving that we will behave ourselves. We need to grow into our brains, so to speak.

I am so impressed by evolution that I cannot believe that we have been given the extraordinary gifts to accomplish what we have—produce vaccines, write books, create beautiful music, fly to the moon—and then are not expected to use them. It makes no sense to me, and I think that evolution is far too wise for such waste. I believe that we are meant to have these gifts—for example, our technological ability—and we are meant to utilize them. But we must be ever mindful that technology is a thing, and like all things it is amoral. The morality lies in how we use it. And that's the catch; that's where the ultimate paradox comes in.

I read of this paradox several years ago (I think it was in the book *The Hidden Brain*, by Shankar Vedantam). In my opinion, the ultimate paradox is this: evolution has used the principle of survival of the fittest to develop a species with full consciousness that recoils at the very idea of survival of the fittest.

Think about it. Most of us abhor the idea of bullying, of taking advantage of the vulnerable, of unfair apportionment of goods, and of getting what you want at all costs. But that's exactly how nature works: you snooze, you lose. In fact, the whole discipline of medicine, of which I am pleased to be a member, is founded on principles contradictory to survival of the fittest: care for the weakest and most defenceless and give them the best life you can.

That is simply astounding! How can we account for this complete and utter reversal of billions of years of a survival-of-the-fittest mentality? Why has evolution used this principle so thoroughly for so long only to do a total about-face when it reached the zenith of full consciousness? What on earth is going on?

Conscience. That's what's going on. Consciousness is a fundamental reality of the universe; even the atoms of the physiosphere, in a primitive way, are "aware" of atoms around them and interact via gravitational and other forces. Consciousness evolved to a higher level of intensity with the arrival of life. In the biosphere, all life is aware and interacts with its surroundings and other life forms. The evolution of life to self-awareness—the full consciousness of the noosphere—led to the ability to know right from wrong. But conscience is not just the *ability* to know right from wrong, to be mindful and act morally, but the *desire* to do so. A desire so strong that it countermands the very foundation upon which it is built. Now that's a paradox of cosmic proportions and significance.

In this book, we've explored a lot about the mind. As we become more mindful, we learn to declutter, as the Eastern spiritual scholars say, our "busy monkey brains." We struggle to focus less on the past and future in order to manage better the present moment. Reflecting upon the past in order to learn from it aids growth; wallowing in guilt or anger generated from the past impedes our growth. Some planning for the future is essential for growth; wallowing in worry hampers it.

We also try to observe the various inputs from the different parts of our brains—the rational, nonrational, and irrational parts—so as to guide our behaviours. But simply observing, focusing, and reflecting are not sufficient. Life is about learning to balance the opposite ends of the spectrum to find the sweet spot. But what is it that helps us to balance all of the spectra in our lives?

The great mystical masters teach that there is a part of us even deeper than the mind or the observer self—something that defines our very essence. Different spiritual belief systems use different names for this essence—Buddha nature, atman, soul, for example. This essence is united with a universal essence, variably referred to as "nature," "universal consciousness," "Supreme Being," "the Creator," "the Tao," "the way," "Allah," "Brahman," "Yahweh," and "God" (and, I am sure, many more).

It's profoundly difficult to comprehend, which paradoxically explains why many of us are drawn to it: as children of the universe, we have always been attracted by the mystery, the awe, the infinite potential of the unknown, even unknowable. It's why we like puzzles or magic or whodunits, and why we visit places like the Grand Canyon. It's what spurs physicists and cosmologists to probe the secrets of the universe.

We also feel it when two people wed: we celebrate the union of two individuals and the unpredictable and inscrutable potential that such a relationship generates. We feel it when we hold a newborn child: we celebrate the infinite possibilities that exist in the tiny life we cradle so preciously.

These are the windows into the level Ken Wilber refers to as the "theosphere." It is this level where we transcend the noetic self of the noosphere, going beyond the mind to something even grander. The great Buddhist sages refer to this level when explaining meditation. We are not just our thoughts, which are neurochemical impulses; they reside in the physical realm. We are not just the thinker of our thoughts—the brain; that resides in the biological realm. We are not even just the observer of the thinker of the thoughts—the mind; that lies in the noetic realm. We transcend that.

Evolution wants nothing less than a full conscience.

That's where love comes in: *willing* the good and growth of the other as other. This is not just awareness or self-awareness but an awareness profound enough to fully grasp our intrinsic interconnectedness. This intertwining starts right down at the subatomic level with the entanglement of electrons that quantum physicists discovered a century ago and progresses throughout the rest of creation.

This means that a full, human life can never be just about oneself. We are noetic and communal creatures infused with a nascent need to care for one another that must be nurtured. Evolution has designed us to become more interconnected by imbuing within us an ability to reflect on what we should do and a conscience to guide us. That is the nexus of the noosphere and theosphere.

That is where we begin the journey of conquering ourselves. It is where the best in us resides: compassion, empathy, resiliency, forgiveness, selflessness, and humility. True humility, not the false humility we are normally surrounded by, is a sincere admission that our lives are cemented on a foundation of fear, insecurity, and desire for pleasure that cannot be eliminated. They are the clay that evolution has used to mold us. We should not be ashamed of this inescapable fact. Rather, we should reflect upon our heritage and engage the process of evolution to its ultimate destiny.

Are you familiar with the expression "bucket list"? It refers to the list of things you want to do, experience, or accomplish before you kick the bucket—that is, die.

There was a movie several years ago titled *Bucket List* in which the two main characters, played by Morgan Freeman and Jack Nicholson, were dying of cancer. Jack plays a very wealthy womanizer (I always wonder if Nicholson really has to act to play this role?) who befriends Morgan, a patient in the hospital Jack runs, and the two of them spend what little time they have left experiencing myriad adrenaline rushes all over the world. I won't give away any more of their entertaining story except to say that it does capture to some degree the present-day thinking regarding how we should approach both death and life.

A similar theme is captured in the motto YOLO—you only live once—which seems nearly omnipresent in Western culture. Now don't get me wrong, I am all in favour of living in the present moment and reflecting more on your life so that you don't wander through it aimlessly and mindlessly. My issue is more with the content of most bucket lists and YOLO activities than with the ideas themselves.

If you have a bucket list, what's on it? If you don't, what would be on it? How did/do you develop it?

I suspect that we develop our bucket lists based on our deepest, maybe even unrecognized, beliefs about what life is all about. In other words, our values.

As we explored earlier in the book, we can value things for two reasons: they make us feel good or they make others feel good. In other words, there are aesthetics, what we find pleasurable, and there are ethics, how we treat other people, including safeguarding their rights to safety, freedom, and the pursuit of their full potential.

Most often when I discover the content of a bucket list, it is replete with purely aesthetic pursuits. That is understandable when we are younger; we are testing out our newly acquired minds and bodies to see what they can do as we discover the world around us. But I seldom see bucket lists that talk about personal growth or conquering ourselves: becoming more patient, more compassionate, humbler, wiser, more generous, more resilient, and more anitfragile.

As we age, we are offered the opportunity to mindfully introspect, and often when we do, we find that aesthetic pursuits are fleeting and not fully satisfying. For that reason, we may want to declutter our lives, letting go of things, knowing that ultimately we must let go of every thing when we die. We may become more attracted to, and engage more with, animals and children (and grandchildren!) because they keep life simple. We begin to see stuff that was too close to see before.

In other words, we are frequently drawn more to the being than to the doing, pensively reflecting on the meaning of our lives, asking why bad things happen to good people, why there is suffering in the world, and what has happened to those who have gone before us.

We come to realize that problems are most often managed not solved, that the experts don't have all of the answers, that we have to pull together as a species and not rely on technology to fix things, and that rights always entail obligations.

Because the universe is such a complex place, where everything interacts with everything else, it means that each of us matters. We must learn to balance the tension of being individuals and being part of a collective simultaneously. We each must contribute to the collective and not wait for the leaders to do so because we are all leaders. The collective grows because its constituents grow; but the constituents need the collective to help them fully grow. There is an inherent reciprocity in living. There is no view from nowhere; none of us is outside of the human experiment.

We are facing a lot of challenges at the moment, but we must never forget that we are a supremely relational species. As Nassim Taleb has stated so correctly, technological problems cannot be solved with more technology; financial problems cannot be solved with more money; drug addictions cannot be solved with more drugs; legal problems cannot be solved with more laws; political problems cannot be solved with more politics; hate cannot be solved with more hate, and so forth.

More technology, money, drugs, laws, politics, and hate cannot solve our problems; they simply up the ante. Only by nurturing our consciences and caring for one another can we manage to make better choices. I am of the conviction that our physical, biological, and noetic selves are capable of making the world a better place, but only when guided by a sufficiently mature conscience. I think it is what evolution has intended all along.

This means that the greatest problem facing humanity, and planet earth, is not even each other, but our own selves. I have always been impressed by Luke 6:41: "Why do you look at the speck that is in your brother's eye, but do not notice the log that is in your own eye?"

Each of us needs to grow our own conscience and be part of the solution. We start by acknowledging and accepting that each one of us is scared and insecure. When we do, we can let go of the need to be special; we are all scared, but we are all *sacred* as well. We abandon the childish concept that there are Übermensch among us (maybe even ourselves) who will rescue us. It has not worked because it can't. As we come to peace with being ordinary and thus ontological equals, we let go of the need to worry about our place in the world. We accept that we have a place in the world that matters like everyone else's place in the world matters. We realize that the only way to make the world the best place it can be for all of us is when each of us uses our gifts and talents to will the good and growth of all others as others. Becoming more loving; that is the only thing truly worthy of being on a bucket list. It is the only desire that does not court suffering.

There is a wonderful Buddhist koan that tells of a woman lamenting the death of her son. In her sorrow, she seeks the counsel of a wise sage. He tells her to visit everyone in her village and collect a mustard seed from each person who has not lost someone they loved and bring all of the seeds back to him. She does so, but no matter which home she visits, everyone has had a loss similar to hers. After much travel, she returns to the sage empty handed and recounts her experience. As he smiles gently at her, she realizes the lesson. We have all been hurt, and we are all broken. But we continue to grow and share our gifts regardless.

So how do we rise above our fear, our insecurity, and our pain to live out this bucket list goal? It's not easy, and I personally have a long way to go. But I am reminded of Saint Paul in Romans 7:15: "I do not understand what I do. For what I want to do I do not do, but what I hate I do." It's never been easy, even for a saint.

I read a story centuries old of a very powerful samurai warrior, the most powerful warrior in all of his land, who sought the insights of a learned teacher. He approached the old and frail man and asked to be told of heaven and hell. The meek sage surprised the warrior by yelling at him and telling him that he was far too dull and stupid to understand something as profound as heaven and hell.

The warrior became enraged, pulled his sword out, and stood over the old man screaming, "I am the most powerful warrior in this land. You have spoken to me disrespectfully. Do you not realize that I can kill you instantly with one strike of my mighty sword?"

The tiny man looked gently up at him and said, "That, my friend, is hell." The warrior fell to his knees and wept, ashamed of his arrogance. "And that, my friend, is heaven," uttered the sage.

Hopefully, having written this book, I understand a little better why I do what I do, even though, like Saint Paul, I still often do what I wish I hadn't. I hope understanding myself a little better will help, provided that I, like the samurai warrior, learn to be humble and forgive myself. See, I told you this was a self-help book!

Where do we start? Look, there is nothing wrong with wanting a good life or developing our talents and enjoying them; I think it is what evolution intends for us. But we must resist the narcissistic tendency to want a lot more than we need, to have it be all about us. The problems of the world will be solved when we listen to our conscience.

From a practical perspective, what does that look like?

If you have been lucky enough to own a business or run a company, treat your employees well. You are not only responsible for making a profit, but also for taking care of them and their loved ones.

Be transparent in how you behave; minimize hidden agendas. Treat people like ends in themselves, not a means to your ends. Don't let privilege of any kind go to your head; none of us completely deserves all of the good things nor bad things that happen to us.

Be generous with your blessings. Many people are engaged in work where they rely on tips for a substantial part of their income. Thank people when they help you and tip well, even if they are having a bad day. They are people, not slaves.

Let go of "us and them" thinking. We are all "us." In particular, abandon the hierarchy of the blue-collar and white-collar mentality. All work that aids the collective is important. If you don't believe me, wait until your sanitation workers go on strike.

At meetings, encourage everyone to participate and develop their leadership skills. The loudest or most charming person in the room is seldom the wisest. The Tao states, "Sincere words are not fine; fine words are not sincere." Ineloquent people often have much to teach. Sometimes wisdom is too close to hear, so don't be duped by charisma.

Address bullying, for the sake of the person being bullied and the bully. Both are scared; help both to grow. Beware people driven to high levels of success; they are frequently very narcissistic and need our help to mature. We have much to learn from those less fortunate; they can teach us about humility and resiliency.

Have enough, but not too much. He with the most toys does not win. Support the idea of a minimum wage that allows people the opportunity to have a full and satisfying life.

Be thankful when you make enough money that you can pay taxes to support the less fortunate (even though I know governments don't always use your money wisely!). You will still have lots left over; likely more than you truly need. Many people go through tough times, and social assistance can help them rise above it. Only a very small percentage of individuals collecting social assistance do so on a chronic basis. Most have a good reason for it, and their stories are often complicated and tragic. They are to be pitied, not scorned.

We should prioritize children and child-rearing. When children are not nurtured well, we all suffer. We need to advocate more for children because they have no power of their own. Resources allocated in early life reap rewards for the rest of life. We should value having parents raise their children and adopt social measure to facilitate it. We should provide adequate assistance for children with health issues, physical and mental, especially learning disorders. The evidence is overwhelming that unfortunate individuals with untreated learning and mental health disorders occupy our jails and prisons.

As we explored earlier, addictions are very common. As much as it is important to adopt measures for harm reduction in those suffering from addictions, if we truly love them we must try to understand the causes of their addictions. The courage of mature intimacy will allow us to judge the behaviours not the person and in so doing foster their ability to regain control of their lives.

That doesn't mean we don't hold people accountable. Our goal is to love, which means not just their good but their growth as well: in order to grow, they must be willing to learn to fish. There is a wide spectrum of desire and ability to grow, and that may frustrate us, but it should not deter us from doing our best to help others grow beyond their narcissism and selfishness. No one can feel truly human nor reach their full potential until they are able to engage with others in a mutually supportive fashion. Love requires both giving and receiving, leadership and followership.

However, I am reminded of a quote from theologian Thomas Merton:

> *He who attempts to act and do things for others or for the world without deepening his own self-understanding, freedom, integrity and capacity to love, will not have anything to give others. He will continue to communicate nothing but the*

> *contagion of his own obsessions, his aggressiveness, his ego-centered ambitions, his delusions about ends and means, his doctrinaire prejudices and ideas. There is nothing more tragic in the modern world than the misuse of power and action to which men are driven by their own Faustian misunderstandings and misapprehensions.*

In other words, there are no pure motives this side of heaven. So often the very rich are applauded for giving away large sums of money to the disenfranchised. However, often the reason that there are impoverished people who need handouts is that the economic system being utilized produces extremes of wealth. In so many societies, those in privileged positions continue to amass more privilege because of their prosperity and power, and they use their vast resources to protect it. Wealth and impoverishment are intimately related; they occur when economics is missing conscience.

We may feel better about ourselves, and look like heroes, for giving a large donation, but when we are still left with far more than we need and the power hierarchies and social inequities remain, we have not truly loved. When we let go of our fears and admit that much of our lives is attributable to luck, good and bad, we will begin the process of conquering ourselves.

That is not to say that we can make everything and everyone identical in the world, because we can't. Spectra will always exist. We all have different and varying talents and gifts, ways of looking at the world, priorities and values. We are all at varying and different stages of maturity and have different rates of growth. But we can make things more equitable and avoid the extremes of the spectra. We should try to ensure that everyone has enough before some have far too much and that everyone has the opportunity and support to grow.

Although the discussion above could go on for pages, I suspect that many of you may find my examples and suggestions naive and unattainable. If you say it can never happen, then ponder this.

When I was a much younger brontosaurus, companies packaged food in containers that contained virtually no information about the contents. As the public became a little more sophisticated and more concerned with what they put into their bodies, they demanded to know more. At first, companies just listed vague ingredients like "beef." We demanded more, so they documented the quality of the beef, often in the process upgrading from beef by-products. Then we wanted to know about the other ingredients and then about the nutritive contents of those ingredients, including calories. The industry grew and became more transparent and accountable.

However, for the consumer, it was still only about the consumer. As we matured, we started to care at a deeper level. We left our narcissism and selfishness and realized that we also cared about how the animals that we consume are treated and how the people making the products are treated too. Our altruism grew to the point that ethical treatment of animals and fair trade are now priorities for consumers.

We care about animals, and we care about people we do not know who work halfway across the world. We are prepared to hold companies responsible for fair treatment of animals and our fellow humans, and pay more for products and services in doing so.

That's conscience and it does work. It has to or else we are in big trouble. I don't think we have a choice any longer; our world is too complicated and complex not to be guided by conscience. So, never say never.

Just as peace is not simply the absence of war, love is not simply the absence of hate. Love involves growth. Each of us must take some responsibility for our own growth and for the growth of others.

Perhaps evolution itself is evolving too. When evolution transcended the physiosphere to produce the biosphere with the arrival of life, new laws, like survival of the fittest, arose. The same was true when evolution transcended the biosphere to give rise to the noosphere: *Homo sapiens* leapt past the awareness of their fellow creatures to self-awareness.

New laws, discovered by these fully conscious beings, changed the playing field; humans began to dominate everything.

Over the time that humans have inhabited the planet, we have seen a rise in the presence of the theosphere: the rise of not just self-awareness, but the awareness of each other and the consciousness of everything else in the universe. We call it "conscience," and it manifests as willing the good and growth of the other as other. Unlike the individual survival of the fittest in the biosphere, survival of the fittest in the noosphere cannot be about individuals but rather about our entire species and beyond. We are starting to understand the deep interconnectedness, the oneness, the nonduality of all things in the universe.

That's why we are searching the heavens for signs of life elsewhere; even the most skeptical among us is excited about the possibility. Evolution may well be a universal phenomenon, and if so, the question must be asked: is *Homo sapiens* a species in the universe that can grow enough to continue to be fit to survive? Can we discover the new laws of the theosphere and enact them in order transcend our physiospheric, biospheric, and noospheric levels? Will we evolve to conquer ourselves and learn to love sufficiently before it is too late? Will we be around long enough to discover and contact life elsewhere in the universe if it has been fit to survive as well?

Evolution has given humans all of the tools that we need, and our communal bucket list has been provided as well. The rest is up to us; *each and everyone one of us.*

The Greek philosopher Seneca wrote over two thousand years ago: "Things can be taken away from us, but good deeds and acts of virtue cannot."

I wish us good luck and peace.

Acknowledgements

I want to thank a number of people who have guided and supported me in writing this book:

Stacey Atkinson, my editor, whose advice and guidance were invaluable. Iqbal Rahemtulla, my good friend and mentor, for his encouragement and wisdom.

My good friends, Carol Brodkin-Sang and Murray Sang. Carol's cover art truly captured the essence of my book and exceeded all of my expectations. Murray's humour, insights, and marketing savvy were inspiring and reassuring.

My wife, Nancy, for her constant companionship and unwavering belief that this book was worth writing. I could not and would not have written it without her. It is as much her book as it is mine.

About the Author

Barry graduated from the University of Toronto School of Medicine in 1982 and completed his residency in Family Medicine at Queen's University in Kingston, Ontario in 1985. After spending three years in Fort Frances, Ontario, he and his wife, Nancy, settled in the Orangeville, Ontario area to raise their three children.

As a rural family doctor he has delivered hundreds of babies and given thousands of anaesthetics in addition to working in the emergency department and doing palliative care.

With a passion for medical ethics, he obtained a master's degree in bioethics at the University of Toronto in 2006 prior to moving back to the Ottawa Valley (he was born in Renfrew, Ontario) where he now works.

When not practising medicine, he and Nancy can be found enjoying the outdoors in Aylmer, Quebec where they now reside. Rumour has it that he still dons his goalie equipment in a local Aylmer 'old boys' hockey league.

Other books by the author:
───────

Moment of Grace, by J. Barry Engelhardt, 2012, ISBN: 9780991757411

Author's website: www.jbarryengelhardtbooks.com

Appendix 1

Fifty Things I've Learned So Far in Medicine

(and I Am Still Working on All of Them)

THE FOLLOWING IS a list of suggestions for medical students to contemplate during their training. Some deal with what I would refer to as the "mechanics" of our discipline—the physiospheric and biospheric realms. But the majority of them deal with the noetic realm—the more complex one involving interrelationships.

1. Try to understand the human body; don't just memorize a lot of mnemonics.

2. Every symptom, disease, and illness, has a psychological component—you have to figure out how much.
3. Pain and suffering are different.
4. Admit when you don't know, and look it up—your patients will thank you.
5. Common things are common.
6. Usually people only get one disease at a time. But not always.
7. Learn to look for patterns of disease and to recognize when things do not fit those patterns. You can't know about all of the black swans and canaries out there, but you'll know that you are dealing with one if it doesn't fit the usual patterns. Get help when you have to.
8. You don't need to know the exact diagnosis when you see a patient, but you must rule out the lethal ones before you let the person go home. Recognize when things are getting worse. Learn to recognize when people are really sick.
9. Medical error can be divided into two types generally: errors of commission and errors of omission. The first can be minimized by not doing stuff you are not comfortable doing; the second by being open-minded and not putting on blinders. We need to learn to think outside the box by not building the box to begin with.
10. Sometimes doing nothing and waiting, as difficult as it is, is the right thing to do. Doing something is not always better.
11. Nature does most of the healing, not us, so try not to get in the way. Don't take credit for stuff nature does.
12. Analogies are helpful to a degree—use them, but they are only rough approximations.
13. Be sceptical, question everything, but don't become cynical.

14. Avoid binary thinking and concrete, mechanical thinking. Linear relationships are uncommon. Understand deductive and inductive reasoning. Learn about fallacies, and avoid falling into them.
15. Learn how to think critically, understand what an argument is, and learn the difference between debate and dialogue. Stick to dialogue.
16. Realize that algorithms and guidelines have severe limitations.
17. Learn more about practical statistics and probabilities. Become familiar with NNT and NNH.
18. Explain things to patients in ways that they will understand. Being well-rounded helps. That doesn't mean being an expert; in fact, being a novice is often very helpful.
19. Read outside of medicine.
20. If you can't explain something to a reasonably intelligent ten-year-old, then you don't understand it yourself.
21. Learn more about the ethics underpinning the patient-physician relationship.
22. Sometimes you are the medicine. Don't underestimate the value of your humanity when shared.
23. Work only so hard as to still enjoy what you are doing—you are likely in it for the long haul. You will be a better doctor and better person if you enjoy what you do.
24. Don't lose your sense of awe and wonder, especially when you see a newborn.
25. Cultivate a sense of humour.
26. Learn how to manage time well; be organized but flexible.
27. Be respectful of your patients' time.

28. You are allowed to be wrong, so forgive yourself when you are wrong. Then do something about it.
29. You are not allowed to lie.
30. Make this a vocation, not a job. Balance techne and episteme.
31. Be yourself.
32. Be humble.
33. You will probably be surprised at the end of your career how much of what you learned is wrong.
34. If you view every patient interaction as a new experience you won't get bored. See past the symptoms and the diseases.
35. Nurture creativity—it will help you think better.
36. True leadership means helping those around you grow to their full potential, nurturing the growth of everyone on the team.
37. You are part of a team. Respect the other members of the team, even though they may not have as many letters after their name as you do.
38. True leadership is not about being the most important person or being centre of attention. Sometimes your place is in the background. We need to be followers a lot of the time; learn to be a good follower.
39. Don't let money run your life. Avoid addictions.
40. Dress respectfully for patients. Address them respectfully, too.
41. Appreciate the business of medicine, but don't let it blind you to the art that you practise.
42. You bring your humanity, foibles, and idiosyncrasies to your work—it is unavoidable—but nurture mindfulness to

minimize the negative impact on your patients. Remember that objectivity is a myth: there is no view from nowhere.

43. There is a difference between information and wisdom; learn to distinguish the two. Cultivating discernment will help.

44. You will reduce stress in your work the sooner you come to peace with uncertainty, which means you can't fix everything, so don't make that your goal.

45. Our job is to love our patients. That means willing the good and growth of the other as other. We want to help them, but we want them to help themselves and grow. Give them a fish, but mostly teach them to fish. In other words, transcend and include.

46. Take responsibility for your share of helping a patient get better, but no more. The patient owns most of the responsibility.

47. Balance being and doing. Being too busy doesn't make you more important; it just makes you tired.

48. Take care of yourself. Model the lifestyle you suggest to your patients.

49. Never stop growing.

50. Read the poem "Desiderata" by Max Ehrmann.

Appendix 2

Thoughts for Patients

HAVING BEEN INVOLVED in perhaps a hundred thousand patient-physician interactions, mostly as a physician, I thought I would offer some observations and suggestions about medical encounters.

1. There is a limit to how many problems a doctor can deal with in one visit—start with the most important first and don't expect to get through all of them necessarily.
2. If you have forms to complete, say so early in your appointment; fill out your parts of the form first, and expect to pay something for this service because it is often not considered part of our usual fee.
3. Forms are not our favourite thing to do, so cut us some slack and don't expect them to be done instantly.

4. Keep an eye on your medications—don't wait until you have run out to do something about it. (Kind of like keeping an eye on the gas tank of your car.)

5. Try to be on time for appointments. For the most part, the two major reasons I get behind are patients presenting with unexpected problems (which is an understandable and often unavoidable part of the business) and patients being late (which is perhaps more avoidable).

6. Understand the patient-physician relationship—generally the deliberative model works best.

7. The internet has lots of data; some is better than others, so be sceptical and critically analytical.

8. Lots of people who will never be held accountable for advice they give you will give you advice—doctors have to back up what they say, and that makes a world of difference.

9. Medicine has a lot to offer, but there are risks to everything, even tests.

10. Tests should be done to answer very specific questions with very specific goals. Blindly fishing is seldom helpful.

11. Talking is the most important part of any visit, so don't underestimate the importance of being a good historian. The better detective you are and the more clues you bring, the better the results.

12. We have bad days, too.

13. It's hard to think on your feet—the more prepared you are the better.

14. Physicians try to pick up on nonverbal cues, but we are not mind readers. The more honest and straightforward you are, the easier it is for us to help you.

15. If you want to know the complete truth, even the bad stuff, say so.

16. Be nice to our staff—they have a tough job, and they tell us when you are not nice, and we remember that. Never forget: we have a lot more patients than we have staff, and good staff are much harder to find than patients.

17. We know you don't like to be disappointed, but we cannot tell you what you want to hear if it isn't the truth—our Hippocratic oath gets in the way of that. And try to resist the temptation to shoot the messenger.

18. Every symptom or illness has a psychological component. Don't be offended when we want to explore that too.

19. Seeing you for a prescription renewal is about monitoring the condition the medication is treating—it is not about the piece of paper.

20. Unless I gave you your illness, you own your illnesses. I can only try to help you with it.

21. We look for patterns, and you should, too. It is usually reassuring to some degree when things are not getting worse.

22. Limit the use of denial. As scary as it may be, if things are bad or getting worse, get them checked out.

23. No doctor has all skill sets. Sometimes their skill sets are more intellectual or technical, not social.

24. Although your symptoms may be new and fascinating for you, it is less likely that they are as new and fascinating for us. Don't misinterpret our lack of excitement as disinterest necessarily.

25. Read the poem "Desiderata" by Max Ehrmann.

Appendix 3

POEMs

THE FOLLOWING ARE brief excerpts from the Patient-Oriented Evidence that Matters (POEM) articles I receive daily. I could list hundreds, but I just picked these as representative of the challenges that we face in trying to find definitive answers to medical problems.

Don't be too disappointed or disillusioned. After all, the world is a complicated and complex place! (Sorry, I couldn't resist.)

1. **Steroid disc injection of little benefit in treating chronic low back pain**

   Clinical question

   Is disc injection with a corticosteroid an effective way to decrease pain in patients with low back pain and active discopathy?

Bottom line

"Refer for invasive procedure" is usually at the bottom of the low back pain treatment algorithm. In this study, one invasive procedure, an injection of prednisolone acetate 25 mg following discography, produced a short-term reduction in, but not elimination of, pain as compared with no treatment. However, the benefit was gone within a year. The process of discography, though, seemed to improve both pain and function in patients whether or not they received an injection. That benefit could be simply due to participation in a research study

2. **The effect of liraglutide in delaying type 2 diabetes mellitus diagnosis is unclear after three years**

   Clinical question

   Is liraglutide more effective than placebo in delaying the diagnosis of type 2 diabetes mellitus in patients with prediabetes?

   Bottom line

   After three years, obese patients with prediabetes who were taking liraglutide were less likely to develop diabetes and experienced a three-month delay in the time to diagnosis compared with those who were taking placebo. However, since half the patients in this study dropped out before its conclusion, these findings are not reliable.

3. **Dexamethasone may reduce sore throat symptoms in adults at forty-eight hours**

   Clinical question

   Are oral steroids effective in the treatment of acute sore throat in adults?

   Bottom line

   A single dose of oral dexamethasone is no more effective than placebo in resolving acute sore throat symptoms at twenty-four hours in adults who do not receive immediate antibiotic therapy. However, among a multitude of exploratory secondary outcomes, the authors found that dexamethasone compared with placebo did increase the proportion of patients with symptom resolution at forty-eight hours (number needed to treat [NNT] = 12; 95% CI 7–146).

4. **No mobility benefit with in-patient rehab added to home-based program after total knee arthroplasty**

   Clinical question

   Does in-patient rehabilitation improve long-term mobility for patients who have undergone total knee arthroplasty?

   Bottom line

   As compared with a home-based rehabilitation program alone, the addition of intensive in-patient rehabilitation for ten days following an uncomplicated total knee arthroplasty does not improve mobility in the long term nor decrease the time to return to work. The home-based program was fairly light, consisting mostly of monitoring and education with an average of only three physical therapy visits. The lack of meaningful clinical benefit as well as the added cost of in-patient rehabilitation should discourage this option for patients who would otherwise recover well at home.

5. **Bisphosphonates decrease vertebral fractures but not clinically important fractures in men**

   Clinical question

   Are bisphosphonates effective in decreasing the rate of fractures in men with osteoporosis?

Bottom line

In this meta-analysis of randomized trials that were generally at high risk of bias, bisphosphonates decreased the rate of all vertebral fractures and nonvertebral fractures in men with osteoporosis. However, the rate of clinically important fractures was not significantly reduced. The authors provide no data on the potential harms of treatment, especially with long-term use

6. High false-positive rate with lung cancer screening

Clinical question

What can patients expect when they undergo computed tomography to screen for lung cancer?

Bottom line

If you are thinking about adding lung cancer screening to your delivery of preventive care, be sure to prepare patients. They are likely to receive a positive result, most of the positive results will not be lung cancer, and one in four patients will require additional tracking (i.e., follow-up scans). In this study, more than half (59.7%) of the current or former smokers screened for lung cancer using low-dose computed tomography (CT) had a positive result of some sort. However, 97.5% of them were falsely positive, and half of the patients who screened positive were identified as needing to undergo additional monitoring.

7. Arthroscopic meniscal surgery = nonoperative management

Clinical question

Is arthroscopy better than nonsurgical treatment for patients with meniscal tears?

Bottom line

The existing research base, with biases that typically make interventions look better, is unable to demonstrate that arthroscopy for meniscal injuries is any better than nonoperative approaches. Since this is a costly intervention, and is being used more frequently, perhaps insurance companies should reevaluate whether to continue paying for it.

8. **8) Prostate cancer screening: no mortality benefit after fifteen years of follow-up**

   Clinical question

   Does screening of asymptomatic men for prostate cancer improve mortality?

   Bottom line

   After nearly two decades of follow-up from the Prostate, Lung, Colorectal, and Ovarian Cancer Screening Trial, there appears to be no mortality benefit to screening asymptomatic men for prostate cancer.

9. **Better outcomes for hospitalized patients treated by female physicians**

   Clinical question

   Are there differences in outcomes for hospitalized patients who are treated by female physicians versus male physicians?

   Bottom line

   Patients hospitalized for medical conditions who are treated by female physicians are less likely to die or be readmitted within thirty days than those treated by male physicians. Although the effects shown in this study were modest, at less than a percentage point reduction for both outcomes, the difference may be clinically meaningful when applied to more than ten million annual Medicare hospitalizations.

10. Antibiotics may equal surgery for children with appendicitis

Clinical question

Can children with appendicitis be treated with antibiotics instead of surgery?

Bottom line

Another shibboleth has toppled, or is at least teetering. Antibiotic treatment appears to be effective for children with uncomplicated appendicitis without evidence of perforation or rupture, with 97% of children discharged without surgery. Approximately one in seven children will eventually have recurrence and require surgery. A couple of days of intravenous antibiotics is an option before surgery.

11. Screening for prediabetes: neither HbA1c nor fasting glucose results are very accurate

Clinical question

Are screening tests for prediabetes accurate?

Bottom line

"What's in a name?" Juliet pondered…to her detriment, as it turned out. So, too, with the diagnosis of prediabetes. In this analysis, an elevated (by various criteria) HbA1c or fasting plasma glucose level only sometimes lines up with impaired glucose tolerance testing results via a glucose tolerance test. If we take an abnormal two-hour glucose tolerance test result to be the true harbinger of eventual type 2 diabetes, an HbA1c level is neither sensitive or specific, and a fasting glucose is specific (can accurately rule in risk) but not sensitive. Depending on the screening test you use (or are required to use), many people will receive an incorrect diagnosis, while others will be falsely reassured.

12. Dietary improvement decreases symptoms of depression

Clinical question

Does dietary improvement help adults with moderate to severe major depression?

Bottom line

In addition to standard pharmacology and psychotherapy, dietary advice aimed at improving dietary consumption in adults with moderate to severe major depression and "poor" dietary quality resulted in a significantly increased rate of clinical remission after twelve weeks (number needed to treat [NNT] = 4.1; 95% CI 2.3–27.8). This study reveals an important group of patients for whom a detailed dietary history may result in improved patient outcomes.

13. One-third of adults with diagnosed asthma can be weaned off all asthma meds

Clinical question

How many adults with physician-diagnosed asthma can safely taper off their asthma medications?

Bottom line

This study found that current asthma was ruled out after repeated testing in one-third of adults with physician-diagnosed asthma. Patients ruled out for current asthma were less likely to be using asthma medications or daily-controlling medications and less likely to have undergone testing for airflow limitation at the time of initial diagnosis. After one year of follow-up, 2.9% of the patients who tapered off their asthma medications presented with respiratory symptoms and resumed treatment.

14. **Percutaneous coronary intervention has more benefits and harms than coronary artery bypass grafting for selected patients with left main coronary disease**

    Clinical question

    For selected patients with left main coronary artery disease, is percutaneous coronary intervention with a drug-eluting stent an option to replace coronary artery bypass grafting?

    Bottom line

    The authors of this study—which was sponsored by the manufacturer of stents—argue that the results prove that percutaneous coronary intervention (PCI) is just as good as coronary artery bypass grafting for many patients with a left main lesion. A deeper dive into the data suggests that it's not quite so clear. Patients undergoing PCI had fewer early myocardial infarctions, but more later deaths and later myocardial infarctions. There are other benefits to PCI, including shorter hospital stay, lower cost, and faster recovery. But patients should be informed of the trade-offs, and it is important to look at longer-term outcomes than three years (which the investigators promise to do).

15. **Nut consumption associated with a lower risk of many bad things**

    Clinical question

    What are the health benefits of nut consumption?

    Bottom line

    There is a consistent association between increased consumption of nuts and improved health outcomes. Unmeasured confounding may explain part of this difference, as persons who consume nuts are less likely to smoke, be obese, or be sedentary, and they tend to eat a better diet in general.

16. Mass abdominal aortic aneurysm screening in Australia was ineffective in decreasing mortality, even in smokers

Clinical question

Is mass screening of older men effective in preventing deaths due to abdominal aortic aneurysm?

Bottom line

A population-based screening approach to detecting and treating abdominal aortic aneurysm (AAA) in (relatively younger) old men in Australia did not find a pronounced benefit. That doesn't mean that no one benefited; among those men who took advantage of screening, the risk of AAA-related death was lower (0.26% vs. 0.82%), though this could be in part explained by a compliance effect. Other studies have found a benefit, but it might be that the rate of AAA is decreasing, following a decrease in smoking. A Canadian task force concluded that screening programs are effective (*J Vasc Surg* 2016; 64:1855–68).

17. Placebo plus message of benefit decreases chronic low back pain

Clinical question

Can simply telling patients that a medicine works, even if it is placebo, decrease pain and improve disability in patients with chronic low back pain?

Bottom line

Building on the received wisdom of Sir William Osler that "The desire to take medicine is perhaps the greatest feature which distinguishes man from animals," these investigators gave twice daily placebo to patients with chronic back pain and told them it was placebo. They also told them that placebos can have a pronounced effect (which is true). The addition of placebo to usual care improved patients' pain and disability scores over the three weeks of the study. Although we probably won't start prescribing placebo, this study emphasizes the great value of conveying one's confidence in the treatment to bolster its effect.

18. Placebo more effective than glucosamine plus chondroitin sulfate for knee degenerative joint disease

Clinical question

How effective is glucosamine plus chondroitin sulfate in improving moderate to severe pain and function in patients with symptomatic knee degenerative joint disease?

Bottom line

This is one of many studies showing that, after six months of treatment, glucosamine plus chondroitin sulfate is no better than placebo in improving pain and function in patients with symptomatic knee degenerative joint disease. In fact, this is one of the first studies to suggest that placebo is better.

References

I have listed below the most important books I have read in developing my book. They are all great reads, and I would recommend all of them.

Many thanks to all of the authors of these books; you have helped me to grow.

A Brief History of Everything, by Ken Wilber, ISBN: 9781570627408

A Briefer History of Time, by Stephen Hawking, ISBN: 9780553385465

A Theory of Everything, by Ken Wilber, ISBN: 9781570628559

An Appetite for Wonder, by Richard Dawkins, ISBN: 9780062315809

Antifragile, by Nassim Nicholas Taleb, ISBN: 9780812979688

Arguably, by Christopher Hitchens, ISBN: 9781455502783

Asking the Right Questions, by M. Neil Browne and Stuart M. Keeley, ISBN: 9780132203043

Being Wrong, by Kathryn Schultz, ISBN: 0780061176050

Beyond the Self, by Thich Nhat Hanh, ISBN: 9781935209416

Bhagavad Gita: A New Translation, by Stephen Mitchell, ISBN: 9780609810347

Blindspot, by Mahzarin R. Banaji and Anthony G. Greenwald, ISBN: 9780345528438

Brain Wars, by Mario Beauregard, ISBN: 9780062071224

Chances Are...: Adventures in Probability, by Michael Kaplan, ISBN: 9780143038344

Comfortable with Uncertainty, by Pema Chödrön, ISBN: 9781590300787

David and Goliath, by Malcolm Gladwell, ISBN: 9780316204378

Denial, by Ajit Varki and Danny Brower, ISBN: 9781455511914

Descartes' Error, by Antonio Damasio, ISBN: 9780143036277

Everyday Zen, by Charlotte J. Beck, ISBN: 9780061285899

Fear, by Thich Nhat Hanh, ISBN: 9780062004734

Finding Peace, by Jean Vanier, ISBN: 9780887846830

Flow, by Mihaly Csikszentmihalyi, ISBN: 9780061339202

From Socrates to Sartre: The Philosophic Quest, by T. Z. Levine, ISBN:9780553251616

God in All Worlds: An Anthology of Contemporary Spiritual Writing, by Lucinda Vardey, ISBN: 9780679745433

Less Medicine, More Health, by Dr. H. Gilbert Welch, ISBN: 9780807077580

Metaphysics as a Guide to Morals, by Iris Murdoch, ISBN: 9780140172324

Mindless, by Simon Head, ISBN: 9780465018444

Mindsight, by Daniel J. Siegel, ISBN: 9780553386394

Mindware, by Richard Nisbett, ISBN: 9780374536244

Nine Essential Things I've Learned about Life, by Harold S. Kushner, ISBN: 9780804173452

Nothing Special, by Charlotte J. Beck and Steve Smith, ISBN: 9780062511171

Plato and a Platypus Walk into a Bar, by Thomas Cathcart and Daniel Klein, ISBN: 9780143113874

Probability for Dummies, by Deborah Rumsey, ISBN: 9780471751410

Quiet, by Susan Cain, ISBN: 9780307352156

Science Set Free, by Rupert Sheldrake, ISBN: 9780770436728

Subliminal, by Leonard Mlodinow, ISBN: 9780307472250

Superforecasting, by Philip E. Tetlock and Dan Gardner, ISBN: 9780804136716

Tao Te Ching, by Lao-Tzu, Stephen Addiss and Stanley Lombardo, ISBN: 9780872202320

The Anatomy of Hope, by Jerome Groopman, ISBN: 9780375757754

The Art of Mindful Living, by Tobin Giblin, ISBN: 9781427650948

The Art of Thinking Clearly, by Rolf Dobelli, ISBN: 9780062219695
The Bed of Procrustes, by Nassim Nicholas Taleb, ISBN: 9780812982404
The Black Swan, by Nassim Nicholas Taleb, ISBN: 9780812973815
The Brain and Emotional Intelligence, by Daniel Goleman, ISBN: 9781934441152
The End of Leadership, by Barbara Kellerman, ISBN: 9780062069160
The Essence of the Bhagavad Gita, by Bernd Helge Fritsch, ISBN: 9783738626278
The Ethical Imagination, by Margaret Somerville, ISBN: 9780773534896
The Fabric of the Cosmos, by Brian Greene, ISBN: 9780375727207
The Grand Design, by Stephen Hawking and Leonard Mlodinow, ISBN: 9780553384666
The Hidden Brain, by Shankar Vedantam, ISBN: 9780385525220
The Hidden Reality, by Brian Greene, ISBN: 9780307278128
The Holy Bible: New International version, ISBN: 9781563297211
The Invisible Gorilla, by Christopher Chabris and Daniel Simons, ISBN: 9780307459664
The Power of Silence, by Horatio W. Dresser, ISBN: 9781544043517
The Psychopath Test, by Jon Ronson, ISBN: 9781594485756
The Rise of Early Modern Science, by Toby E. Huff, ISBN: 9781107571075
The Road Less Traveled, by M. Scott Peck, ISBN: 9780743243155
The Quantum Universe, by Brian Cox and Jeff Forshaw, ISBN: 9780306821448
The Seven Story Mountain, by Thomas Merton, ISBN: 9780156010863
The Signal and the Noise, by Nate Silver, ISBN: 9780143125082
The Tao of Emerson, by Ralph Waldo Emerson and Lao Tse, ISBN: 9780677963395
The Tell, by Matthew Hertenstein, ISBN: 9780465036592
The Tipping Point, by Malcolm Gladwell, ISBN: 9780316346627
The Trouble with Physics, by Lee Smolin, ISBN: 9780618551057
The White Man's Burden, by William Easterly, ISBN: 9780143038825
The Wisest One in the Room, by Thomas Gilovich and Lee Ross, ISBN: 9781451677553
Time Reborn, by Lee Smolin, ISBN: 9780544245594
Walden, by Henry David Thoreau, ISBN: 9781619493919
What Dying People Want, by David Kuhl, ISBN: 9781586481971

What the Dog Saw, by Malcolm Gladwell, ISBN: 9780316076203
What Would Confucius Do?, by Evelyn Berthrong, ISBN: 9781569243497
Your Money or Your Life, by Joe Dominguez and Vicki Robin, ISBN: 9780140167153

www.ingramcontent.com/pod-product-compliance
Lightning Source LLC
Chambersburg PA
CBHW020721180526
45163CB00001B/57